ESSENTIALS IN OPHTHALMOLOGY: Oculoplastics and Orbit

R. Guthoff · J. A. Katowitz (Eds.)

ESSENTIALS IN OPHTHALMOLOGY

G. K. Krieglstein · R. N. Weinreb
Series Editors

Glaucoma

Cataract and Refractive Surgery

Uveitis and Immunological Disorders

Vitreo-retinal Surgery

Medical Retina

Oculoplastics and Orbit

Pediatric Ophthalmology, Neuro-Ophthalmology, Genetics

Cornea and External Eye Disease

Editors Rudolf Guthoff
James A. Katowitz

Oculoplastics and Orbit

With 145 Figures, Mostly in Color, and 20 Tables

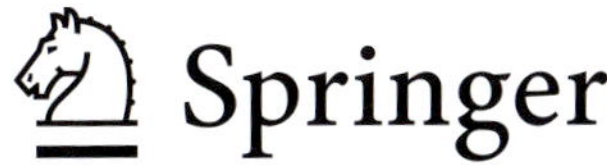

Series Editors

Guenter K. Krieglstein, MD
Professor and Chairman
Department of Ophthalmology
University of Cologne
Joseph-Stelzmann-Straße 9
50931 Cologne
Germany

Robert N. Weinreb, MD
Professor and Director
Hamilton Glaucoma Center
Department of Ophthalmology – 0946
University of California at San Diego
9500 Gilman Drive
La Jolla, CA 92093-0946
USA

Volume Editors

Rudolf Guthoff, MD
Professor of Ophthalmology
University of Rostock
Department of Ophthalmology
Doberaner Straße 140
18057 Rostock, Germany

James A. Katowitz, MD
Professor of Ophthalmology
University of Pennsylvania
Children's Hospital of Philadelphia
Division of Ophthalmology
R.D. Wood Ambulatory Care Building
34th Street Civic Center Blvd.
Philadelphia, PA 19104, USA

ISBN-10 3-540-22599-4
Springer Berlin Heidelberg New York

ISBN-13 978-3-540-22599-4
Springer Berlin Heidelberg New York

ISSN 1612-3212

Library of Congress Control Number: 2005928345

Springer is a part of Springer Science + Business Media

springeronline.com

Printed in The Netherlands

Cover picture "Cataract and Refractive Surgery" from Kampik A, Grehn F (eds) Augenärztliche Therapie. Georg Thieme Verlag Stuttgart, with permission.

Editor: Marion Philipp, Springer-Verlag Heidelberg, Germany
Desk editor: Martina Himberger, Springer-Verlag Heidelberg, Germany
Production: ProEdit GmbH, Elke Beul-Göhringer, Heidelberg, Germany
Cover design: Erich Kirchner, Heidelberg, Germany
Typesetting and reproduction of the figures: AM-productions GmbH, Wiesloch, Germany
Printing: Krips, HV Meppel, The Netherlands
Binding: Litges & Dopf Buchbinderei GmbH, Heppenheim, Germany

Printed on acid-free paper
24/3151beu-göh 5 4 3 2 1 0

Foreword

Essentials in Ophthalmology is a new review series covering all of ophthalmology categorized in eight subspecialties. It will be published quarterly; thus each subspecialty will be reviewed biannually.

Given the multiplicity of medical publications already available, why is a new series needed? Consider that the half-life of medical knowledge is estimated to be around 5 years. Moreover, it can be as long as 8 years between the description of a medical innovation in a peer-reviewed scientific journal and publication in a medical textbook. A series that narrows this time span between journal and textbook would provide a more rapid and efficient transfer of medical knowledge into clinical practice, and enhance care of our patients.

For the series, each subspecialty volume comprises 10–20 chapters selected by two distinguished editors and written by internationally renowned specialists. The selection of these contributions is based more on recent and noteworthy advances in the subspecialty than on systematic completeness. Each article is structured in a standardized format and length, with citations for additional reading and an appropriate number of illustrations to enhance important points. Since every subspecialty volume is issued in a recurring sequence during the 2-year cycle, the reader has the opportunity to focus on the progress in a particular subspecialty or to be updated on the whole field. The clinical relevance of all material presented will be well established, so application to clinical practice can be made with confidence.

This new series will earn space on the bookshelves of those ophthalmologists who seek to maintain the timeliness and relevance of their clinical practice.

G. K. Krieglstein
R. N. Weinreb
Series Editors

Preface

Ophthalmologists working in the subspecialty of oculoplastic and facial reconstructive surgery often cooperate with other surgical and non-surgical disciplines in managing complex patient problems. The present volume of "Essentials in Ophthalmology" provides valuable information which will enhance the links between ophthalmologists and other specialists by sharing the latest information and experiences with a number of challenging problems. The subjects covered include: the risks of infectious disease transmission through use of allografts, current concepts in the management of conjunctival neoplasms, including the latest imaging technology, and the specific role that sentinel node biopsy can play in the management of malignant disorders in the periorbital area.

The discussion regarding the paradox of "success" in lacrimal drainage surgery will stimulate "lateral thinking" and offers a new systematic approach for understanding patient problems with tear overflow.

Recent advances in endoscopy, including microendoscopic techniques, demonstrate how ophthalmology continues to evolve as an innovative surgical discipline. While the enigma of thyroid-related orbitopathy is still unsolved, nevertheless, advances in medical and surgical management are presented that can offer considerable benefits to patients and contribute significantly to improving their quality of life.

The field of esthetic surgery has also been advanced by innovations developed by oculofacial plastic surgeons, including the application of lasers, endoscopic brow lift techniques, and midface reconstruction methods for facial rejuvenation. Those treating patients with acquired disorders such as facial paralysis and congenital problems such as micro-/anophthalmos are also offered new approaches which can at least improve a patient's appearance if not completely solve their functional deficiencies.

The editors have selected specific topics in an effort to provide an overview of what is new in the areas of orbital, lid and lacrimal surgery. The variety and speed of innovation requires more space than any one volume can cover. We plan to offer the readers more new information in subsequent volumes and hope that we may have stimulated their curiosity sufficiently to look forward to further publication of the rapid developments occurring in our surgical discipline.

R. Guthoff
J.A. Katowitz

Contents

General Considerations

Chapter 1
Risk of Infectious Disease Transmission Through Use of Allografts
Robert H. Kennedy, C. Randal Mills, Paul Brown

1.1 Introduction 4
1.2 Reports of Infectious Disease Transmission 4
1.2.1 Hepatitis C Virus (HCV) 5
1.2.2 Human Immunodeficiency Virus (HIV) 6
1.2.3 Other Conventional Infectious Diseases 7
1.2.4 Creutzfeldt-Jakob Disease (CJD) 8
1.3 Sources of Risk for Allograft Contamination 9
1.3.1 Living Donors and Cadaveric Tissue 10
1.3.2 Donor Screening and Testing 11
1.3.3 Aseptic Processing of Donor Tissue 12
1.4 Estimated Risk of Allograft Contamination 14
1.4.1 HIV 14
1.4.2 HCV and HBV 15
1.5 Human Error in Donor Screening and Testing 15
1.6 Conclusions and Recommendations 16
References 17

Oncology

Chapter 2
Current Concepts in the Management of Conjunctival Neoplasms
Carol L. Shields, Jerry A. Shields

2.1 Introduction 21
2.2 Conjunctival Anatomy 21
2.3 Diagnostic Techniques 22
2.4 Management 22
2.5 Diagnostic Categories of Conjunctival Tumors 25
2.6 Papilloma 26
2.7 Ocular Surface Squamous Neoplasia (OSSN) 27
2.7.1 Conjunctival Intraepithelial Neoplasia (CIN) 27
2.7.2 Squamous Cell Carcinoma 27
2.8 Nevus 28
2.9 Primary Acquired Melanosis (PAM) 29
2.10 Malignant Melanoma 31
2.11 Lymphoid Tumors 32
2.12 Caruncular Tumors 32
References 33

Chapter 3
Sentinel Lymph Node Biopsy for Conjunctival and Eyelid Malignancies
Dominick Golio, Bita Esmaeli

3.1 Introduction ... 38
3.2 Historical Perspective and Rationale for Sentinel Lymph Node Biopsy ... 38
3.3 Sentinel Lymph Node Biopsy for Conjunctival and Eyelid Tumors ... 39
3.3.1 Patient Selection and Indications ... 40
3.3.2 Anatomic Considerations ... 40
3.3.3 Technical Considerations ... 40
3.3.4 Histopathologic Analysis of Sentinel Lymph Nodes ... 43
3.3.5 Lymphatic Basins at Risk ... 44
3.4 Care of Patients with a Positive Sentinel Lymph Node ... 44
3.4.1 Potential Complications and Limitations ... 44
3.5 Conclusions and Future Directions ... 46
References ... 46

Lacrimal Surgery

Chapter 4
The Apparent Paradox of "Success" in Lacrimal Drainage Surgery
Geoffrey E. Rose

4.1 Introduction ... 51
4.2 The "Lacrimal Paradox" and the Dichotomy of Lacrimal Characteristics ... 52
4.3 The Three-Compartment Model of Lacrimal Drainage ... 55
4.4 Osteotomy Size and the Soft-Tissue Anastomosis After Dacryocystorhinostomy ... 57
References ... 59

Chapter 5
Microsurgery of the Lacrimal System: Microendoscopic Techniques
Karl-Heinz Emmerich, Hans-Werner Meyer-Rüsenberg

5.1 Introduction ... 61
5.2 Dacryoendoscopy ... 62
5.2.1 Technical Equipment ... 62
5.2.2 Performing Endoscopy ... 64
5.2.3 Transcanalicular Endoscopic Procedures ... 66
5.3 Conclusions ... 69
Citation and References ... 70

Chapter 6
Techniques in Endonasal Dacryocystorhinostomy
Peter J. Dolman

6.1 Introduction ... 71
6.2 History ... 71
6.3 Preoperative Considerations ... 72
6.3.1 Clinical Assessment of Epiphora ... 72
6.3.2 Indications for Surgery ... 72
6.3.3 Special Considerations in Endonasal DCRs ... 73
6.4 Perioperative Considerations ... 73
6.4.1 Hemostasis ... 73
6.4.2 Anesthesia ... 73
6.4.3 Antibiotics ... 74
6.4.4 Set-up ... 74
6.5 Operative Techniques ... 74
6.5.1 Illumination Source ... 74
6.5.2 Viewing Systems ... 74
6.5.3 Formation of the Osteotomy ... 75
6.5.4 Fenestrating the Lacrimal Sac ... 77
6.5.5 Mitomycin-C ... 78
6.5.6 Stenting ... 78
6.6 Postoperative Care ... 78
6.7 EN-DCR for Specific Conditions ... 78
6.7.1 Pediatric EN-DCR ... 78
6.7.2 EN-DCR with Canalicular Stenosis ... 79
6.8 Complications ... 79
6.9 Comparison of EN-DCR and EX-DCR ... 80
6.10 Transition to EN-DCR ... 80
References ... 81

CHAPTER 7
Monocanalicular Lacrimal Pathway Intubation with a Stable Punctal Attachment
BRUNO FAYET, JEAN-MARC RUBAN

7.1 Introduction 83
7.2 Description and Fitting for Monocanalicular Stenting: The Mono-Ka® Device 83
7.2.1 Description of the Superior Fixation Device (SFD) 83
7.2.2 Monocanalicular Intubation: Technique for Insertion 84
7.2.3 Limitations of the Mono-Ka® Device 84
7.2.4 Indications and Contraindications for the Mono-Ka® 84
7.2.5 Caution 84
7.3 The Mini-Mono-Ka® Device 84
7.4 Supervision and Removal of the Mono-Ka® 85
7.5 Complications 85
7.5.1 Complications Related to the Insertion of the Mono-Ka® .. 85
7.6 Undesirable Side Effects of the Mono-Ka® After Placement in the Lacrimal Pathways 86
7.6.1 Dyeing of the Silicone 86
7.6.2 Itching 86
7.6.3 Impermeability 86
7.7 Late Complications of the Mono-Ka® After Insertion in the Lacrimal Drainage Pathway . 87
7.7.1 Externalization or Extrusion 87
7.7.2 Intracanalicular Migration 87
7.8 Prevention of Intracanalicular Migration of the Mono-Ka® 87
7.9 Complications of the Mini- Mono-Ka® Device 88
References 88

Graves' Ophthalmopathy

CHAPTER 8
The Role of Orbital Radiotherapy in the Management of Thyroid Related Orbitopathy
MICHAEL KAZIM

8.1 Introduction: Historical Background 91
8.2 Biological Effects of Radiotherapy . 93
8.3 Safety 94
8.4 Pre-treatment Analysis 94
8.4.1 10- vs. 20-GY Dose Treatment 94
8.5 Recommendations and Future Developments 94
References 95

CHAPTER 9
Bony Orbital Decompression Techniques
K.E. MORGENSTERN, PAUL PROFFER, JILL A. FOSTER

9.1 Introduction 97
9.2 History of Bony Decompression ... 98
9.3 Indications 98
9.4 Characterizing Decompressive Surgery 99
9.5 Surgical Approach 99
9.6 Bony Decompression Techniques .. 100
9.6.1 Anterior and Posterior Lateral Wall 100
9.6.2 Medial Wall..................... 102
9.6.3 Floor 103
9.6.4 Roof 104
9.7 Alternative Approaches to Orbital Decompression 104
9.7.1 Transantral 104
9.7.2 Endoscopic 105
9.7.3 Orbital Fat Decompression........ 106
9.7.4 Potential Complications 106
9.8 Conclusion 107
References 107

Chapter 10
Orbital Decompression Using Fat Removal Orbital Decompression
Jean-Paul Adenis, Pierre-Yves Robert

10.1 Introduction ... 109
10.2 Description ... 110
10.2.1 The Upper Eyelid ... 110
10.2.2 The Lower Eyelid ... 112
10.2.3 The Volume of Resection ... 113
10.2.4 Treatment Program ... 113
10.3 Our Experience ... 114
10.3.1 Patients ... 114
10.3.2 Surgical Procedure ... 114
10.3.3 Clinical Data ... 114
10.3.4 Statistics ... 114
10.4 Results ... 114
10.4.1 Proptosis ... 114
10.4.2 Visual Field ... 115
10.4.3 Intraocular Pressure ... 116
10.4.4 Volume of Excised Fat ... 116
10.4.5 Diplopia ... 116
10.5 Discussion ... 116
10.5.1 Types of Bone Removal Orbital Decompression (BROD) Performed ... 116
10.5.2 FROD or BROD? ... 117
10.6 Conclusion ... 119
References ... 119

Esthetic and Lid Surgery

Chapter 11
Update on Upper Lid Blepharoplasty
Markus J. Pfeiffer

11.1 Introduction ... 123
11.2 Surgical Anatomy of the Upper Lid and Upper Orbit ... 123
11.2.1 Relationship of Aperture Plane, Lid Crease and Skin Fold ... 124
11.2.2 The Aperture Plane ... 124
11.2.3 The Upper Lid Crease ... 125
11.2.4 The Skin Fold ... 125
11.2.5 The Eyelid Skin ... 126
11.2.6 The Relationship of the Anterior and the Posterior Lid Lamella ... 126
11.2.7 The Pretarsal Orbicularis Muscle ... 126
11.2.8 The Preseptal Orbicularis Muscle ... 127
11.2.9 The Orbital Part of the Orbicularis Muscle ... 127
11.2.10 The Suborbicularis Oculi Fat (SOOF) ... 127
11.2.11 The Orbital Septum ... 128
11.2.12 The Orbital Fat ... 128
11.2.13 The Eyebrow ... 129
11.2.14 The Frontalis Muscle and Its Antagonists ... 129
11.2.15 The Posterior Lid Lamella ... 130
11.3 The Preoperative Evaluation and Surgical Planning ... 130
11.3.1 The Patient's Expectation ... 130
11.3.2 The Evaluation of the Lid Crease Symmetry ... 131
11.3.3 Preoperative Examination ... 131
11.3.4 Differentiation of Simple and Complicated Cases ... 132
11.3.5 Planning Blepharoplasty According to the Typology of Cases ... 132
11.4 Surgical Technique of the Most Frequent Types of Upper Lid Blepharoplasty ... 134
11.4.1 Marking the Outlines of Incisions ... 134
11.4.2 Local Anaestesia ... 135
11.4.3 Skin Incision ... 135
11.4.4 Skin Excision ... 135
11.4.5 Orbicularis Separation ... 135
11.4.6 Orbicularis Excision ... 135
11.4.7 Identification of the Septum ... 135
11.4.8 Dissection of the Septum ... 136
11.4.9 Management of the Preaponeurotic Fat ... 136
11.4.10 Management of the Intermedial Orbital Fat ... 136
11.4.11 Exposure of the Medial Orbital Fat ... 136
11.4.12 Resection of the Medial Orbital Fat ... 137
11.4.13 Resection of the Medial Subcutaneous Fat ... 137
11.4.14 SOOF Resection ... 137
11.4.15 Sutures ... 138
11.4.16 Laser Blepharoplasty ... 138
11.5 Complications in Upper Lid Blepharoplasty: Prevention and Management ... 138
11.5.1 Undercorrection ... 138
11.5.2 Overcorrection ... 139
11.5.3 Excessive Skin Resection ... 139

11.5.4 Excessive Orbicularis Muscle Resection 139
11.5.5 Excessive SOOF Resection 140
11.5.6 Excessive Resection of Preaponeurotic Fat 140
11.5.7 Excessive Resection of Medial Orbital Fat 140
11.5.8 Asymmetry 140
11.5.9 Double Skin Fold 141
11.5.10 Posterior Lamella Lacerations 141
11.5.11 Failure to Correct Associated Pathology 141
11.5.12 Hemorrhage, Edema and Scar Formation 141
References 141

CHAPTER 12
Update on Lasers in Oculoplastic Surgery
JULIE A. WOODWARD, AERLYN G. DAWN

12.1 Introduction 144
12.2 Incisional Laser Surgery 145
12.2.1 CO_2 Laser 145
12.2.2 Erbium: YAG Laser 148
12.2.3 Neodymium: YAG Laser 149
12.3 Laser Skin Resurfacing 149
12.3.1 CO_2 Laser Skin Resurfacing 151
12.3.2 Erbium: YAG Laser Skin Resurfacing 152
12.3.3 Combined CO_2 and Erbium Laser Resurfacing 153
12.3.4 Non-ablative Resurfacing 153
12.4 Laser Treatment of Cutaneous Vascular Lesions 156
12.5 Laser Treatment of Tattoos 157
12.6 Laser Hair Removal 158
12.7 Laser Dacryocystorhinostomy 158
12.7.1 Holmium Laser 159
12.7.2 Potassium Titanyl Phosphate Laser 159
References 160

CHAPTER 13
Update on the Endoscopic Brow Lift: Pearls and Nuances
BHUPENDRA C.K. PATEL

13.1 Introduction 163
13.2 Number of Scalp Incisions 164
13.3 Sites of Scalp Incisions 164
13.4 Forehead Dissection 165
13.5 Release of Periosteum 166
13.6 Weakening of the Forehead Muscles 167
17.7 Fixation of the Mobilized Forehead: How Long Is Fixation Necessary? .. 168
13.8 Methods of Fixation 168
13.9 Simplified Technique of Bone Tunneling 169
13.10 Method of Elevation 170
13.11 Buried Screw and Suture 171
13.12 Endotine Fixation 173
13.13 Closure 173
13.14 Postoperative Care 175
13.15 Conclusion 175
References 179

CHAPTER 14
The SOOF Lift in Midface Reconstruction and Rejuvenation
ROBERT M. SCHWARCZ, NORMAN SHORR

14.1 Introduction 181
14.2 Anatomy of the Midface 182
14.3 Age Related Changes of the Midface 183
14.4 Patient Selection 183
14.5 Surgical Technique 184
14.5.1 Transconjunctival Approach 185
14.5.2 Sublabial Approach 187
14.5.3 Closed Cable Lift 188
References 189

CHAPTER 15
Facial Paralysis: A Comprehensive Approach to Current Management
ROBERTA E. GAUSAS

15.1 Introduction 191
15.2 Diagnosis 191
15.2.1 Patient History 192
15.2.2 Anatomy and Function 193
15.3 Facial Nerve: Physical Examination 195
15.3.1 Brow Complex 196
15.3.2 Periorbital Complex 196
15.3.3 Midface and Perioral Complex 197
15.4 Treatment Strategies 198
15.4.1 Supportive Care 198
15.4.2 Surgical Strategies 199
15.5 Aberrant Regeneration 203
References 203

Chapter 16
Self-inflating Hydrogel Expanders for the Treatment of Congenital Anophthalmos
Michael P. Schittkowski, James A. Katowitz, Karsten K.H. Gundlach, Rudolf F. Guthoff

16.1 Introduction ... 205
16.1.1 Clinical Features ... 205
16.1.2 Epidemiology ... 205
16.1.3 Definition of Terms ... 206
16.1.4 Etiology ... 206
16.1.5 Treatment ... 206
16.2 Patients and Method ... 207
16.2.1 Osmotic Expanders ... 207
16.2.2 Patients ... 208
16.3 Results ... 209
16.3.1 Treatment Course ... 209
16.3.2 Expander Failures/Complication ... 212
16.3.3 Number of Operations ... 212
16.3.4 Treatment Results ... 213
16.3.5 Acceptance ... 215
16.4 Discussion ... 215
16.4.1 Introduction ... 215
16.4.2 Pathogenesis ... 215
16.4.3 Existing Therapy Concepts – Pros and Cons ... 216
References ... 220

Chapter 17
Methods to Improve Prosthesis Motility in Enucleation Surgery Without Pegging and With Emphasis on Muscle Pedunculated Flaps
Rudolf F. Guthoff, Michael P. Schittkowski, Artur Klett

17.1 Introduction ... 223
17.2 Short History of Alloplastic Implants ... 223
17.3 Evisceration/Enucleation – Pros and Cons ... 224
17.3.1 Intraocular Malignancy ... 224
17.3.2 Endophthalmitis ... 224
17.3.3 Blind and Painful Eye ... 225
17.3.4 Sympathethic Ophthalmia ... 225
17.4 Orbital Implants – Materials, Shape, Implantation Technique ... 225
17.4.1 Non-integrated Implants ... 225
17.4.2 Integrated Implants ... 227
17.5 Wrapping Materials ... 228
17.6 Indications for Pegging ... 228
17.7 Motility Evaluation ... 228
17.8 Strategies to Improve Prosthesis Motility Without Pegging ... 229
17.9 Suggestions for an Effective Compromise Between Enucleation and Evisceration: Muscle Pedunculated Scleral Flaps ... 232
References ... 234

Chapter 18
Current Management of Traumatic Enophthalmos
Richard C. Allen, Jeffrey A. Nerad

18.1 Introduction ... 238
18.1.1 Anatomy ... 238
18.2 Enophthalmos ... 239
18.2.1 Non-traumatic Causes of Enophthalmos ... 239
18.2.2 Traumatic Enophthalmos ... 240
18.2.3 Mechanism of Traumatic Enophthalmos ... 240
18.2.4 Fractures Associated with Enophthalmos ... 241
18.2.5 Evaluation of the Patient with Traumatic Enophthalmos ... 242
18.3 Treatment of Traumatic Enophthalmos ... 244
18.3.1 Non-surgical Treatment of Traumatic Enophthalmos ... 244
18.3.2 Surgical Treatment of Traumatic Enophthalmos ... 244
18.4 Enophthalmos Associated with the Anophthalmic Socket ... 248
18.4.1 Mechanism ... 248
18.4.2 Treatment of Enophthalmos in the Anophthalmic Socket ... 249
References ... 249

Subject Index ... 253

Contributors

Jean-Paul Adenis, MD
Service d'Ophthalmologie
C.H.V. Dupuytren
2, Ave. Martin-Luther-King
87042 Limoges, France

Richard C. Allen, MD, PhD
Department of Ophthalmology
and Visual Sciences, Oculoplastic, Orbital,
and Oncology Service
University of Iowa Hospitals and Clinics
200 Hawkins Drive
Iowa City, IA 52242–1091, USA

Paul Brown, PhD
The National Institute of Health
9000 Rockville Pike
Bethesda, MD 20892, USA

Aerlyn G. Dawn, MD, MBA
Duke University School of Medicine
Durham, NC 27710, USA

Peter J. Dolman, MD, FRCSC
Eye Care Center, Section 1
2550 Willow Street, Vancouver
British Columbia V5Z 3N9, Canada

Karl-Heinz Emmerich, Dr.
Augenklinik des Klinikums Darmstadt
Heidelberger Landstraße 379
64297 Darmstadt, Germany

Bita Esmaeli, MD, FACS
Associate Professor and Chief
Section of Ophthalmology
Department of Plastic Surgery
M. D. Anderson Cancer Center
1515 Holcombe Boulevard
Houston, TX 77030, USA

Bruno Fayet, MD
70, Av. de Breteuil
75007 Paris, France

Jill A. Foster, MD
Department of Ophthalmology
Division of Oculoplastic Surgery
The Ohio State University
340 East Town Street
Columbus, OH 43215, USA

Roberta E. Gausas, MD
Department of Ophthalmology
Scheie Eye Institute, University of Pennsylvania
Medical School, 51 North 39th Street
Philadelphia, PA 19104, USA

Dominick Golio, MD
Section of Ophthalmology
Department of Plastic Surgery
The University of Texas
M. D. Anderson Cancer Center
1515 Holcombe Boulevard
Houston, TX 77030, USA

KARSTEN K.H. GUNDLACH, Dr.
Department of Oro-Maxillofacial
and Facial Plastic Surgery, Rostock University
Strempelstraße 13
18057 Rostock, Germany

RUDOLF F. GUTHOFF, MD
Professor of Opthalmology
Department of Ophthalmology
Rostock University
Doberaner Straße 140
18057 Rostock, Germany

JAMES A. KATOWITZ, MD
Professor of Ophthalmology
University of Pennsylvania
Children's Hospital of Philadelphia
Division of Ophthalmology
R.D. Wood Ambulatory Care Building
34th Street Civic Center Blvd.
Philadelphia, PA 19104, USA

MICHAEL KAZIM, MD
Associate Clinical Professor of Ophthalmology
and Surgery, Columbia University
and Edward S. Harkness Eye Institute
635 W. 165th Street
New York, NY 10032, USA

ROBERT H. KENNEDY, MD, PhD
910 North Davis #400
Arlington, TX 76012, USA

ARTUR KLETT, MD
Central Hospital
Department of Ophthalmology
Ravi 18
10138 Tallinn, Estonia

HANS-WERNER MEYER-RÜSENBERG, MD
Augenklinik am St. Josefs-/
St. Marienhospital Hagen
Dreieckstraße 17
58097 Hagen, Germany

C. RANDAL MILLS, PhD
Osiris Therapeutics, Inc.
2001 Alecianna Street
Baltimore, MD 21231-3043, USA

K.E. MORGENSTERN, MD
Department of Ophthalmology
Division of Oculoplastic Surgery
The Medical College of Virginia
and The Ohio State University
340 East Town Street
Columbus, OH 43215, USA

JEFFREY A. NERAD, MD, FACS
Department of Ophthalmology
and Visual Sciences, Oculoplastic, Orbital,
and Oncology Service
University of Iowa Hospitals and Clinics
200 Hawkins Drive
Iowa City, IA 52242–1091, USA

BHUPENDRA C.K. PATEL, MD
Professor & Chief
Division of Facial Plastic Reconstructive
and Cosmetic Surgery, Moran Eye Center
University of Utah, 825 Northview Drive
Salt Lake City, Utah 84103, USA

MARKUS J. PFEIFFER
Augenklinik "Herzog Carl Theodor"
Nymphenburger Straße 43
80335 München, Germany

PAUL PROFFER, MD
Department of Ophthalmology
Division of Oculoplastic Surgery
The Medical College of Virginia
and The Ohio State University
340 East Town Street
Columbus, OH 43215, USA

PIERRE-YVES ROBERT, MD
Service d'Ophthalmologie 2ET
C.H.V Dupuytren
2, Rue Martin-Luther-King
87000 Limoges, France

GEOFFREY E. ROSE, FRCS, MD
Consultant Surgeon, Orbital, Lacrimal
and Oculoplastic Service, Moorfields
Eye Hospital, City Road
London EC1V 2PD, UK

Jean Marc Ruban, MD
70, Av. de Breteuil
75007 Paris, France

Michael P. Schittkowski, Dr.
Department of Ophthalmology
Rostock University
Doberaner Straße 140
18057 Rostock, Germany

Robert M. Schwarcz, MD
Jules Stein Eye Institute
Division of Orbito-Facial Plastic
& Reconstructive Surgery
UCLA School of Medicine
Los Angeles, CA, USA

Carol L. Shields, MD
900 Walnut Street
Philadelphia, PA 19107, USA

Jerry A. Shields, MD
900 Walnut Street
Philadelphia, PA 19107, USA

Norman Shorr, MD, FACS
Jules Stein Eye Institute
Division of Orbito-Facial Plastic
& Reconstructive Surgery
UCLA School of Medicine
Los Angeles, CA, USA

Julie A. Woodward, MD
Department of Ophthalmology
Duke University School of Medicine
Box 3802
Durham, NC 27710, USA

General Considerations

Risk of Infectious Disease Transmission Through Use of Allografts

1

Robert H. Kennedy, C. Randal Mills, Paul Brown

Core Messages

- The number of musculoskeletal and other allografts implanted in patients continues to increase because of the desirable characteristics of such grafts for use in plastic and reconstructive surgery. Allografts, however, can harbor pathogens and pose at least some risk for transmission of infectious diseases to recipients.
- Case reports document that bacterial, viral, and prion diseases (Creutzfeldt-Jakob disease or CJD) have been transmitted through implantation of contaminated allografts. Though transmission of disease is infrequent, it can, in some cases, lead to considerable morbidity or death.
- Transmission of CJD through implantation of the types of donor tissue used most frequently in eyelid and orbital reconstruction (fascia lata, pericardium, dermis, sclera, and bone) has not been reported. Because sclera is linked to the optic nerve, a tissue with infectivity that should be considered to be as high as brain, we favor the use of substitute materials such as fascia lata, pericardium, or dermis. Surgeons who prefer to use donor sclera should strongly consider selecting Tutoplast-processed sclera because such processing may reduce the risk of transmitting CJD.
- Screening of donors and testing for human immunodeficiency virus and hepatitis are necessary to identify and eliminate contaminated tissue. Those procedures are not 100% sensitive, however, and some contaminated tissue is processed, fashioned into allografts, and distributed for implantation in patients.
- Aseptic processing represents the current standard for promoting allograft safety. It includes procedures to minimize the introduction of pathogens, but does not require steps to eliminate pathogens that may already be present in donor tissue. Therefore, aseptic processing alone is not sufficient to ensure allograft sterility.
- FDA data concerning allograft recalls indicate that human error in following standard donor screening and testing practices represents an important source of risk for allograft contamination.
- Recently, methods of sterilizing allografts during processing have been introduced. The BioCleanse process offered by Regeneration Technologies, Inc., has been validated to sterilize tissue by inactivating and removing all pathogens. Another method introduced by Clearant, Inc., involves use of high doses of gamma irradiation as well as a free-radical scavenging solution to prevent adverse biomechanical effects.
- Until soft tissue grafts documented to be sterile become widely available for use in eyelid and orbital reconstruction, we recommend the selection of allografts that have undergone irradiation or Tutoplast processing rather than those that have undergone aseptic processing alone.
- Surgeons should consider the potential risks for infectious diseases to be transmitted through allografts and should report to local and state health authorities any case of postoperative infection that may have been due to use of a contaminated allograft.

1.1 Introduction

Use of allografts in plastic and reconstructive surgery has grown rapidly in recent years because of the desirable biomechanical and biocompatibility characteristics offered by donor tissue. The number of musculoskeletal allografts distributed in the U.S. has grown to about 1,000,000 per year [1, 2]. Although many of those grafts are implanted in patients with bone, joint, and spine abnormalities, ophthalmic plastic and reconstructive surgeons frequently place tissue grafts in patients with eyelid and orbital disorders. The types of tissue used most commonly for eyelid and orbital reconstruction include fascia lata, pericardium, dermis, sclera, and bone.

In weighing the benefits and risks associated with use of donor tissue, the possibility for transmission of infectious disease should be considered. Case reports and other information document that bacterial and viral diseases as well as prion disease (Creutzfeldt-Jakob disease or CJD) have been transmitted through implantation of contaminated allografts [1–16]. Overall, the frequency of transmission of infectious diseases to recipients seems to be quite low. However, current methods of screening, testing, and processing donor tissue have limitations that result in some contaminated allografts being distributed in the U.S. each year. Also, the possibility of tissue contamination with new or emerging pathogens poses at least some risk, particularly because such pathogens may not be identified and eliminated through current methods of donor screening and tissue processing. Consequently, it is important for surgeons who recommend allografts to their patients to be aware of those limitations and to adopt procedures for minimizing recipient exposure to pathogens.

1.2 Reports of Infectious Disease Transmission

We are not aware of any reports of allograft-associated transmission of human immunodeficiency virus (HIV), hepatitis B virus (HBV), hepatitis C virus (HCV), or prion disease during eyelid, orbit, or lacrimal system procedures. Transmission of prion disease (CJD) following cornea transplantation has been reported in one patient in the U.S. [13], and possible transmission has been reported in one patient in Japan [14] and one patient in Germany [15]. One of the authors (RHK) and other ophthalmic plastic surgeons have treated patients with postoperative bacterial infection involving donor fascia lata used to repair congenital ptosis (Fig. 1.1). It is quite possible that the infections in those patients may have occurred through wound contamination rather than through contamination of the donor fascia lata. The lack of case reports of disease transmission suggests that the overall risk for patients who have eyelid or orbital procedures is quite low. For several reasons though, identification of patients who have developed infectious diseases from contaminated allografts is likely incomplete.

Diseases such as HIV and forms of viral hepatitis such as HCV may not become evident in the recipient until many weeks or months after implantation of an allograft. At that time, the possibility of graft contamination may not be considered, and even if it is, it may not be possible to document whether the graft had been contaminated. Also, unless the patient had been tested for HIV or viral hepatitis previously, it may not be possible to determine whether the disease developed before or after placement of the allograft. This is particularly true with regard to HCV because many patients with the disease do not know that they are infected and the prevalence rate of the disease in the general population is relatively high. Even when bacterial infection occurs during the early postoperative period, investigation to determine whether graft contamination could have played a role is generally not conducted. Unfortunately, limitations of commonly used methods for screening donors and culturing tissue grafts may preclude identification of the specific causes of bacterial infection in recipients. For example, if graft contamination were suspected as the cause of bacterial infection in a recipient, the tissue bank that supplied the graft could be notified and the records concerning screening and testing of the donor could be reviewed. Typically, only the

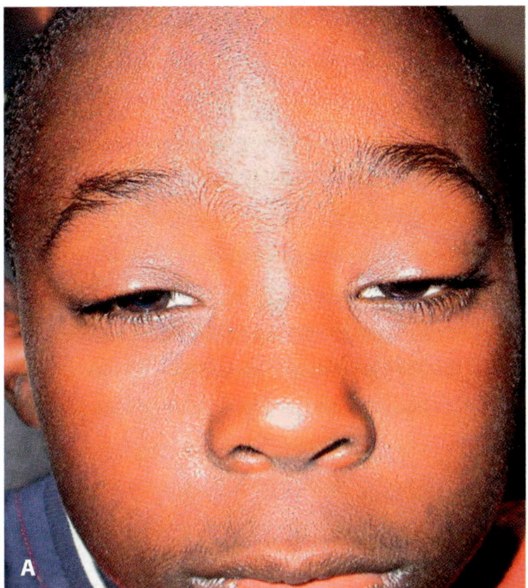

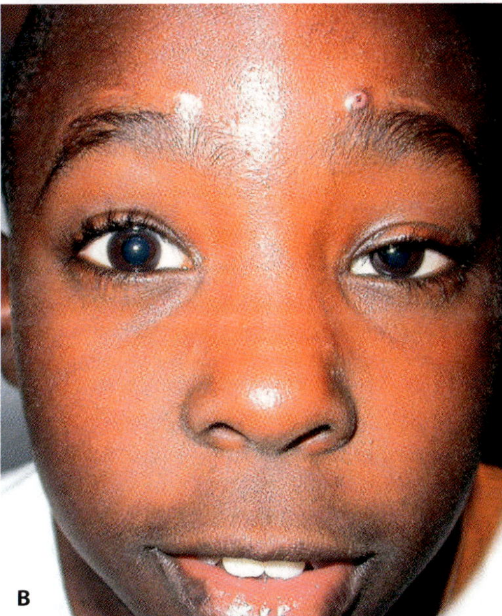

Fig. 1.1. **A** Congenital ptosis with poor levator function (preoperative). **B** Postoperative bacterial infection with recurrence of ptosis and purulent discharge from wound above left brow following bilateral ptosis repair with frontalis suspension with donor fascia lata

surfaces of allografts are cultured, sometimes after the surfaces have been exposed to solutions that contain antibiotics. Consequently, if the culture results were reported as negative (as would be expected for donor tissue that had been released for distribution), the question of whether contamination with bacteria or spores had been present within the inner matrices of the allograft might remain unanswered.

The following case reports demonstrate that infectious disease transmission through implantation of contaminated allografts has occurred with donor tissue similar to that used in eyelid and orbital reconstruction. Although the overall risk for disease transmission seems quite low, factors such as the specific methods used to process donor tissue do influence risk. For donor tissue obtained and processed under similar conditions, however, there is no evidence to suggest that risk varies according to whether an allograft is used for spine or joint reconstruction or is placed in the eyelids or orbit. The total number of allografts used in procedures on the spine and joints is much greater than the volume implanted by ophthalmic plastic surgeons. This may be one reason for the lack of case reports of disease transmission in the ophthalmic literature. Also, the relatively small tissue grafts implanted in eyelids and orbits may not transmit disease as readily as the larger allografts used in other reconstructive procedures.

1.2.1 Hepatitis C Virus (HCV)

The introduction of a new test for HCV (HCV 2.0 assay) provided an opportunity to re-test frozen sera from donors that had previously been determined not to have had HCV based on the results of testing with the HCV 1.0 assay [7]. Allografts from those donors had already been processed, distributed, and implanted in patients. Of 470 specimens tested, two were found to be positive for HCV based on the HCV 2.0 assay.

A total of 23 tissue grafts had been produced from one of those donors shown to have actually been positive for HCV. Thirteen of the allografts had been implanted in 12 patients. Only six recipients were found and included in a follow-up study. All allografts implanted in those recipients had been irradiated during processing. One recipient tested positive for HCV, but exposure to the allograft may not have led to transmission because the patient had other risk factors for HCV and sequence analysis demonstrated non-identity between the donor and recipient HCV isolates.

Five recipients were identified who had received allografts from the second donor found to be positive with the HCV 2.0 assay and all five were clinically asymptomatic with regard to HCV. The donor tissue had been cryopreserved, but had undergone minimal processing and had not been irradiated before distribution. Four of the five recipients tested positive for HCV. Of those four recipients, three had received donor patellar ligament and one had received bone. The investigators concluded that transmission of HCV had occurred through exposure to the contaminated allografts.

In 2003, investigators at the Centers for Disease Control and Prevention (CDC) reported that HCV had been transmitted to recipients of allografts from a donor who had tested negative with the HCV 2.0 assay [3]. A recipient of a patellar tendon with bone allograft was diagnosed as having HCV about 6 weeks postoperatively. This led to additional testing of stored frozen serum that had been obtained from the donor before death. It tested positive for HCV RNA, confirming that the donor had HCV. A total of 91 organs and tissues had been obtained from the donor, and 44 had already been transplanted into 40 recipients. Six recipients received organs, two received corneas, and 32 received other tissues (saphenous vein, tendon, bone, and skin). Three of three organ recipients who were tested had developed HCV. Of the 32 who received other tissues, HCV was known to have been present in three before placement of the contaminated allografts and test results were not available for another two recipients. Five of the 27 other recipients of tissue grafts tested positive for HCV (one of two recipients of saphenous vein; one of three recipients of tendon; and three of three recipients of tendon with bone). Transmission of HCV was not observed among recipients of skin (zero of two recipients) or among recipients of bone that had been irradiated during processing (zero of 16 recipients). One cornea recipient had HCV before transplantation and the other remained negative for HCV (but HCV RNA testing had not been completed).

Investigation of the cause of HCV in the patient who had received an allograft 6 weeks earlier was initiated by the patient's physician [3]. The clinician's suspicion that the infection may have been due to allograft contamination and his or her prompt action in alerting health authorities might well have prevented transmission of HCV to others. It led to identification of the source of infection and to recall of many contaminated allografts before they could be implanted in other patients. This emphasizes that physicians should maintain an awareness of the risk for transmission of HCV and other infectious diseases through use of allografts and should report possible allograft-related infections to local or state health departments promptly.

1.2.2 Human Immunodeficiency Virus (HIV)

In 1985, organs, musculoskeletal tissue, and other tissues were obtained from an adult male donor who had been tested for HIV and was incorrectly found to be negative [8]. It seems likely that the donor had been exposed to HIV only a short time before his death due to a gunshot wound and had not yet developed antibodies that could be detected through the serological testing available at that time. HIV was transmitted to four of four organ recipients and to three of four recipients of fresh-frozen bone. A total of 50 other allografts including bone, soft tissue, and cornea from the same donor were processed in various ways and distributed. Serum samples from 33 recipients of those tissue grafts were tested for HIV and all were found to be negative. The authors noted that avascular tissues and those processed by lyophilization, ethanol extraction, irradiation, or the mechanical removal of blood were not associated with HIV transmission in this particular case. All of the allografts that led to transmission of HIV were relatively large and had been processed in a manner that involved immersion in various chemical solutions. Unfortunately, immersion in solutions does not provide any assurance of complete penetration of the inner matrices of bone and removal of all blood, pathogens, and other possible contaminants.

1.2.3 Other Conventional Infectious Diseases

Other diseases including HBV [9], human T-lymphotropic virus [11], rabies [16], and tuberculosis [17] have been transmitted through use of contaminated allografts. Although it remains unknown how frequently bacterial diseases are transmitted, there is considerable evidence to suggest that contamination of allografts with bacteria or spores is not uncommon. Based on direct and swab culturing of 1,999 musculoskeletal tissue grafts obtained from 200 donors, Deijkers and associates reported that 50 % of grafts were contaminated with low virulence organisms and 3% were contaminated with high virulence organisms such as streptococci, *Staphylococcus aureus*, and *Escherichia coli* [18]. The relatively high prevalence of allograft contamination with bacteria may be a consequence of most donor tissue being contributed by cadaveric donors rather than living donors. Following death, bacteria from the gut can gain access to the blood and contaminate other tissues [1, 2]. The low oxygen environment in cadaveric tissue may especially promote persistence of spore-forming organisms such as clostridia. Also, bacterial contamination can be introduced during donor tissue harvesting or processing.

A report from the CDC in 2001 drew attention to the serious consequences of allograft-related transmission of infectious disease [5, 6]. A young man who had received an osteochondral graft during knee reconstruction reported pain around the wound, rapidly developed shock, and died 4 days postoperatively. An investigation conducted by staff from the CDC found that the patient had been infected with *Clostridium sordellii* (an anaerobic spore- and toxin-forming organism) and documented that the infection had been transmitted through use of a contaminated allograft. Following that investigation, the CDC solicited additional reports of allograft-associated infection. Within several weeks, a total of 26 reports of bacterial infections associated with musculoskeletal tissue allografts had been received [4].

All of the contaminated allografts associated with transmission of bacterial infections had been processed aseptically. That is, the tissue had been harvested under controlled conditions according to standard protocols used in tissue banks. Additionally, some of the grafts had been frozen; and three patients received grafts that were reported to have been treated with gamma irradiation [4].

In 2004, investigators from the CDC expanded on their previous findings concerning the transmission of clostridium infection through musculoskeletal allografts [1]. A total of 14 recipients developed such infections following transplantation of tissue from nine contaminated donors processed by a single tissue bank. Aseptic technique was used at the tissue bank and processing included immersion of tissue in a proprietary solution containing imipenem, vancomycin, amikacin, amphotericin B, and fluconazole. Validation studies of the effectiveness of the process in eliminating clostridia and other spore-forming organisms were not provided. The types of contaminated allografts included nine patellar tendons, four femoral condyles, and one meniscus. One recipient died of infection and the others required hospitalization and intravenous antimicrobial therapy. The infections resulted in considerable morbidity including additional surgical procedures to remove the allografts (n=10) and knee-replacement surgery (n=3). Some tissue from the contaminated donors was provided to other tissue banks and was either exposed to irradiation (n=25: bone, tendon, and fascia lata allografts) or processed with a recently introduced method (the BioCleanse process from Regeneration Technologies, Inc.) for sterilizing musculoskeletal tissue (n=65: bone allografts). The allografts processed by those methods were not associated with transmission of clostridium infection.

The investigators concluded that standards for testing and processing need to be strengthened to prevent allograft-related transmission of infectious diseases [1]. They made several recommendations about procedures related to culturing and handling of donor tissue and emphasized the need for widespread use of processing methods that can kill bacterial spores and sterilize tissue.

Summary for the Clinician

- **Allograft-associated transmission of HIV, HBV, HCV, human T-lymphotropic virus, rabies, and tuberculosis has occurred during various plastic and reconstructive surgical procedures. Although we are not aware of any reports of transmission during eyelid, orbit, or lacrimal system procedures, the risk for such an occurrence is present. Transmission of bacterial infection (e.g., clostridium infection) through use of contaminated allografts has resulted in considerable morbidity or death in some patients. In the future, it should be possible to prevent most recipients from being exposed to infectious diseases through widespread adoption of currently available processing methods that are capable of sterilizing allografts.**

1.2.4 Creutzfeldt-Jakob Disease (CJD)

Prion diseases, such as CJD, are rare, fatal neurodegenerative disorders that generally terminate within 1 year of initial symptoms. Many reports document that CJD can be transmitted through contaminated dura mater and anterior pituitary hormones [12]. However, there has never been recognized transmission of CJD through transplantation of fascia lata, pericardium, dermis, sclera, or bone, the donor tissues most commonly used by ophthalmic plastic surgeons, or in association with human musculoskeletal tissue, or organs peripheral to the central nervous system. Despite several decades of epidemiological investigation, no disease transmission has ever been documented to occur in recipients of labile blood components or therapeutic proteins derived from plasma pools to which patients later dying of the sporadic form of CJD had contributed [19]. However, two British patients with the variant form of CJD (vCJD) resulting from exposure to bovine spongiform encephalopathy (BSE or mad-cow disease) have very likely been responsible for secondary transmissions via transfusions of packed red blood cells donated 18 months and 3 years before the onset of their symptoms [20, 21].

The risk of prion disease transmission from connective tissue, skin, and bone has been classified as theoretical only (Table 1.1) [22]. Findings from several studies provide confidence that the risk of transmitting CJD through use of donor fascia lata, pericardium, dermis, or bone, if not zero, must be exceedingly low. The findings include: (1) epidemiological information from five case-control studies involving more than 600 patients with CJD shows no evidence that blood transfusion increases the risk for CJD; (2) recipients of blood components from known CJD donors have not developed the disease (the studies are limited by small sample sizes of subjects followed for long periods); (3) patient populations with increased exposure to blood or blood products (e.g., patients with hemophilia) are not at increased risk for CJD; (4) transfusion of blood units from three patients with CJD failed to transmit the disease to chimpanzees; and (5) skeletal muscle (n=5), heart muscle (n=4), and adipose tissue (n=1) from patients with CJD have been inoculated intracerebrally into primates and no transmission of CJD has occurred [22, 23]. Another factor is that more than eight million musculoskeletal tissue grafts have been distributed in the U.S. in the past 15 years without identification of allograft-related transmission of CJD in any recipient.

In the U.S., a single case report provides strong evidence of transmission of CJD through cornea transplantation [13]. This raises concerns about the safety of implanting donor sclera in patients who need eyelid or orbital reconstruction. Donor sclera often includes a small segment of optic nerve (Fig. 1.2), a tissue that should be considered to have the same potential infectivity as brain (Table 1.1). Although there have been no reports to implicate the use of donor sclera as the cause of disease in a patient with CJD, this does not confirm that such transmission could not occur. Several factors would make it difficult to identify an association between donor sclera and development of CJD (if it really does exist). Those include the relatively low prevalence rate of CJD among donors who have been screened for the disease, the relatively low volume of scleral grafts implanted in patients in the U.S., the long average duration of the incubation period for development of CJD, and the difficulty in establishing an association

Table 1.1. Distribution of infectivity in patients with Creutzfeldt-Jakob disease (CJD)

Infectivity category	Tissues, secretions, and excretions
High infectivity	Brain, spinal cord, eye
Medium infectivity	Reticuloendothelial system including spleen, tonsil, and lymph nodes; cerebrospinal fluid, ileum, proximal colon, adrenal gland, pituitary gland, dura mater, pineal gland, placenta
Low infectivity	Thymus, peripheral nerves, bone marrow, liver, lung, pancreas, nasal mucosa, blood (in vCJD)
No detectable infectivity	Skeletal muscle, heart, bone, mammary gland, colostrum, milk, serum, urine, feces, bile, kidney, thyroid, salivary gland, saliva, ovary, uterus, testis, seminal testis, fetal tissue, connective tissue, cartilaginous tissue, hair, skin

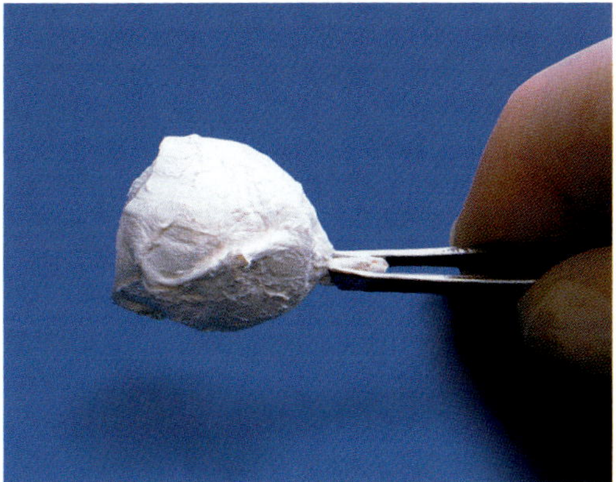

Fig. 1.2. Donor sclera following Tutoplast processing. The attached segment of optic nerve may pose risk for transmission of Creutzfeldt-Jakob disease (CJD) even though Tutoplast processing may reduce any such risk. (Photograph courtesy of IOP, Inc.)

even if a recipient later developed CJD [24]. For those reasons, we favor use of donor tissues other than sclera (e.g., fascia lata, pericardium, or dermis) for eyelid and orbital reconstruction. Surgeons who believe the benefits of donor sclera outweigh the risks, however, should consider using Tutoplast-processed tissue (Fig. 1.2). Although we are not aware of any published validation studies to confirm that the Tutoplast process inactivates or eliminates prions from sclera, the process includes immersion in a solution of sodium hydroxide that may reduce the risk for transmission of CJD. Also, it would seem prudent to excise and discard any attached segment of optic nerve and a small rim of surrounding sclera before implanting scleral grafts.

Summary for the Clinician

- **The risk of transmitting CJD through implantation of donor fascia lata, pericardium, dermis, or bone is either exceedingly low or non-existent. Use of donor sclera raises concerns because it is closely associated with the optic nerve, a tissue that should be considered to have the same high risk for transmission of CJD as brain.**
  For this reason, we prefer to use substitute materials rather than donor sclera. If sclera is selected, however, we recommend Tutoplast-processed sclera because processing may reduce the risk of transmitting CJD.

1.3 Sources of Risk for Allograft Contamination

Unfortunately, each step in current procedures for selecting tissue donors and applying aseptic processing has inherent limitations and is less than completely effective in eliminating contamination (Table 1.2). Also, human errors in applying those procedures and handling test results contribute to the risk of allograft contamination with pathogens. Consequently, the relative safety of allografts depends on applying a combination of several different screening and testing methods that when used together eliminate most contaminated tissue. An understanding of the weaknesses of current procedures as described in this section should be helpful in discussing with patients the risks and benefits of using allografts as well as possible alternatives.

Table 1.2. Sources of risk for allograft contamination and recipient exposure to pathogens

Most donor tissue obtained from cadaveric donors, not living persons
Prevalence rates of infectious disease generally higher in cadavers than in living persons
Prolonged time interval from death to tissue harvest
Complete medical records not always available for review
Medical and social history provided by someone other than donor
Contamination of tissue from sources already present within the donor (after death, bacteria may spread from the gut to the blood and tissue)
Break of sterile technique during tissue harvesting or processing with the introduction of pathogens
Low sensitivity of tissue culturing to detect bacterial contamination (bacteria present in graft inner matrices may not be detected by culturing of graft surface)
Infectious window periods for HIV, HBV, and HCV when infection will not be detected by currently used tests
False negative test results for viral infection
Emergence of new pathogens that would not be detected and eliminated through current screening, testing, and tissue processing (e.g., emergence of West Nile virus)
Processing methods that sterilize allografts not required by FDA regulations and not widely used by tissue banks; label claims about graft sterility not currently regulated by FDA
Human error in following standard practices for screening and testing donors and for processing tissue

1.3.1 Living Donors and Cadaveric Tissue

Several factors contribute to the risk of pathogens remaining in donor tissue that has been screened, tested, and processed for distribution. One of those factors – whether the donor tissue was obtained from a cadaver or a living donor – has an important impact on the risk of contamination, but is not usually recognized by surgeons as a variable that should be considered. The difference in risk by source of donor tissue arises from the generally greater prevalence rates of infectious diseases and CJD among cadavers than among living persons. Clostridia and other bacteria that can pass from the gut into the blood and tissue following death and that can persist and form spores in a low oxygen environment, for example, may be much more common in cadaveric tissue than in tissue obtained from living donors [1, 2]. This is important because unlike blood and blood products that are obtained from living donors, almost all donor fascia lata, pericardium, dermis, sclera, and bone are obtained from cadavers.

The annual mortality rate of CJD in the U.S. has been reported to be about 1 per 1,000,000 persons [25]. Also, the prevalence rate of symptomatic CJD among living persons at any given point in time can be estimated to be approximately 1 per 1,000,000. For comparison, the prevalence rate of CJD among cadavers can be calculated by dividing the total number of deaths due to CJD by the total number of deaths due to all causes. In the U.S., this yields a rate of about 1 per 10,000 [24, 26]. Thus, CJD is about 100 times more frequent among cadavers (potential tissue donors) than symptomatic CJD is among living persons. Kennedy and associates have reported that after all screening of potential cornea donors (medical record reviews and interviews of medical staff and family members), about 1 in 35,000 donors selected for processing might be expected to have CJD [24].

Similar considerations apply with regard to HIV, HCV, and other infectious diseases. For example, the prevalence rate of HCV has been reported to be 0.4% among first-time blood donors [27], but data from tissue banks show a rate of 1.06% among potential donors [28]. If screening were completely effective in identifying and excluding infected donors or if tissue processing were completely effective in eliminating pathogens from donor tissue, the generally higher prevalence rates of infectious diseases among cadavers than among living persons would not be of particular concern. Because donor screening and tissue processing are not completely effective, however, the higher prevalence rates of infectious diseases among cadavers contribute directly to higher rates of contamination of allografts than if donor tissue were obtained primarily from living persons.

1.3.2 Donor Screening and Testing

Screening of each potential donor for the presence of transmissible disease involves a review of the medical records, completion of a medical and social history questionnaire (generally based on an interview of a family member or acquaintance), and physical examination of the body for any evidence of infectious disease, disease processes indicative of infectious disease such as Kaposi's sarcoma, or high-risk behaviors such as use of intravenous drugs. Although screening serves an important function in eliminating potential donors who are obviously unacceptable, it has several limitations. For cadaveric donors, someone other than the donor must provide the medical and social history information. Because the social history involves questions about behaviors and activities that are not widely considered to be socially acceptable, the person responding to the interviewer may not know whether the donor engaged in any such activities. Also, family members and acquaintances may be reluctant to share information concerning behaviors that they consider to be embarrassing or to reflect poorly on the potential donor.

If initial screening yields no disqualifying information, blood is drawn and tested for various infectious diseases. The U.S. Food and Drug Administration (FDA) requires that all donors be tested for HIV, HBV, and HCV, but most tissue banks conduct additional tests for diseases such as syphilis and human T-lymphotropic virus. Tissue banks are required to conduct additional testing on tissue to be distributed in certain states such as New York and Florida that have more stringent regulations than those enforced by the FDA. Such testing does not completely eliminate the possibility of disease transmission because a donor may have been exposed to the pathogen only recently and still be within what is termed the infectious window period (the time interval from exposure to a pathogen to when the infectious particles or antibodies to the pathogen can be detected by testing). Also, false negative test results can occur even when disease has been present for longer than the duration of the infectious window period. The total risk of an allograft harboring a particular virus, therefore, is related to the combined risks arising from both the infectious window period and false negative test results.

With regard to HIV, the currently required HIV types 1 and 2 antibody screening assay for cadaveric blood samples (Genetic Systems Human Immunodeficiency Virus Types 1 and 2 Peptide EIA) has very high sensitivity, reported to be 99.84–100% (95% confidence interval). Similarly, the sensitivity of testing for HBV (Genetic Systems Antibody to Hepatitis B Surface Antigen EIA) approaches 100%. An analysis of the sensitivity of third-generation diagnostic tests for HCV provided a sensitivity estimate of 97.2% (95% confidence interval: 92–99%) [29]. Although this level of sensitivity seems quite high, it suggests that about three of every 100 potential donors who have HCV (and pass the medical record and other screening) are found to have negative test results for the disease. Based on the negative test results, tissue from those infected donors is accepted, processed, and distributed for implantation in patients. Recently, the Procleix HIV type 1 and HCV test (Gen-Probe, Inc.) based on nucleic-acid amplification has been approved by the FDA for use on cadaveric blood samples. The sensitivity of this test for HIV and HCV approaches 100%, and it allows earlier detection of infection, resulting in considerably shorter infectious window periods for both HIV and HCV.

There is at present no practical method capable of identifying prion infection during the pre-clinical (asymptomatic) phase of disease. However, several tests designed to detect the pathognomonic prion protein in circulating blood are under investigation. Preliminary data for two such test methods presented at recent scientific meetings suggest that a successful blood screening test may become available in the future.

Summary for the Clinician

- **Incorrectly diagnosed causes of death and the generally higher prevalence rates of infectious diseases among cadavers than among living persons contribute to the risk of tissue donors having unsuspected infectious diseases. Screening and testing are useful in identifying donor tissue that harbors pathogens, but are not effective in eliminating all contaminated tissue due to the limitations of test sensitivity in detecting infection during pre-clinical stages of disease, and the occurrence of false negative test results.**

1.3.3 Aseptic Processing of Donor Tissue

The current standard for ensuring the safety of donor tissue is termed aseptic processing (Table 1.3). This involves conducting the required donor screening and testing. Also, tissue must be harvested and allografts must be packaged under controlled conditions. (That is, the harvesting and packaging should be conducted in a manner to minimize the risk of contamination being introduced, but this does not address the problem of contamination due to pathogens that are already present in the donor tissue.) It is assumed (erroneously) that these procedures will result in the selection of donor tissue that harbors no pathogens.

Table 1.3. Aseptic processing of donor tissue

Represents the current standard method for tissue processing used throughout much of the industry
Relies completely on donor screening and testing to eliminate already contaminated tissue from being processed and distributed
Involves conducting tissue harvesting and processing under controlled conditions to prevent the introduction of pathogens
Does not require any processing steps to inactivate or remove pathogens already present in the tissue

Currently, the FDA does not require the application of any procedures to inactivate or eliminate pathogens that might remain in donor tissue that has passed the required screening and testing. Many tissue banks go beyond what is required, however, and apply processing methods that involve immersion of donor tissue in various chemical solutions or exposure to ethylene oxide or irradiation. Because the use of liquid chemical germicides or other processing methods directed at reducing or eliminating pathogens is entirely optional, it is not necessary for tissue banks to conduct and provide the results of validation studies to confirm that any of the processing methods are actually effective in eliminating pathogens. Historically, the FDA has not regulated the claims that tissue banks and other providers of allografts make about tissue products. (A new regulation has recently been published by the agency that will allow the FDA to regulate label claims in the future.) This has led to a situation where many providers offer a range of confusing information to suggest that their allograft products are clean, pure, or even sterile. In some cases, a claim of product sterility has been made on a product package even when there is no evidence that the provider uses any sterilization process. (For the contents to be sterile in those cases, it would have to be assumed that donor screening and testing are 100% effective in eliminating contaminated donor tissue. Based on what is known about the limitations of donor screening and testing, that is not a reasonable assumption.)

In March 2000, Regeneration Technologies, Inc., introduced a validated process (BioCleanse) for sterilizing musculoskeletal allografts (Fig. 1.3). Initially, it was applied to bone, but the company has since validated the process for use on tendon and some other soft tissues. Currently, BioCleanse is not used to sterilize fascia lata, pericardium, dermis, or sclera for eyelid or orbital reconstruction. Unfortunately, the market for allograft products that are used in

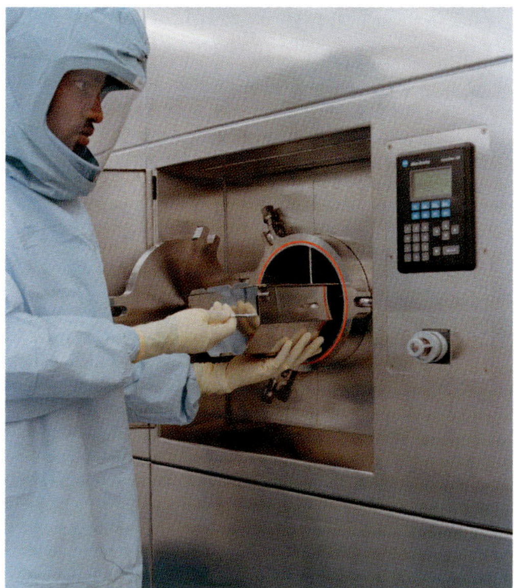

Fig. 1.3. The BioCleanse sterilization process involves use of various chemical solutions, cycles of pressure and vacuum, and serial dilution to inactivate and remove pathogens including bacteria, viruses, spores, and fungi. (Photograph courtesy of Regeneration Technologies, Inc.)

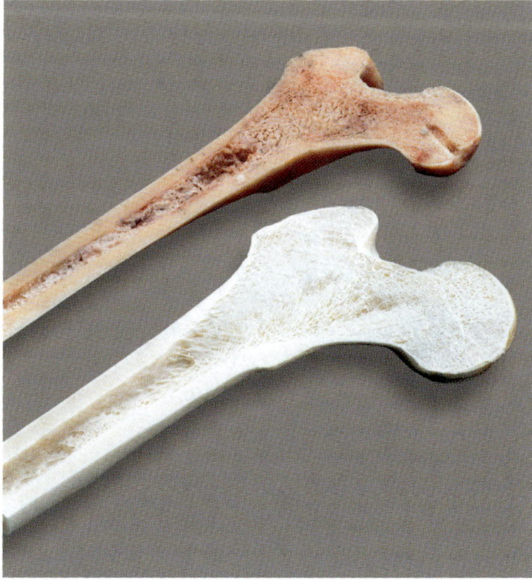

Fig. 1.4. Blood, contaminants, and pathogens that may remain in tissue following aseptic processing (*above*) are removed during BioCleanse processing (*below*). (Photograph courtesy of Regeneration Technologies, Inc.)

eyelid and orbital reconstruction is much smaller than other markets for allografts (e.g., spine, bone, and joint reconstruction). The BioCleanse process involves the introduction and removal of various chemical solutions, the application of cycles of pressure and vacuum to facilitate complete penetration of tissue matrices, and serial dilution with inactivation and removal of pathogens. It has sufficient redundancy to fully compensate for the possibility of a process failure and includes continuous process monitoring. Testing has documented that BioCleanse ensures the sterility of processed allografts and that it has no harmful effects on graft biocompatibility or biomechanical properties (Fig. 1.4). Clearant, Inc., has introduced another method for sterilizing allograft tissue, the Clearant Process. It involves use of high doses of gamma irradiation (50 kGy) as well as a free-radical scavenging solution to minimize or prevent adverse biomechanical effects.

Hopefully, validated methods for sterilizing allografts will be applied in the future to process the types of soft tissue (fascia lata, pericardium, dermis, and sclera) used in eyelid and orbital reconstruction. Current methods that involve use of chemical germicides known to inactivate bacteria and viruses must be shown to fully penetrate the tissue matrices and sterilize not just the surface of a graft, but the entire graft. Sterilization of bone and soft tissue can be achieved with gamma irradiation, but it must be applied at sufficiently high doses. Compared to other pathogens, HIV is somewhat resistant to inactivation by irradiation. Reports indicate that inactivation of HIV requires greater than 35 kGy of irradiation [30, 31], but most tissue banks that use irradiation expose the tissue to a dose of only 5–30 kGy. Doses higher than 30 kGy can be associated with significant loss of tissue strength [32, 33], a particularly important consideration for some types of allografts and clinical applications. The Clearant Process involves use of a free-radical scavenging solution that minimizes or prevents loss of tissue strength even when a dose of 50 kGy is applied. The sterility and biomechanical integrity of processed half round sections of bovine femur up to 20 cm in length have been validated (unpublished data). Although use of chemical germicides and other processing methods may reduce allograft contamination and enhance safety relative to the use of standard aseptic processing alone, any claims of graft sterility should be supported by an extensive set of validation studies that confirm allograft sterility as well as the absence of any harmful effects on graft biocompatibility or biomechanical properties.

Summary for the Clinician

- **Aseptic processing involves donor screening and testing as well as procedures for minimizing contamination of donor tissue during harvesting and processing. Although it represents the current standard for promoting allograft safety, it does not require any procedures for inactivating and removing pathogens that sometimes remain in donor tissue after screening and testing. Aseptic processing, therefore, is not sufficient to ensure allograft sterility.**
- **The BioCleanse process (Regeneration Technologies, Inc.) is a recently introduced tissue sterilization process that has been validated to inactivate and remove all pathogens from musculoskeletal allografts. Currently, it is not used to sterilize fascia lata, pericardium, dermis, or sclera for eyelid or orbital reconstruction. Another method for sterilizing allografts, the Clearant process (Clearant, Inc.) involves the application of high doses of gamma irradiation and use of a free-radical scavenging solution to prevent adverse biomechanical effects.**

1.4 Estimated Risk of Allograft Contamination

The limitations of aseptic processing that contribute to the risk of allograft contamination include less than 100% sensitivity of donor screening and testing to eliminate contaminated tissue and the lack of any requirement that a validated sterilization process be applied. With regard to bacterial contamination, Deijkers and associates reported that 50% of musculoskeletal grafts were contaminated with low virulence organisms and 3% with high virulence organisms [18]. The frequency of contamination with HIV, HBV, and HCV due to false negative test results can be estimated from the sensitivity of tests used to detect those diseases and from epidemiological information concerning the prevalence rates of disease among potential donors who have passed the initial screening of medical records and the interview of a family member or acquaintance [28]. Similarly, data concerning the prevalence rates of viral infection among first-time and repeat blood donors provide a basis for estimating the risk of contamination associated with the infectious window period among tissue donors [34].

1.4.1 HIV

The risk of a living donor giving blood during the infectious window period for HIV (the time interval from donor exposure to HIV to when antibodies have formed that could be detected by testing) has been reported to be 1 in 493,000 among serial or repeat blood donors [35]. Koerner and associates have reported that the risk of disease among first-time blood donors is about 10 times greater than among repeat donors based on a study of HCV [34]. Because of the decreased effectiveness of screening tissue donors for infectious disease compared to that of blood donors (due to reliance on family members and acquaintances for medical and social history information), it seems likely that the prevalence rates of viral diseases among tissue donors are at least as great as among first-time blood donors. Based on this assumption, it can be estimated that the risk of HIV associated with the infectious window period among tissue donors would be about 1 in 49,000. Because the sensitivity of testing for HIV is very high (about 99.9%) and the prevalence rate of HIV among potential tissue donors is very low (about 1 per 3,300), false negative test results should occur quite infrequently. Consequently, the risk of tissue contamination with HIV after all screening and testing has been completed is due almost entirely to risk associated with the infectious window period; and the overall risk of allograft contamination with HIV is estimated to be about 1 in 49,000 with use of the currently required HIV types 1 and 2 antibody screening assay. Because tests based on nucleic acid testing (Procleix HIV type 1 and HCV test, Gen-Probe, Inc.) are associated with a much shorter infectious window period (reduced by as much as half), the risk of allograft contamination with HIV following such testing might be as low as about 1 in 100,000.

1.4.2 HCV and HBV

False negative test results for HCV are a much greater problem than for HIV because the prevalence rate of HCV among potential tissue donors is considerably higher at approximately 1 in 94 and the sensitivity of the third-generation diagnostic test for HCV commonly used by tissue banks is lower (97.2%) [28, 29]. Using those figures, it can be calculated that about 1 in every 3,260 donors who passes all screening and testing and is accepted for tissue processing would be expected to actually have HCV (but would have had a false negative test result). After adjustment for risk associated with the infectious window period (based on the assumption that this risk is the same as that among first-time blood donors) [34, 35], the overall risk of allograft contamination with HCV is estimated to be about 1 in 2,500. Again, use of nucleic acid testing should lower this risk considerably, possibly to a level of about 1 in 40,000 based on the reported sensitivity of 100% and much shorter infectious window period associated with this test. Because the sensitivity of testing for HBV is reported to be 100%, the overall risk of HBV arises entirely from the infectious window period and is estimated to be about 1 in 6,300 with use of currently required tests [34, 35].

1.5 Human Error in Donor Screening and Testing

Even when the procedures involved in donor screening and testing are applied properly, some contaminated allografts are distributed and implanted in patients because of the inherent limitations of those methods (e.g., less than 100% sensitivity of testing for contamination). Another important factor that contributes to risk is human error in following standard screening and testing practices. Although it is not possible to estimate precisely how frequently human error leads to recipient exposure to pathogens or transmission of disease, data from the FDA indicate that human error represents an important source of risk. The FDA has regulated tissue products since 1994 and reports information about allograft recalls [36]. A recall occurs when it becomes apparent after allograft distribution that standard donor screening and testing procedures were not followed or that the tissue was contaminated. For example, subsequent discovery of mishandled serology results that were positive for HIV, HBV, or HCV would trigger recalls of all allografts from the affected donor tissue.

Table 1.4. Number of musculoskeletal tissue grafts recalled by the U.S. Food and Drug Administration, 1994–October 2004 [36]

Reason for recall	No.	%
Improper donor evaluation	11,490	43.0
Positive culture	10,007	37.5
Positive serology or improper donor evaluation	3,140	11.8
Positive serology	1,506	5.6
Other	569	2.1
Total	26,712	100.0

The reports provided by the FDA concerning individual recalls vary with regard to the amount of detail provided. For example, in some cases, the numbers of donors rather than grafts are listed. Also, the reason for each recall is not always described in sufficient detail to determine the exact reason. Information shown in Table 1.4 indicates, however, that human error is not uncommon. A total of 26,712 musculoskeletal tissue grafts have been recalled during a period of about 10 years. It is concerning that large numbers of recalls involved tissue associated with positive culture or serology results. The FDA does not provide information about the intended clinical applications of recalled musculoskeletal grafts (i.e., what proportion was prepared for eyelid and orbital applications and what proportion for other types of reconstruction) or even how many of the recalled grafts had already been implanted in patients.

Summary for the Clinician

- **Human errors in following standard donor screening and testing procedures are not uncommon and often lead to the recall of allografts that have been distributed for use in patients. This represents a major source of risk for recipient exposure to pathogens. The FDA does not report how many recalled tissue grafts had already been implanted in patients at the time of recall initiation. This source of risk emphasizes the need for widespread use of processing methods that have been validated to sterilize donor tissue.**

1.6 Conclusions and Recommendations

Factors that influence the risk of recipient exposure to contaminated allografts include the prevalence rates of disease among cadavers (potential donors), effectiveness of screening and laboratory testing, duration of the infectious window periods before disease can be detected, effectiveness of tissue processing in eliminating pathogens, type of tissue graft, and human error in conducting screening, testing, and processing (Table 1.2). Improvements in testing for HIV and viral hepatitis (such as nucleic acid testing) have shortened the infectious window periods for those diseases and should reduce the number of false negative test results. Data published by the FDA concerning allograft recalls suggest that human error remains a major source of risk for allograft contamination. Because the annual volume of musculoskeletal allografts used in the U.S. is about 1,000,000 [1, 2], human error and the other sources of contamination risk likely account for the distribution of many allografts (perhaps in the hundreds) contaminated with HIV, HCV, or HBV each year. A much larger number of allografts are likely contaminated with bacteria.

Clearly, recipient exposure to contaminated allografts does not always lead to disease transmission. With regard to blood products, the risk of transmission after recipient exposure to HCV, HBV, or HIV has been estimated to be about 90% [35]. Based on the limited case reports of disease transmission to allograft recipients, the corresponding risk associated with large or vascular bone or tendon allografts that have not been processed with BioCleanse or exposed to irradiation (such as with the Clearant Process) may be just as high [3, 7–9]. The risk of disease transmission associated with exposure to small or thin contaminated fascia lata, pericardium, or dermis grafts (such as the grafts used in eyelid and orbital reconstruction) remains unknown, but is almost certainly much lower. Also, processing that includes immersion of small or thin grafts in various liquid chemical germicides may be more effective in eliminating pathogens than similar processing of large allografts. Large allografts may not be fully penetrated by the solution and may continue to harbor pathogens.

The need for reliable methods of sterilizing allografts has been recognized by investigators at the CDC and the FDA [1, 4]. Recently, they have encouraged the development and widespread implementation of processing methods that will sterilize tissue without producing any harmful effects on graft biocompatibility or biomechanical properties. Although the introduction of the BioCleanse process demonstrates that this is possible, other methods of tissue sterilization such as exposure to irradiation or ethylene oxide can be associated, in certain circumstances, with unsatisfactory adverse effects on biocompatibility or biomechanical properties [32, 33, 37, 38].

A new regulation will allow the FDA to regulate product label claims about allograft sterility in the future. This should reduce the amount of confusing information offered by allograft providers concerning the safety of tissue products. Currently, the BioCleanse process is validated to sterilize bone and some soft tissues. Although it has not been applied to the soft tissue allografts used in eyelid and orbital reconstruction (fascia lata, pericardium, and dermis), it may be in the future. The Clearant Process involves use of a tissue radioprotectant solution and, therefore, offers a promising method for sterilizing allografts without producing the harmful effects generally associated with doses of gamma irradiation as high as 50 kGy. Though the results of validation studies have not been shared with us, a review of the Tutoplast process suggests that the fascia lata and pericardium processed in this manner and offered by IOP, Inc. are likely sterile.

Until soft tissue grafts that are documented to be sterile become available for use in eyelid and orbital reconstruction, we recommend the selection of allografts that have undergone irradiation or Tutoplast processing rather than those handled according to the current standard of aseptic processing alone (Table 1.3). Also, other materials such as autografts may provide an acceptable alternative in certain situations. Of course, use of an autograft is not without risk as it may prolong the duration of the surgical procedure and can lead to wound infection and other complications at the graft harvest site. Similarly, synthetic materials may not function as well as a tissue graft and may have other disadvantages.

Because of the close association between optic nerve and sclera, consideration should be given to the risk for transmission of CJD through transplantation of sclera (Table 1.1). For this reason, we favor the use of substitute materials such as fascia lata, pericardium, or dermis. Ophthalmic plastic surgeons who believe the benefits of using sclera outweigh the risks should strongly consider selecting Tutoplast-processed sclera because such processing may reduce the risk of transmitting CJD. Also, the risk may be lowered further by excising any attached segment of optic nerve together with a small rim of surrounding sclera before implanting the graft. The risk of transmitting non-variant forms of CJD through implantation of donor fascia lata, pericardium, dermis, or bone is exceedingly low and may be non-existent. However, there may be greater risk of disease transmission from patients incubating the variant form of CJD, based on the greater amount of prions in the peripheral tissues of such patients and the already documented infectivity in blood [20, 21].

Finally, all surgeons should maintain an awareness of the potential for infectious diseases to be transmitted through allografts and should report to local and state health authorities any case of postoperative infection that may have been due to implantation of a contaminated allograft. This could prevent additional cases of disease transmission if other allografts from the same donor have already been distributed, but not yet implanted, in patients.

References

1. Kainer MA, Linden JV, Whaley DN, et al. (2004) Clostridium infections associated with musculoskeletal-tissue allografts. N Engl J Med 350: 2564–2571
2. Patel R, Trampuz A (2004) Infections transmitted through musculoskeletal-tissue allografts. N Engl J Med 350:2544–2546
3. Morb Mortal Wkly Rep (2003) Hepatitis C virus transmission from an antibody-negative organ and tissue donor – United States, 2000–2002. MMWR Morb Mortal Wkly Rep 52:273–276
4. Morb Mortal Wkly Rep (2002) Update. Allograft-associated bacterial infections – United States, 2002. MMWR Morb Mortal Wkly Rep 51:207–210
5. Morb Mortal Wkly Rep (2001) Unexplained deaths following knee surgery – Minnesota, November 2001. MMWR Morb Mortal Wkly Rep 50:1035–1036
6. Morb Mortal Wkly Rep (2001) Update: unexplained deaths following knee surgery – Minnesota, 2001. MMWR Morb Mortal Wkly Rep 50:1080
7. Conrad EU, Gretch DR, Obermeyer KR, et al. (1995) Transmission of the hepatitis-C virus by tissue transplantation. J Bone Joint Surg Am 77: 214–224
8. Simonds RJ, Holmberg SD, Hurwitz RL, et al. (1992) Transmission of human immunodeficiency virus type 1 from a seronegative organ and tissue donor. N Engl J Med 326:726–732
9. Shutkin NM (1954) Homologous-serum hepatitis following the use of refrigerated bone-bank bone. J Bone Joint Surg Am 36:160–162
10. Morb Mortal Wkly Rep (2001) Septic arthritis following anterior cruciate ligament reconstruction using tendon allografts – Florida and Louisiana, 2000. MMWR Morb Mortal Wkly Rep 50:1081–1083
11. Lennart S, Carlsson A (1997) Transmission of human T-cell lymphotropic virus type 1 by a deep-frozen bone allograft. Acta Orthop Scand 68:72–74

12. Brown P, Preece M, Brandel J-P, et al. (2000) Iatrogenic Creutzfeldt-Jakob disease at the millennium. Neurology 55:1075–1081
13. Duffy P, Wolf J, Collins G, DeVoe AG, Streeten B, Cowen D (1974) Possible person-to-person transmission of Creutzfeldt-Jakob disease. N Engl J Med 290:692–693
14. Uchiyama K, Ishida C, Yago S, Kuramaya H, Kitmoto T (1994) An autopsy case of Creutzfeldt-Jakob disease associated with corneal transplantation. Dementia 8:466–473
15. Heckmann JG, Lang CJG, Petruch F, et al. (1997) Transmission of Creutzfeldt-Jakob disease via a corneal transplant. J Neurol Neurosurg Psychiatry 63:388–390
16. Houff SA, Burton RC, Wilson RW, et al. (1979) Human-to-human transmission of rabies virus by corneal transplant. N Engl J Med 300:603–604
17. James JIP (1953) Tuberculosis transmitted by banked bone. J Bone Joint Surg Br 35:578
18. Deijkers RL, Bloem RM, Petit PL, Brand R, Vehmeyer SB, Veen MR (1997) Contamination of bone allografts: analysis of incidence and predisposing factors. J Bone Joint Surg Br 79:161–166
19. Wilson K, Code C, Ricketts MN (2000) Risk of acquiring Creutzfeldt-Jakob disease from blood transfusions: systematic review of case-control studies. BMJ 321:17–19
20. Llewelyn CA, Hewitt PE, Knight RSG, et al. (2004) Possible transmission of variant Creutzfeldt-Jakob disease by blood transfusion. Lancet 363: 417–421
21. Peden AH, Head MW, Ritchie DL, Bell JE, Ironside JW (2004) Autopsy detection of pre-clinical vCJD transmission following blood transfusion from a *PRNP* codon 129 heterozygous patient. Lancet 364:527–529
22. Brown P, Gibbs CJ, Rodgers-Johnson P, et al. (1994) Human spongiform encephalopathy: the National Institutes of Health series of 300 cases of experimentally transmitted disease. Ann Neurol 35:513–529
23. Food and Drug Administration (1999) Revised precautionary measures to reduce the possible risk of transmission of Creutzfeldt-Jakob disease (CJD) and new variant Creutzfeldt-Jakob disease (nvCJD) by blood and blood products. Food and Drug Administration, Rockville, MD
24. Kennedy RH, Hogan RN, Brown P, et al. (2001) Eye banking and screening for Creutzfeldt-Jakob disease. Arch Ophthalmol 119:721–726
25. Holman RC, Khan AS, Belay ED, Schonberger LB (1996) Creutzfeldt-Jakob disease in the United States, 1979–1994: using national mortality data to assess the possible occurrence of variant cases. Emerg Infect Dis 2:333–337
26. Brown P, Gajdusek DC, Gibbs CJ Jr, Asher DM (1985) Potential epidemic of Creutzfeldt-Jakob disease from human growth hormone therapy. N Engl J Med 313:728–731
27. Glynn SA, Kleinman SH, Schreiber GB, et al. (2000) Trends in incidence and prevalence of major transfusion-transmissible viral infections in US blood donors, 1991 to 1996. JAMA 284:229–235
28. Archibald LK (2003) Risk of HCV-infected allografts. Infectious Diseases Society of America, 41st Annual Meeting: Poster 372. Presented October 10, 2003, San Diego, CA
29. Colin C, Lanoir D, Touzet S, Meyaud-Kraemer L, Bailly F, Trepo C and the Hepatitis Group (2001) Sensitivity and specificity of third-generation hepatitis C virus antibody detection assays: an analysis of the literature. J Viral Hepat 8:87–95
30. Campbell DG, Li P (1999) Sterilization of HIV with irradiation: relevance to infected bone allografts. Aust N Z J Surg 69:517–521
31. Fideler BM, Vangsness CT, Moore T, Li Z, Rasheed S (1994) Effects of gamma irradiation on the human immunodeficiency virus: a study in frozen human bone-patellar ligament-bone grafts obtained from infected cadavera. J Bone Joint Surg Am 76:1032–1035
32. Hamer AJ, Stockley I, Elson RA (1999) Changes in allograft bone irradiated at different temperatures. J Bone Joint Surg Br 81:342–344
33. Hamer AJ, Strachan JR, Black MM, Ibbotson CJ, Stockley I, Elson RA (1996) Biochemical properties of cortical allograft bone using a new method of bone strength measurement: a comparison of fresh, fresh-frozen and irradiated bone. J Bone Joint Surg Br 78:363–368
34. Koerner K, Cardoso M, Dengler T, Kerowgan M, Kubanek B (1998) Estimated risk of transmission of hepatitis C virus by blood transfusion. Vox Sang 74:213–216
35. Schreiber GB, Busch MP, Kleinman SH, Korelitz JJ (1996) The risk of transfusion-transmitted viral infections. N Engl J Med 334:1685–1690
36. Food and Drug Administration. Enforcement Report, 1994–2004. Food and Drug Administration, Rockville, MD
37. Jackson DW, Windler GE, Simon TM (1990) Intraarticular reaction associated with the use of freeze-dried, ethylene oxide-sterilized bone-patella tendon-bone allografts in the reconstruction of the anterior cruciate ligament. Am J Sports Med 18:1–10
38. Thoren K, Aspenberg P (1995) Ethylene oxide sterilization impairs allograft incorporation in a conduction chamber. Clin Orthop 318:259–264

Oncology

Current Concepts in the Management of Conjunctival Neoplasms

2

Carol L. Shields, Jerry A. Shields

Supported by the Eye Tumor Research Foundation, Inc., Philadelphia, PA.

Core Messages

- The most common conjunctival tumor is the nevus
- Conjunctival nevi can be pigmented or non-pigmented and often display cysts
- Conjunctival melanoma is rare but is slightly more common nowadays, similar to cutaneous melanoma
- Conjunctival melanoma can arise from a conjunctival nevus, conjunctival primary acquired melanosis, or de novo
- In the USA, squamous cell carcinoma most often occurs in elderly Caucasian males
- Topical chemotherapy is most useful for conjunctival squamous cell carcinoma or intraepithelial neoplasia and it is less effective for primary acquired melanosis. Topical chemotherapy is not effective for conjunctival melanoma
- Amelanotic melanoma and pagetoid invasion of eyelid sebaceous carcinoma can simulate conjunctival squamous cell carcinoma and differentiation histopathologically is important
- Lymphoid tumors tend to occur in the fornix of the conjunctiva and, if bilateral, strongly suggest the presence of systemic lymphoma

2.1 Introduction

Tumors of the conjunctiva and cornea occupy a large spectrum of conditions ranging from benign lesions such as conjunctival nevus or papilloma to aggressive, life-threatening malignancies such as malignant melanoma or Kaposi's sarcoma. The clinical differentiation of these tumors is based on the patient's medical background as well as certain typical clinical features of the tumor. The recognition and proper management of such tumors requires an understanding of the anatomy of the conjunctiva and cornea and knowledge of general principles of tumor management.

2.2 Conjunctival Anatomy

The conjunctiva is a continuous mucous membrane that covers the anterior portion of the globe. It extends from the eyelid margin onto the back surface of the eyelid (palpebral portion), into the fornix (forniceal portion), onto the surface of the globe (bulbar portion), and up to the corneoscleral limbus (limbal portion). The conjunctiva comprises epithelium and stroma. The epithelium consists of both stratified squamous and columnar epithelium. The squamous pattern is found near the limbus and the columnar pattern is found near the fornix. The stroma comprises fibrovascular connective tissue that thickens in the fornix and thins at the limbus.

Special regions of the conjunctiva include the plica semilunaris and caruncle. The plica semilunaris is a vertically oriented fold of conjunctiva, located in the medial portion of the bulbar conjunctiva. It is speculated that the plica semilunaris represents a remnant of the nictitating membrane found in certain animals. The caruncle is located in the medial canthus between the upper and lower punctum. It contains both conjunctival and cutaneous structures such as non-keratinized stratified squamous epithelium overlying the stroma of fibroblasta, melanocytes, sebaceous glands, hair follicles, and striated muscle fibers.

Neoplasms can arise in the conjunctiva from both its epithelial and stromal structures [1–4]. These are similar clinically and histopathologically to tumors that arise from other mucous membranes in the body. However, unlike other mucous membranes in the body, the conjunctiva is partially exposed to sunlight, which may be a factor in the development of some tumors. Similarly, the cornea can develop epithelial tumors, but corneal stromal tumors are uncommon. The caruncle, with its unique composition of both mucous membrane and cuta- neous structures, can generate tumors found both in mucosa and skin [5, 6].

2.3 Diagnostic Techniques

Unlike many other mucous membranes in the body, the conjunctiva is readily visible. Thus, tumors and related lesions that occur in the conjunctiva are generally recognized at a relatively early stage. Since many of these tumors have typical clinical features, an accurate diagnosis can often be made by external ocular examination and slit lamp biomicroscopy, provided that the clinician is familiar with their clinical characteristics. A diagnostic biopsy is not usually necessary in cases of smaller tumors (≤4 clock hours limbal tumor or ≤15 mm basal dimension) that appear benign. If a smaller tumor does require a biopsy, it is often better to completely remove the lesion in one operation (excisional biopsy). In cases of larger lesions (>4 clock hour limbal tumor or >15 mm basal dimension), it may be appropriate to remove a portion of the tumor (incisional biopsy) to obtain a histopathologic diagnosis prior to embarking upon more extensive therapy. Occasionally, exfoliative cytology [7] and fine needle aspiration biopsy can provide useful information on the basis of a few cells.

In addition to evaluation of the conjunctival lesion, meticulous slit lamp examination of the cornea is essential in patients with suspected conjunctival tumors. Invasion of squamous cell carcinoma and melanoma into the peripheral cornea may appear as a subtle, gray surface opacity. It is important to completely outline such corneal involvement prior to surgery, since it is often less visible through the operating microscope than it is with slit lamp biomicroscopy in the office.

2.4 Management

Depending on the presumptive diagnosis and the size and extent of the lesion, management of a conjunctival tumor can consist of serial observation, incisional biopsy, excisional biopsy, cryotherapy, chemotherapy, radiotherapy, modified enucleation, orbital exenteration or various combinations of these methods [1–4]. If large areas of conjunctiva are removed, mucous membrane grafts from the conjunctiva of the opposite eye, buccal mucosa, or amniotic membrane may be necessary [8, 9].

Observation is generally the management of choice for most benign, asymptomatic tumors of the conjunctiva. Selected examples of lesions that can be observed without interventional treatment include pingueculum, dermolipoma, and nevus. External or slit lamp photographs are advisable to document all lesions and are important for the more suspicious lesions. Most patients are examined every 6–12 months looking for evidence of growth, malignant change, or secondary effects on normal surrounding tissues.

Incisional biopsy is reserved for extensive suspicious tumors that are symptomatic or suspected to be malignant. Examples include large squamous cell carcinoma, primary acquired melanosis, melanoma, and conjunctival invasion by sebaceous gland carcinoma. It should be understood that if tumors occupy 4 clock hours or less on the bulbar conjunctiva, excisional biopsy is generally preferable to incisional biopsy. However, larger lesions can be approached by incisional wedge biopsy or punch biopsy. Definitive therapy would then be planned based on the results of biopsy. Incisional biopsy is also appropriate for conditions that are ideally treated with radiotherapy, chemotherapy, or other topical medications. These lesions include lymphoid tumors, metastatic tumors, extensive papillomatosis, and some cases of squamous cell carcinoma and primary acquired melanosis. Incisional biopsy should generally be avoided for melanocytic tumors, especially melanoma, as this can increase the risk for numerous tumor recurrences [10].

Primary excisional biopsy is appropriate for smaller tumors (≤4 clock hours limbal tumor or ≤15 mm basal dimension) that are symptomatic or suspected to be malignant. In these situations, excisional biopsy is preferred over incisional biopsy to avoid inadvertent tumor seeding. Examples of benign and malignant lesions that are ideally managed by excisional biopsy include symptomatic limbal dermoid, steroid-resistant pyogenic granuloma, squamous cell carcinoma and melanoma. When such lesions are located in the conjunctival fornix they can be completely excised and the conjunctiva reconstructed primarily with absorbable sutures, sometimes with fornix deepening sutures or symblepharon ring to prevent adhesions. If the defect cannot be closed primarily, then a mucous membrane graft can be inserted. The surgical technique for limbal tumors is different than that for forniceal tumors [11, 12]. Limbal neoplasms possibly can invade through the corneal epithelium and sclera into the anterior chamber. Thus, it is often necessary to remove a thin lamella of sclera to achieve tumor-free margins and decrease the chance for tumor recurrence. In this regard, we employ a partial lamellar sclerokeratoconjunctivectomy with primary closure for such tumors [11, 12]. Because cells from these friable tumors can seed into adjacent tissues, a gentle technique without touching the tumor (no touch technique) is advised. Additionally, the surgery should be performed using microscopic technique and the operative field should be left dry so that cells adhere to the resected tissue. It is wise to avoid wetting the field with balanced salt solution until after the tumor is completely removed to minimize seeding of cells.

The technique for resection of limbal tumors is performed under retrobulbar anesthesia. Under the operating microscope, the corneal epithelial component is approached first and the conjunctival component is dissected second, with the goal of excising the entire specimen completely in one piece. Absolute alcohol soaked on an applicator is applied to the corneal tumor component [11, 12]. This devitalizes the epithelial cells and allows easier release of the tumor cells from Bowman's layer. A beaver blade is used to gently sweep the affected corneal epithelium into a scroll that rests on the limbal tumor. Next, a conjunctival incision based at the limbus is made 4–5 mm outside the tumor margin down to bare sclera. Flat dissection of a thin underlying scleral lamella is performed to achieve tumor free base. In this way, the entire tumor with tumor-free margins is removed in one piece without touching the tumor itself (no touch technique). The removed specimen is then placed flatly on a piece of cardboard from the surgical tray, placed in fixative, and submitted for histopathologic studies. The used instruments are then replaced with fresh instruments for subsequent steps, to avoid contamination of healthy tissue with possible tumor cells. Double freeze-thaw cryotherapy is applied to the margins of the remaining bulbar conjunctiva. It is not necessary to treat the corneal margins with cryoapplication. The tumor bed is treated with absolute alcohol wash on cotton tip applicator and bipolar cautery, avoiding cryotherapy directly to the sclera. Using clean instruments, the conjunctiva is mobilized for closure of the defect by loosening the intermuscular septum with Steven's scissor spreading and creation of transpositional conjunctival flaps. Closure is completed with interrupted absorbable 6-0 or 7-0 sutures. The patient is treated with topical antibiotics and corticosteroids for 2 weeks.

In the management of conjunctival tumors, cryotherapy can be used as a supplemental treatment to excisional biopsy as described above to eliminate subclinical, microscopic tumor cells and prevent recurrence of malignant tumors like squamous cell carcinoma and melanoma. Cryotherapy can also be used as a principal treatment for primary acquired melanosis and pagetoid invasion of sebaceous gland carcinoma. Cryotherapy can cause temporary conjunctival chemosis and long lasting dry eye symptoms. If inadvertent freezing of the globe occurs, cataract, uveitis, scleral and corneal thinning, and phthisis bulbi can occur.

Topical chemotherapy comprising mitomycin C, 5-fluorouracil, or interferon can be effective in treating epithelial malignancies such as squamous cell carcinoma, primary acquired melanosis, and pagetoid invasion of sebaceous gland carcinoma [13–18]. Mitomycin C or 5-fluorouracil is employed most successfully for squamous cell carcinoma, especially after tumor recurrence following previous surgery. This medication is prescribed topically 4 times daily for a 1-week period followed by a 1-week hiatus to allow the ocular surface to recover. This cycle is repeated once again so that most patients receive a total of 2 weeks of the chemotherapy topically. Both mitomycin C and 5-fluorouracil are most effective for squamous cell carcinoma and less effective for primary acquired melanosis and pagetoid invasion of sebaceous gland carcinoma. Caution should be used with this medication as it is ineffective for tumors deep to the epithelium. Toxicities include dry eye, superficial punctate epitheliopathy, punctal stenosis, corneal melt, scleral melt, and cataract.

Two forms of radiotherapy, external beam radiotherapy and custom designed plaque radiotherapy, can be used for conjunctival tumors. External beam radiotherapy to a total dose of 3,000–4,000 cGy is used to treat conjunctival lymphoma and metastatic carcinoma when they are too large or diffuse to excise locally. Side effects of dry eye, punctate epithelial abnormalities and cataract should be anticipated.

Custom designed plaque radiotherapy to a dose of 3,000–4,000 cGy can be used to treat conjunctival lymphoma or metastasis. A higher dose of 6,000–8,000 cGy is employed to treat the more radiation resistant melanoma and squamous cell carcinoma. In general, plaque radiotherapy is reserved for those patients who have diffuse tumors that are incompletely resected and for those who display multiple recurrences.

In rare instances, modified enucleation is used for tumors that have invaded through the limbal tissues into the globe. This can be found with squamous cell carcinoma (mucoepidermoid variant and spindle cell variant) and melanoma. At the time of enucleation, the involved conjunctiva should be removed intact with the globe. Orbital exenteration is the treatment of choice for primary malignant conjunctival tumors that have invaded the orbit or some that exhibit complete involvement of the conjunctiva [19, 20]. Either an eyelid-removing or eyelid-sparing exenteration is employed, depending on the extent of eyelid involvement. The eyelid-sparing technique is preferred in that the patients have better cosmetic appearance and heal within 2 or 3 weeks. Specifically, if the anterior lamella of the eyelid is uninvolved with tumor, an eyelid-sparing (eyelid-splitting) exenteration may be accomplished.

Mucous membrane grafts are occasionally necessary to replace vital conjunctival tissue after removal of extensive conjunctival tumors. The best donor sites include the forniceal conjunctiva of the ipsilateral or contralateral eye and buccal mucosa from the posterior aspect of the lower lip or lateral aspect of the mouth. Such grafts are usually removed by a freehand technique, fashioned to fit the defect, and secured into place with cardinal and running absorbable 6–0 or 7–0 sutures. In other cases, donor amniotic membrane can be used to replace lost conjunctiva [8, 9]. The fine, transparent material is laid basement membrane side up and sutured into place with absorbable sutures. Topical antibiotic and steroid ointments are applied following all conjunctival grafting procedures.

Summary for the Clinician

- **Conjunctival tumors arise from either the epithelium or the stromal tissue**
- **Most conjunctival tumors are readily recognized by clinical features and can be categorized as benign or malignant based on these features**
- **When possible, complete excision of a conjunctival tumor is advised so that residual cells are not left for future proliferation. This is especially important for malignant conjunctival tumors. Use of the "no touch" technque is advised**

Table 2.1. Subclassification of conjunctival choristomatous, epithelial, melanocytic, vascular, neural, xanthomatous, myxomatous, fibrous, lipomatous, lacrimal gland, lymphoid, metastatic, and secondary tumors [4]

	% all conjunctival tumors
Choristomatous tumors (n=40)	
Dermolipoma	1
Dermoid	<1
Complex choristoma	<1
Osseous choristoma	<1
Lacrimal gland choristoma	<1
Benign epithelial tumors (n=38)	
Adult papilloma	1
Childhood papilloma	<1
Kerototic plaque	<1
Actinic keratosis	<1
Benign hyperplasia of epithelium	<1
Keratoacanthoma	<1
Premalignant and malignant epithelial tumors (n=181)	
Squamous cell carcinoma	7
Conjunctival intraepithelial neoplasia	4
Basal cell carcinoma of the caruncle	<1
Melanocytic tumors (n=872)	
Nevus	28
Malignant melanoma	13
Primary acquired melanosis	11
Racial melanosis	1
Vascular tumors (n=63)	
Lymphangioma	<1
Pyogenic granuloma	<1
Telangiectasia	<1
Capillary hemangioma	<1
Kaposi's sarcoma	<1
Cavernous hemangioma	<1
Lymphangiectasia	<1
Racemose hemangioma	<1
Neural tumors (n=1)	
Neurofibroma	<1
Xanthomatous tumors (n=1)	
Juvenile xanthogranuloma	<1
Myxomatous tumors (n=1)	
Myxoma	<1
Fibrous tumors (n=7)	
Fibrous histiocytoma	<1
Fibroma	<1
Spindle cell tumor	<1
Lipomatous tumors (n=23)	
Herniated orbital fat	1
Lipoma	<1
Lacrimal gland tumors (n=12)	
Dacryops	<1
Oncocytoma	<1
Lymphoid tumors (n=128)	
Lymphoma	6
Benign reactive lymphoid hyperplasia	2
Plasmacytoma	<1
Metastatic tumors (n=13)	
Breast cancer	<1
Lung cancer	<1
Skin melanoma	<1
Laryngeal cancer	<1
Carcinoid tumor	<1
Unknown primary cancer	<1
Secondary tumors (n=54)	
Extraocular extension of intraocular tumor	3
Eyelid sebaceous gland carcinoma	<1
Eyelid basal cell carcinoma	<1
Malignant mixed tumor of lacrimal gland	<1

2.5 Diagnostic Categories of Conjunctival Tumors

There have been only a few large published series on conjunctival tumors. In 1950, Ash published a major report on 1,120 epibulbar tumors on file at the Army Institute of Pathology in the United States [21]. Based on the clinical information submitted with the specimen, Ash correlated the pathologic diagnosis with patient age, race, and sex. Overall, the clinical diagnoses included epidermidalization (7%), papilloma (12%), carcinoma (17%), pterygium/pingueculum (9%), teratoma/dermoid/dermoid cyst (7%), nevus (26%), melanoma (6%), miscellaneous benign neoplasms (6%), and others (9%).

Since then, other studies on smaller series of epibulbar tumors have been published from Lesotho in Africa [22], Queensland, Australia [23], and Kakindada, India [24]. In 1987, Grossniklaus and coworkers provided a major contribution from the Eye Pathology Laboratory of the Wilmer Ophthalmological Institute over a 61-year period with 2,455 conjunctival lesions in adults over age 15 years [2]. In that series, the most common lesions were pterygium (18%), nevus (8%), dysplasia (7%), inflammation (non-specific non-granulomatous) (7%), and epithelial inclusion cyst (6%). The most common malignancies were squamous cell carcinoma (4%), melanoma (3%), and pagetoid invasion by sebaceous gland carcinoma (<1%).

In 2004, Shields and associates provided the first large clinical series of 1,643 conjunctival tumors [4] (Table 2.1). In their series, the tumor was classified as melanocytic in 872 cases (53%) and non-melanocytic in 771 cases (47%). The non-melanocytic categories included congenital choristoma (2%), epithelial (13%), vascular (4%), fibrous (<1%), neural (<1%), xanthomatous (<1%), myxomatous (<1%), lipomatous (1%), lacrimal gland origin (<1%), lymphoid (8%), leukemic (<1%), metastatic (<1%), secondary (3%), and non-neoplastic lesions simulating a tumor (13%). Of the 872 melanocytic lesions, the specific tumor diagnosis was nevus in 454 cases (52%), melanoma in 215 (25%), and primary acquired melanosis in 180 (21%). Overall, melanocytic tumors, epithelial tumors, and lymphoid tumors accounted for 74% of all cases. These tumors were far more common in Caucasian patients, and epithelial tumors were found more frequently in men.

In this chapter, we will focus on the most common or important conjunctival tumors including squamous lesions (papilloma, conjunctival intraepithelial carcinoma, and squamous cell carcinoma), melanocytic lesions (nevus, primary acquired melanosis, malignant melanoma), lymphoid lesions, and those that occur in the caruncle.

2.6 Papilloma

Squamous papilloma is a benign tumor, documented to be associated with human papillomavirus (subtypes 6, 11, 16, and 18) infection of the conjunctiva [25]. This tumor can occur in both children and adults. It is speculated that the virus is acquired through transfer from the mother's vagina to the newborn's conjunctiva as the child passes through the mother's birth canal. Papilloma appears as a pink fibrovascular frond of tissue arranged in a sessile or pedunculated configuration. The numerous fine vascular channels ramify through the stroma beneath the epithelial surface of the lesion. In children, the lesion is usually small, multiple, and located in the inferior fornix (Fig. 2.1). In adults, it is usually solitary, more extensive, and can often extend to cover the entire corneal surface simulating malignant squamous cell carcinoma.

For a small sessile papilloma in a child, there are several treatment options. Sometimes, periodic observation allows for slow spontaneous resolution of the viral-produced tumor. Larger or more pedunculated lesions are usually symptomatic with foreign body sensation, chronic mucous production, hemorrhagic tears, incomplete eyelid closure, and poor cosmetic appearance. These lesions are managed by surgical excision. Complete removal of the mass without direction manipulation of the tumor (no touch technique) is advisable to avoid spreading of the tumor-related virus. Double freeze-thaw cryotherapy is applied to the remaining conjunctiva around the excised lesion in order to help prevent tumor recurrence. In some instances, the pedunculated tumor is frozen alone and allowed to slough off the conjunctival surface later. For some large unwieldy pedunculated tumors, complete cryotherapy of the mass down its stalk to its base is performed and excision while the mass is in the frozen state is achieved. Topical interferon, mitomycin C, and cidofovir have been employed for conjunctival papillomas [26, 27]. For those lesions that show recurrence, oral cimetidine for sever-

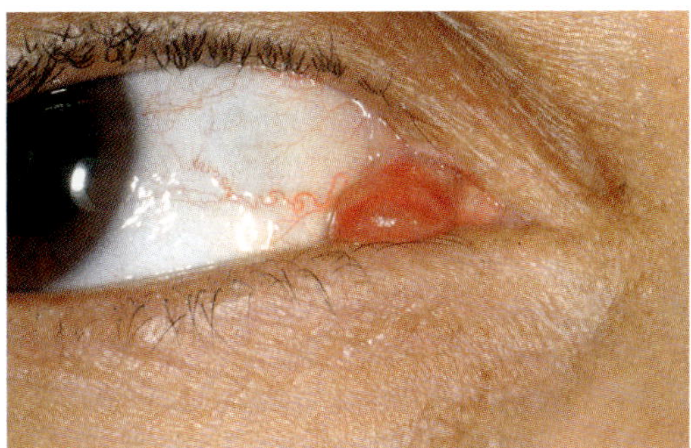

Fig. 2.1. Conjunctival papilloma

al months can resolve the papilloma virus-related tumor by boosting the patient's immune system and stimulating regression of the mass [28].

2.7 Ocular Surface Squamous Neoplasia (OSSN)

Ocular surface squamous cell neoplasia can occur as a localized lesion confined to the surface epithelium (conjunctival intraepithelial neoplasia or dysplasia) or as a more invasive squamous cell carcinoma that has broken through the basement membrane and invaded the underlying stroma. The former has no potential to metastasize but the latter can gain access to the conjunctival lymphatics and occasionally metastasize to regional lymph nodes. It has been found that most squamous cell neoplasia is related to human papillomavirus infection of the conjunctival epithelium [29] and this is most certain in those patients with bilateral squamous cell neoplasia and those immunosuppressed patients who develop this disease.

2.7.1 Conjunctival Intraepithelial Neoplasia (CIN)

Clinically CIN appears as a fleshy, sessile or minimally elevated lesion usually at limbus in the interpalprebal fissure and less commonly in the forniceal or palpebral conjunctiva. The limbal lesion may extend for a variable distance into the epithelium of the adjacent cornea. A white plaque (leukoplakia) may occur on the surface of the lesion due to secondary hyperkeratosis.

Histopathologically, mild CIN (dysplasia) is characterized by a partial thickness replacement of the surface epithelium by abnormal epithelial cells that lack normal maturation. Severe CIN (severe dysplasia) is characterized by a nearly full-thickness replacement of the epithelium by similar cells. Carcinoma-in-situ represents full thickness replacement by abnormal epithelial cells.

2.7.2 Squamous Cell Carcinoma

Squamous cell carcinoma is an extension of abnormal epithelial cells through the basement membrane to gain access to the conjunctival stroma [30]. Clinically, invasive squamous cell carcinoma is generally larger and more elevated than CIN (Fig. 2.2). Leukoplakia may be variable. Uncommonly, lesions that are untreated or incompletely excised can invade through the corneoscleral lamella into the anterior chamber of the eye or they can transgress the orbital septum and invade the soft tissues of the orbit adjacent to the globe [31–34]. A rare variant of squamous cell carcinoma of the conjunctiva is the mucoepidermoid carcinoma. Clinically, this variant occurs in older patients and has a yellow globular cystic component due to the presence of abundant mucus-secreting cells within cysts. It tends to be more aggressive than the standard squamous cell carcinoma and therefore deserves wider excision and closer follow-up [31, 32]. The spindle cell variant of squamous cell carcinoma is likewise aggressive.

Histopathologically, invasive squamous cell carcinoma is characterized by malignant squamous cells that have violated the basement membrane and have grown in sheets or cords into the stromal tissue. As mentioned above, the mucoepidermoid variant contains mucus-secreting cells that often produce mucus-containing cysts within the lesion. Even though the cells of invasive squamous cell carcinoma gain access to the blood vessels and lymphatic channels, regional and distant metastases are both rather

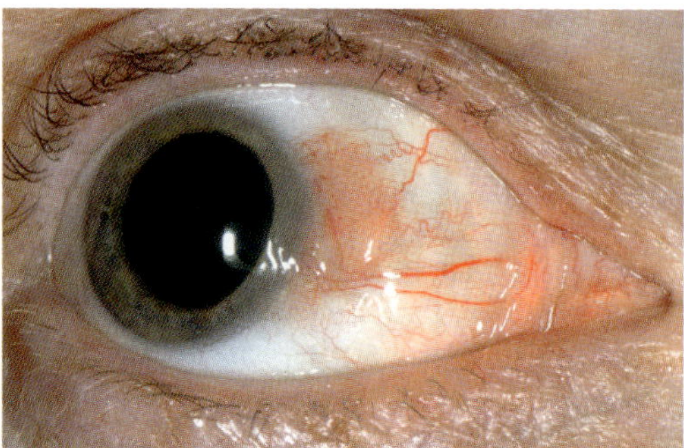

Fig. 2.2. Conjunctival squamous cell carcinoma

uncommon. Patients who are medically immunosuppressed for organ transplantation or those with human immunodeficiency virus are at particular risk to develop conjunctival squamous cell carcinoma. In these cases, the risk for life-threatening metastatic disease is greater.

The management of squamous cell carcinoma of the conjunctiva varies with the extent of the lesion. In general, the management of lesions in the limbal area involves alcohol epitheliectomy for the corneal component and partial lamellar scleroconjunctivectomy with wide margins for the conjunctival component followed by freeze-thaw cryotherapy to the remaining adjacent bulbar conjunctiva, as described above [12]. In some cases, microscopically controlled excision (Mohs surgery) is performed at the time of surgery to ensure tumor-free margins [35]. Those tumors in the forniceal region can be managed by wide local resection and cryotherapy. In cases where excessive conjunctiva is sacrificed, a mucous membrane graft or amniotic membrane graft may be employed for reconstruction. In all cases, the full conjunctival component along with the underlying Tenon's fascia should be excised using the no touch technique as mentioned previously.

For those patients with extensive tumors or those tumors that are recurrent, especially those with extensive corneal component, treatment with topical mitomycin C, 5-fluorouracil, or interferon is advised [13–18]. We generally use mitomycin C for two cycles with close monitoring of the patient.

Summary for the Clinician

- **Squamous epithelial tumors can be benign, premalignant, and malignant**
- **Papilloma is a benign tumor caused by human papilloma virus, but it can be re-current and lead to the development of multiple tumors**
- **Squamous cell carcinoma is a malignant tumor that requires special surgical technique for complete removal. Recurrences can be managed with topical chemotherapy**

2.8 Naevus

The circumscribed nevus is the most common melanocytic tumor of the conjunctiva. It generally becomes clinically apparent in the 1st or 2nd decade of life as a discrete variably pigmented, slightly elevated, sessile lesion that usually contains fine clear cysts on slit lamp biomicroscopy [36–38] (Fig. 2.3). It is typically located in the interpalpebral bulbar conjunctiva near the limbus and remains relatively stationary throughout life with less than 1% risk for transformation into malignant melanoma [36, 38]. Over time, a nevus can become more pigmented and the previously inapparent non-pigmented portions can acquire pigment, simulating growth.

In 2004, Shields and associates reported clinical features of 410 patients with conjunctival nevus [38]. They found anatomic location of the nevus was bulbar conjunctiva (72%), caruncle (15%), plica semilunaris (11%), fornix (1%), tarsus (1%), and cornea (<1%). The bulbar conjunctival lesions most commonly abutted the corneoscleral limbus. The nevus quadrant was temporal (46%), nasal (44%), superior (6%), and inferior (5%). Additional features included intralesional cysts (65%), feeder vessels (33%), and visible intrinsic vessels (38%). Of the 149 patients who returned for periodic observation for a mean of 11 years, the lesion color gradually changed in 13%; the lesion size was larger in 7%; and 3 patients developed malignant melanoma.

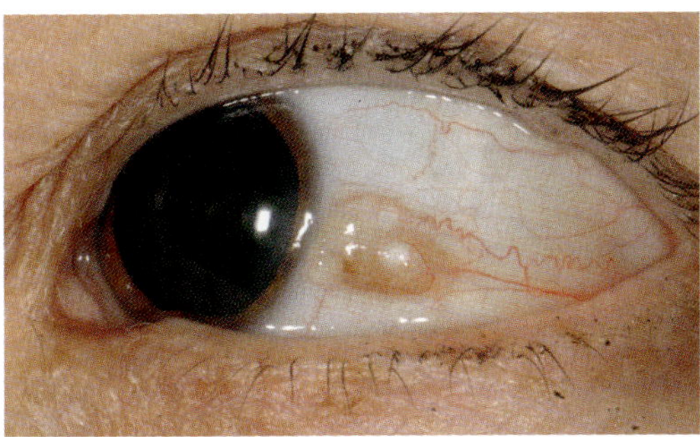

Fig. 2.3. Conjunctival nevus

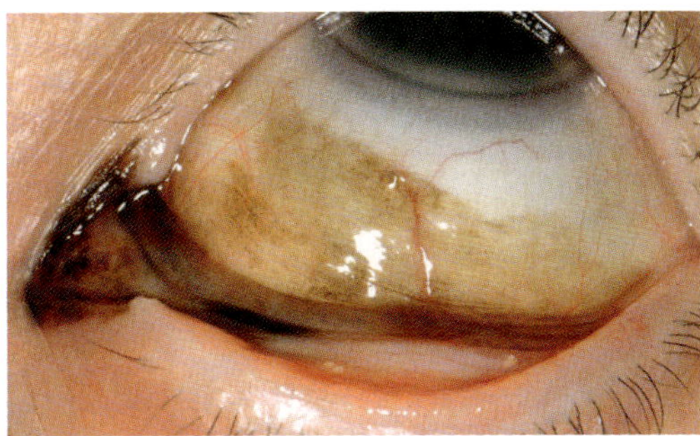

Fig. 2.4. Conjunctival primary acquired melanosis

The best management is usually periodic observation with photographic comparison and if growth is documented then local excision of the lesion should be considered. In some cases, excision for cosmetic reasons is desired. At the time of excision, the entire mass is removed using the no touch technique and if it is adherent to the globe, then a thin lamella of underlying sclera is removed intact with the tumor. Standard double freeze-thaw cryotherapy is applied to the remaining conjunctival margins. These precautions are employed to prevent recurrence of the nevus and also to prevent recurrence should the lesion prove to be a melanoma.

2.9 Primary Acquired Melanosis (PAM)

Primary acquired melanosis is an important benign conjunctival pigmented condition that can give rise to conjunctival melanoma. In contrast to conjunctival nevus, it is acquired in middle age and appears diffuse, patchy, flat, and non-cystic (Fig. 2.4) (Table 2.2). In contrast to ocular melanocytosis, the pigment is acquired, located within the conjunctiva, and appears brown, not gray, in colour. The pigmentation can wax and wane over time. In contrast to racial melanosis, PAM generally is found in fair skinned individuals as a unilateral patchy condition.

Histopathologically, PAM is characterized by the presence of abnormal melanocytes near the basal layer of the epithelium. Pathologists should attempt to classify the melanocytes as having atypia or no atypia based on nuclear features and growth pattern [28, 40]. PAM with atypia carries nearly a 50% risk for ultimate evolution into malignant melanoma whereas PAM without atypia carries nearly a 0% risk for melanoma development.

The management of PAM depends on the extent of involvement and the association with melanoma. If there is only a small region of PAM, occupying less than 3 clock hours of the conjunctiva, then periodic observation or complete excisional biopsy and cryotherapy are options [12]. If the PAM occupies more than 3 clock hours, then incisional map biopsy of all four quadrants is warranted, followed by double freeze-thaw cryotherapy to all affected pigmented sites. If the patient has a history of previous or current conjunctival or cutaneous melanoma or if there are areas of nodularity or vascularity within the presumed PAM that are suspicious for melanoma, then a more aggressive approach is warranted with complete excisional biopsy of the suspicious areas using the no touch technique as described previously. Additional small incisional map biopsies should be performed in the regions of flat PAM and even in the apparently uninvolved quadrants of the bulbar conjunctiva to determine if there are melanocytes with atypia. Cryotherapy should be applied to all remaining pigmented areas. Topical mitomycin C can also be beneficial, especially if there is recurrent corneal PAM [41, 42]; however, mitomycin C is not as effective for PAM as it is for squamous epithelial neoplasia.

Table 2.2. Differential diagnosis of pigmented epibulbar lesions

Condition	Anatomic location	Colour	Depth	Margins	Laterality	Other features	Progression
Nevus	Interpalpebral limbus usually	Brown or yellow	Stroma	Well defined	Unilateral	Cysts	<1 % progress to conjunctival melanoma
Racial melanosis	Limbus >bulbar > palpebral conjunctiva	Brown	Epithelium	Ill defined	Bilateral	Flat, no cysts	Very rare progression to conjunctival melanoma
Ocular melanocytosis	Bulbar conjunctiva	Gray	Episclera	Ill defined	Unilateral more so than bilateral	Congenital, usually 2 mm from limbus, often with periocular skin pigmentation	<1 % progress to uveal melanoma
Primary acquired melanosis (PAM)	Anywhere, but usually bulbar conjunctiva	Brown	Epithelium	Ill defined	Unilateral	Flat, no cysts	Progresses to conjunctival melanoma in nearly 50 % of cases that show cellular atypia
Malignant melanoma	Anywhere	Brown or pink	Stroma	Well defined	Unilateral	Vascular nodule, dilated feeder vessels, may be non-pigmented	32 % develop metastasis by 15 years

2.10 Malignant Melanoma

There is an increasing incidence of conjunctival malignant melanoma [43]. Melanoma most commonly arises from PAM, but it can also arise from a preexisting nevus or de novo. It typically arises in adults at a median age of 62 years, but rare cases of conjunctival melanoma in children have been recognized [10, 44–47]. Conjunctival melanoma shows considerable clinical variability. It is generally a pigmented or tan, elevated conjunctival lesion that can be located on the limbal, bulbar, forniceal, or palpebral conjunctiva (Fig. 2.5). Occasionally, the tumor shows predominance on the cornea, despite origin from the conjunctiva. Often prominent feeder vessels and surrounding flat PAM are present. Conjunctival melanoma can show both local tumor recurrence and distant metastasis (Table 2.3). Multiple recurrences, especially those that occur within the orbit, frequently necessitate orbital exenteration [48, 49]. Metastases to ipsilateral facial lymph nodes, brain, lung, and liver are the most common sites [10, 47, 49].

The management of conjunctival melanoma varies with the extent of the lesion [11, 12]. This malignancy is particularly difficult to treat. Despite excellent microscopic excision of the mass, further disease can develop from associated PAM in 26% of patients by 5 years and 65% of patients by 15 years follow-up [10]. Classic limbal tumors are removed by absolute alcohol epitheliectomy for the flat corneal component and wide no touch technique, partial lamellar scleroconjunctivectomy with 4-mm margins followed by double freeze-thaw cryotherapy for the conjunctival portion. Larger lesions that extend into the forniceal region or orbit may require more extensive excision, always with tumor free margins encapsulating the tumor and with no touch, dry technique. Paridaens and associates found that early exenteration did not improve life prognosis [48].

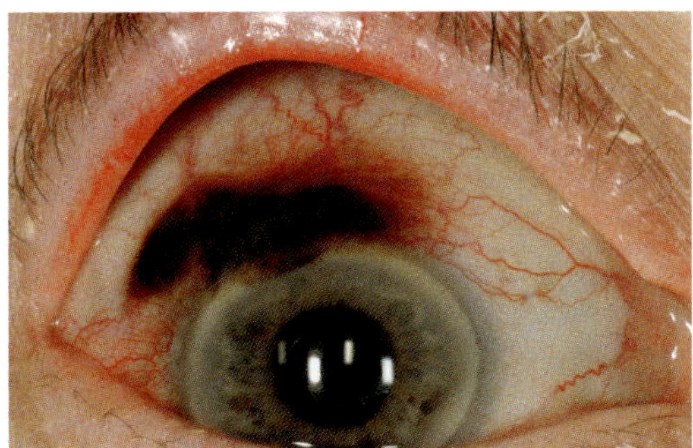

Fig. 2.5. Conjunctival malignant melanoma

Shields and associates found tumor related death occurred in 7% of patients at 5 years and 13% at 8 years [10]. The risk factors for death using multivariate analysis included initial symptoms of a lump and pathology findings of de novo melanoma. The technique of initial surgery, using complete excisional biopsy with the "no touch" technique combined with cryotherapy to remaining tumor free margins, was shown to be an important factor in preventing eventual tumor recurrence, metastasis, and death.

Table 2.3. Risks for local tumor recurrence, exenteration, metastasis, and death in patients with conjunc-tival melanoma [10]

Outcome	Length of follow-up by Kaplan-Meier analysis @ 5 years	@ 10 years	@ 15 years
Recurrence	26%	51%	65%
Exenteration	8%	16%	32%
Metastasis	16%	26%	32%
Death	7%	13%	Not available

Table 2.4. Risks for the development of systemic lymphoma in patients who present with conjunctival lymphoid infiltrate and no sign of systemic lymphoma [52]

	Development of systemic lymphoma by Kaplan-Meier analysis @ 1 years	@ 5 years	@ 10 years
Generally, if conjunctival lymphoid tumor	7%	15%	28%
Specifically, if conjunctival lymphoma	12%	38%	79%

Summary for the Clinician

- **Conjunctival naevus is a common tumor and is most often detected in children**
- **Cysts can be visualized within a conjunctival nevus in nearly two-thirds of cases**
- **Conjunctival melanoma is a potentially lethal tumor with 13% death by 8 years follow-up**
- **The original surgical excision of a conjunctival melanoma is important in prevention of tumor recurrence and metastasis**

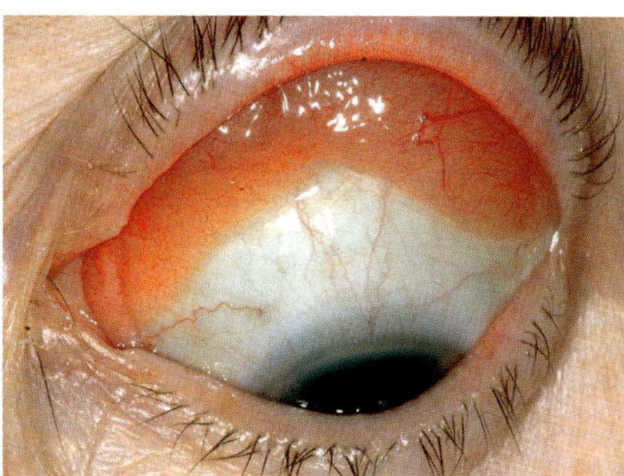

Fig. 2.6. Conjunctival lymphoma

2.11 Lymphoid Tumors

Lymphoid tumors can occur in the conjunctiva as isolated lesions or they can be a manifestation of systemic lymphoma [50–53]. Clinically, the lesion appears as a diffuse, slightly elevated pink mass located in the stroma or deep to Tenon's fascia, most commonly in the forniceal region (Fig. 2.6). This appearance is similar to that of smoked salmon; hence it is termed the "salmon patch". It is not usually possible to differentiate clinically between a benign and malignant lymphoid tumor. Therefore, biopsy is necessary to establish the diagnosis and a systemic evaluation should be done in all affected patients to exclude the presence of systemic lymphoma (Table 2.4). Histopathologically, sheets of lymphocytes are found and classified as reactive lymphoid hyperplasia or malignant lymphoma. Most are B cell lymphoma (non-Hodgkin's type). Treatment of the conjunctival lesion should include chemotherapy if the patient has systemic lymphoma or external beam irradiation (2,000–4,000 cGy) if the lesion is localized to the conjunctiva. Other options include excisional biopsy and cryotherapy, local interferon injections, or observation.

Summary for the Clinician

- **Conjunctival lymphoid tumors appear as a pink mass below the epithelium, usually in the fornix**
- **Most patients with conjunctival lymphoid tumors have excision and low dose radiotherapy**

2.12 Caruncular Tumors

Tumors of the caruncle resemble those on the eyelid and those on the conjunctiva. Reviews of caruncular tumors have revealed that the most common tumors include papilloma (32%), nevus (24%), pyogenic granuloma (9%), epithelial inclusion cyst (7%), chronic inflammation (7%), oncocytoma (4%) and others [4–6]

Table 2.5. Types and frequency of tumors of the caruncle [4]

Category of tumors	%
Choristomatous (n=40)	0
Benign epithelial (n=38)	18
Premalignant and malignant epithelial (n=181)	1
Melanocytic (n=872)	8
Vascular (n=63)	2
Fibrous (n=7)	14
Neural (n=1)	0
Xanthomatous (n=1)	0
Myxomatous (n=1)	0
Lipomatous (n=23)	0
Lacrimal gland (n=12)	33
Lymphoid (n=128)	2
Leukemic (n=3)	0
Metastatic (n=13)	0
Secondary (n=54)	2
Non-neoplastic masses simulating a tumor (n=206)	5

(Table 2.5). Malignancies of the caruncle represent only 5% or less of biopsied caruncular tumors [6].

References

1. Shields JA, Shields CL (1999) Tumors and pseudotumors of the conjunctiva. Atlas of eyelid and conjunctival tumors. Lippincott Williams and Wilkins, Philadelphia, 199–334
2. Grossniklaus HE, Green WR, Luckenbach M, Chan CC (1987) Conjunctival lesions in adults. A clinical and histopathologic review. Cornea 6:78–116
3. Shields CL, Shields JA (2004) Tumors of the conjunctiva and cornea. Surv Ophthalmol 49:3–24
4. Shields CL, Demirci H, Karatza KC, Shields JA (2004) Clinical survey of 1643 melanocytic and nonmelanocytic conjunctival tumors. The John E. Brown Memorial Lecture. Ophthalmology (in press)
5. Luthra CL, Doxanas MT, Green WR (1978) Lesions of the caruncle. A clinicopathologic study. Surv Ophthalmol 23:183–195
6. Shields CL, Shields JA, White D, Augsburger JJ (1986) Types and frequency of lesions of the caruncle. Am J Ophthalmol 102:771–778
7. Spinak M, Friedman AH (1977) Squamous cell carcinoma of the conjunctiva. Value of exfoliative cytology in diagnosis. Surv Ophthalmol 21:351–572
8. Shields CL, Shields JA, Armstrong T (2001) Management of conjunctival and corneal melanoma with combined surgical excision, amniotic membrane allograft, and topical chemotherapy. Am J Ophthalmol 132:576–578
9. Paridaens D, Beekhuis H, van Den Bosch W, Remeyer L, Melles G (2001) Amniotic membrane transplantation in the management of conjunctival malignant melanoma and primary acquired melanosis with atypia. Br J Ophthalmol 85:658–661
10. Shields CL, Shields JA, Gunduz K, Cater J, Mercado GV, Gross N, Lally B (2000) Conjunctival melanoma: risk factors for recurrence, exenteration, metastasis, and death in 150 consecutive patients. Arch Ophthalmol 118:1497–1507
11. Shields JA, Shields CL, De Potter P (1998) Surgical management of circumscribed conjunctival melanomas. Ophthal Plast Reconstr Surg 14:208–215
12. Shields JA, Shields CL, De Potter P (1997) Surgical management of conjunctival tumors. The 1994 Lynn B. McMahan Lecture. Arch Ophthalmol 115:808–815
13. Frucht-Pery J, Rozenman Y (1994) Mitomycin C therapy for corneal intraepithelial neoplasia. Am J Ophthalmol 117:164–168
14. Frucht-Pery J, Sugar J, Baum J, Sutphin JE, Pe'er J, Savir H, Holland EJ, Meisler DM, Foster JA, Folberg R, Rozenman Y (1997) Mitomycin C treatment for conjunctival-corneal intraepithelial neoplasia: a multicenter experience. Ophthalmology 104:2085–2093
15. Shields CL, Naseripour M, Shields JA (2002) Topical mitomycin C for extensive, recurrent conjunctival-corneal squamous cell carcinoma. Am J Ophthalmol 133:601–631
16. Yeatts RP, Engelbrecht NE, Curry CD, Ford JG, Walter KA (2000) 5-Fluorouracil for the treatment of intraepithelial neoplasia of the conjunctiva and cornea. Ophthalmology 107:2190–2195
17. Midena E, Angeli CD, Valenti M, de Belvis V, Boccato P (2000) Treatment of conjunctival squamous cell carcinoma with topical 5-fluorouracil. Br J Ophthalmol 84:268–272
18. Karp CL, Moore JK, Rosa RH Jr (2001) Treatment of conjunctival and corneal intraepithelial neoplasia with topical interferon alpha-2b. Ophthalmology 108:1093–1098

19. Shields JA, Shields CL, Suvarnamani C, Tantasira M, Shah P (1991) Orbital exenteration with eyelid sparing: Indications, technique and results. Ophthalmic Surg 22:292–297
20. Shields JA, Shields CL, Demirci H, Hanovar S, Singh AD (2001) Experience with eyelid-sparing orbital exenteration. The 2000 Tullos O. Coston Lecture. Ophthal Plast Reconstr Surg 17:355–361
21. Ash JE (1950) Epibulbar tumors. Am J Ophthalmol 33:1203–1219
22. Gordon YJ, McLean IW, Mokete M, Lahav M (1981) Incidence of epibulbar tumors in Lesotho. Albrecht Von Graefes Arch Klin Exp Ophthalmol 216:135–143
23. Harrison M, Glasson W (1985) Conjunctival and limbal tumours. Aust N Z J Ophthalmol 13:193–194
24. Reddy SC, Sarma CS, Rao VV, Banerjea S (1983) Tumours and cysts of conjunctiva. A study of 175 cases. Ind J Ophthalmol 31:658–660
25. Sjo NC, Heegaard S, Prause JU, von Buchwald C, Lindeberg H (2001) Human papillomavirus in conjunctival papilloma. Br J Ophthalmol 85:785–787
26. Schechter BA, Rand WJ, Velazquez GE, Williams WD, Starasoler L (2002) Treatment of conjunctival papillomata with topical interferon alfa-2b. Am J Ophthalmol 134:268–270
27. Hawkins AS, Yu J, Hamming NA, Rubenstein JB (1999) Treatment of recurrent conjunctival papillomatosis with mitomycin C. Am J Ophthalmol 128:638–640
28. Shields CL, Lally MR, Singh AD, Shields JA, Nowinski T (1999) Oral cimetidine (Tagamet) for recalcitrant, diffuse conjunctival papillomatosis. Am J Ophthalmol 128:362–364
29. Scott IU, Karp CL, Nuovo GJ (2002) Human papillomavirus 16 and 18 expression in conjunctival intraepithelial neoplasia. Ophthalmology 109:542–547
30. McKelvie PA, Daniell M, McNab A, Loughnan M, Santamaria JD (2002) Squamous cell carcinoma of the conjunctiva: a series of 26 cases. Br J Ophthalmol 86:168–173
31. Brownstein S (1981) Mucoepidermoid carcinoma of the conjunctiva with intraocular invasion. Ophthalmology 88:1126–1130
32. Gunduz K, Shields CL, Shields JA, Mercado G, Eagle RC Jr (1998) Intraocular neoplastic cyst from mucoepidermoid carcinoma of the conjunctiva. Arch Ophthalmol 116:1521–1523
33. Shields JA, Shields CL, Gunduz K, Eagle RC Jr (1999) The 1998 Pan American Lecture. Intraocular invasion of conjunctival squamous cell carcinoma in five patients. Ophthal Plast Reconstr Surg 15:153–160
34. Tunc M, Char DH, Crawford B, Miller T (1999) Intraepithelial and invasive squamous cell carcinoma of the conjunctiva: analysis of 60 cases. Br J Ophthalmol 83:98–103
35. Buus DR, Tse DT, Folberg R, Buuns DR (1994) Microscopically controlled excision of conjunctival squamous cell carcinoma. Am J Ophthalmol 117:97–102
36. Gerner N, Norregaard JC, Jensen OA, Prause JU (1996) Conjunctival naevi in Denmark 1960–1980. A 21-year follow-up study. Acta Ophthalmol Scand 74:334–337
37. McDonnell JM, Carpenter JD, Jacobs P, Wan WL, Gilmore JE (1989) Conjunctival melanocytic lesions in children. Ophthalmology 96:986–993
38. Shields CL, Fasiudden A, Mashayekhi A, Shields JA (2004) Conjunctival nevi: Clinical features and natural course in 410 consecutive patients. Arch Ophthalmol 122:167–175
39. Folberg R, McLean IW, Zimmerman LE (1985) Primary acquired melanosis of the conjunctiva. Hum Pathol 16:136–143
40. Folberg R, McLean IW (1986) Primary acquired melanosis and melanoma of the conjunctiva; terminology, classification, and biologic behavior. Hum Pathol 17:652–654
41. Demirci H, McCormick SA, Finger PT (2000) Topical mitomycin chemotherapy for conjunctival malignant melanoma and primary acquired melanosis with atypia: clinical experience with histopathologic observations. Arch Ophthalmol 118:885–891
42. Shields CL, Demirci H, Shields JA, Spanich C (2002) Dramatic regression of conjunctival and corneal acquired melanosis with topical mitomycin C. Br J Ophthalmol 86:244–245
43. Yu GP, Hu DN, McCormick S, Finger PT (2003) Conjunctival melanoma: is it increasing in the United States? Am J Ophthalmol 135:800–806
44. Seregard S, Koch E (1992) Conjunctival malignant melanoma in Sweden 1969–91. Acta Ophthalmol 70:289–296
45. Seregard S (1998) Conjunctival melanoma. Surv Ophthalmol 42:321–350
46. Shields CL (2002) Conjunctival melanoma (editorial). Br J Ophthalmol 86:127
47. Anastassiou G, Heiligenhaus A, Bechrakis N, Bader E, Bornfeld N, Steuhl KP (2002) Prognostic value of clinical and histopathological parameters in conjunctival melanomas: a retrospective study. Br J Ophthalmol 86:163–167
48. Paridaens AD, McCartney AC, Minassian DC, Hungerford JL (1994) Orbital exenteration in 95 cases of primary conjunctival malignant melanoma. Br J Ophthalmol 78:520–528

49. Paridaens AD, Minassian DC, McCartney AC, Hungerford JL (1994) Prognostic factors in primary malignant melanoma of the conjunctiva: a clinicopathological study of 256 cases. Br J Ophthalmol 78:252–259
50. Cockerham GC, Jakobiec FA (1997) Lymphoproliferative disorders of the ocular adnexa. Int Ophthalmol Clin 37:39–59
51. Knowles DM II, Jakobiec FA (1982) Ocular adnexal lymphoid neoplasms: clinical, histopathologic, electron microscopic, and immunologic characteristics. Hum Pathol 123:148–162
52. Shields CL, Shields JA, Carvalho C, Rundle P, Smith AF (2001) Conjunctival lymphoid tumors: clinical analysis of 117 cases and relationship to systemic lymphoma. Ophthalmology 108:979–984
53. Coupland SE, Hummel M, Stein H (2002) Ocular adnexal lymphomas: five case presentations and a review of the literature. Surv Ophthalmol 47: 470–490

Sentinel Lymph Node Biopsy for Conjunctival and Eyelid Malignancies

3

Dominick Golio, Bita Esmaeli

Core Messages

- Sentinel lymph node (SLN) biopsy is a minimally invasive technique that aims to diagnose microscopic metastasis in the regional lymph nodes
- The value of SLN biopsy has been widely studied for cutaneous melanoma, breast carcinoma, as well as other solid cancers. We have modified SLN biopsy techniques for conjunctival and eyelid tumors, because many of the cancers of the ocular adnexa such as conjunctival melanoma and sebaceous cell carcinoma have the predilection for regional lymph nodes as the site of first metastasis
- An SLN biopsy technique using both isosulfan blue dye (0.2 cc volume) and technetium (0.3 mCi in 0.2 cc volume) was initially used by our group. A smaller volume of these tracers is used than in other anatomic sites, in order to prevent excessive ballooning up of the conjunctiva and the spread of the tracer to non-specific quadrants of the conjunctiva. We have abandoned the use of the isosulfan blue dye in the latter part of our trial as none of the SLNs was found to be blue. We believe this is due to the much smaller volume of the isosulfan dye used for ocular adnexal lesions and the rapid transit of the dye through the lymphatics in the head and neck region
- The regional lymph nodes at the greatest risk for metastasis from conjunctival and eyelid cancers are the parotid, preauricular, and submandibular lymph nodes
- Our experience suggests that SLN biopsy can be safely performed for conjunctival and eyelid cancers and is associated with very few side effects. Only three out of 27 patients enrolled in our trial have had a temporary weakness of the marginal mandibular branch of the facial nerve as a result of sentinel lymph node biopsy in the parotid region. Each has had spontaneous resolution of the facial nerve paresis within a few weeks. Blue discoloration of the ocular surface or periocular skin has not been observed in any of the patients enrolled in our trial so far. No patient in our trial has experienced an anaphylactic shock from the blue dye, although this has been reported in other studies of SLN biopsy
- Two out of 27 patients enrolled in our trial – both with a diagnosis of conjunctival melanoma – have had a histologically positive sentinel lymph node which was clinically (on physical examination) and radiographically negative. This validates the concept that SLN biopsy can identify patients who may harbor microscopic nodal metastasis, thus offering the opportunity for additional treatments earlier in their course
- Two out of 27 patients who had a "negative" SLN later developed clinically detectable metastasis within the regional lymph nodes, suggesting a false negative rate of about 8%
- Careful evaluation of regional lymph nodes is indicated in all patients with conjunctival melanoma, eyelid melanoma, eyelid sebaceous cell carcinoma, Merkel cell carcinoma, or other ocular adnexal cancers with a tendency to metastasize to the regional lymph nodes. Ultrasonography and computed tomography should be utilized at baseline and throughout the course of the disease. If these radiographic modalities fail to find a positive node at baseline, consideration should be given to sentinel lymph node biopsy at the time of initial diagnosis of these ocular adnexal cancers

3.1 Introduction

Sentinel lymph node (SLN) biopsy is a minimally invasive technique for identifying patients with microscopic regional lymph node metastasis, who may benefit from additional regional or systemic treatment [1, 2]. While this technique has been widely used for many solid tumors in the last decade, its potential utility for conjunctival and eyelid tumors is still considered investigational [3–5]. To our knowledge, our trial at The University of Texas M.D. Anderson Cancer Center is the only clinical trial to date of SLN biopsy for conjunctival and eyelid tumors. We herein review the rationale for and technical aspects of SLN biopsy for conjunctival and eyelid malignancies and summarize our experience in the last 4 years with SLN biopsy for eyelid and conjunctival tumors at M.D. Anderson Cancer Center.

3.2 Historical Perspective and Rationale for Sentinel Lymph Node Biopsy

Previous studies examining the implications of regional nodal metastasis for survival resulted in different theories regarding the dissemination of solid tumors. Bartholin, in 1653, was the first to notice the existence of a lymphatic channel. Numerous subsequent investigations elucidated the intricate lymphatic system throughout the body [6, 7]. In the nineteenth century, the idea that lymphatics may filter particulate matter was first introduced. This assumption led to the theory that cancer could potentially be cured at an early stage by achieving local and regional control with adequate surgery, in contradiction to the counterargument that cancer is the local manifestation of a systemic disease and is thus incurable by local or regional surgery.

In the mid 1900s, several investigators injected inanimate particles or tumor cells into afferent lymphatics in animal models to determine the barrier function of lymph nodes [8]. Zeidman and Buss injected stained V_2 carcinoma cells into the afferent lymphatics of popliteal nodes in rabbits [7]. They found that tumor cell emboli are immediately trapped in the subcapsular sinus of the first lymph node and do not spread to the next node for at least 3 weeks. These observations supported en bloc dissection as the guiding principle of cancer surgery. Observations that cancer patients without regional nodal involvement have better survival outcomes supported the idea of a "lymph node barrier" [8].

In the majority of patients with cutaneous melanoma, there seems to be an orderly progression of metastasis to the regional lymph nodes followed by distant metastasis. Conjunctival melanoma has an analogous pattern of metastasis to cutaneous melanoma in that the regional lymph nodes are the first site of metastasis in the majority of patients. Results of prospective randomized clinical trials designed to evaluate the efficacy of elective lymph node dissection in patients with melanoma of the head and neck have shown no survival benefit from early dissection of the regional nodes [9]. Elective regional lymph node dissection can subject many patients without lymph node metastasis to unnecessary surgery. However, selective lymphadenectomy (SLN biopsy) offers important staging information for patients with cutaneous melanoma and can spare the majority of patients with early-stage melanoma from having unnecessary extensive lymph node dissection. The "sentinel" node(s) refers to the first lymph node or the first few lymph nodes reached by metastasizing cells from a primary cancer. SLN biopsy identifies patients who have microscopic nodal metastasis. Patients with micrometastases then undergo therapeutic lymph node dissection, and patients without micrometastasis can be spared this procedure.

The concept of sentinel node biopsy is based on two basic principles: the existence of an orderly and predictable pattern of lymphatic drainage to a regional lymph node basin, and the functioning of a first lymph node as an effective filter for tumor cells [10]. As early as 1960, Gould et al. described a normal-appearing node at the junction of the anterior and posterior facial vein in a patient with melanoma that was sent for frozen section investigation and was found to harbor metastatic disease [11]. Intraoperative histologic examination of this "sentinel" lymph node guided the decision to perform a radical neck dissection. Despite these isolated attempts at using SLN status to guide the management of regional lymph nodes, however, the concept of lymphatic mapping was not widely popularized until the end of the twentieth century.

Beginning in 1977, on the basis of their landmark studies, Morton et al. popularized the concepts of lymphoscintigraphy, intraoperative SLN mapping, and SLN biopsy for cutaneous melanoma [1]. Since then, many other centers have utilized SLN biopsy as an integral part of the management strategies for cutaneous melanomas and for many other solid tumors. With the widespread use of SLN biopsy, a large body of data is now available that supports the concepts of sequential lymphatic dissemination and entrapment of tumor cells in first draining lymph nodes and the value of SLN biopsy as a staging procedure for melanoma patients [10–17]. The histologic status of SLN(s) is now viewed as the most important prognostic factor for recurrence and survival in cutaneous melanoma patients [17]. A few studies have also demonstrated a survival benefit from immediate elective lymph node dissection in cutaneous melanoma patients who harbor microscopic regional nodal metastasis compared with patients in whom the "wait and watch" approach is used and therapeutic lymph node dissection was done only after clinically obvious nodal metastasis was noted [18].

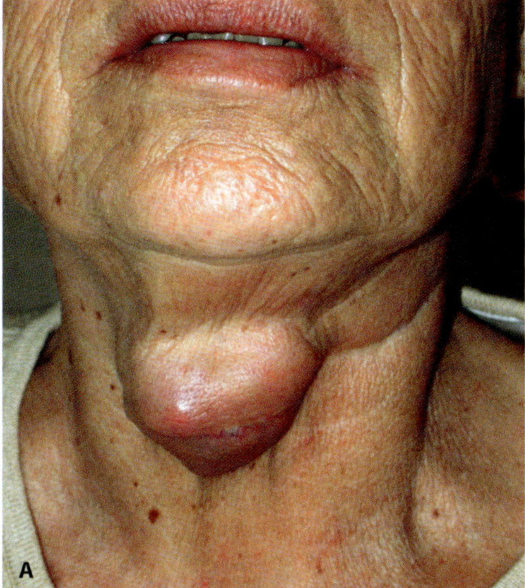

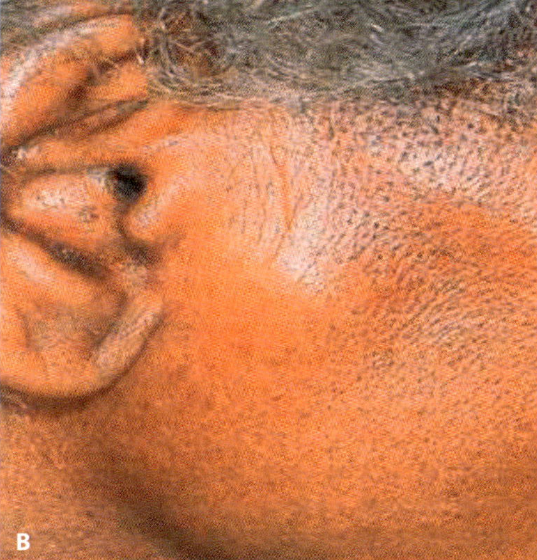

Fig. 3.1. A Patient with conjunctival melanoma with clinically positive regional lymph nodes in the submandibular basin. **B** Patient with sebaceous cell carcinoma of the eyelid with clinically positive regional lymph nodes in the parotid basin

3.3 Sentinel Lymph Node Biopsy for Conjunctival and Eyelid Tumors

With the exception of basal cell carcinoma, all malignant lesions of the eyelid and conjunctiva have a propensity to metastasize to the regional lymph nodes before other sites. Thus, the idea of sentinel node biopsy for patients with these lesions is a natural extension [3]. For conjunctival melanoma, although in a subset of patients the regional nodes may be "skipped" and distant hematogenous spread may be the first manifestation of metastasis [19, 20], several studies suggest that the most common first site of metastasis is the regional nodes. Similarly for other tumors of the ocular adnexa, such as sebaceous cell carcinoma and Merkel cell carcinoma, while the possibility exists of a "skipped" node and hematogenous spread as the first clinical sign of metastasis, the majority of patients have regional nodal metastasis as the first site of spread of their cancer [21, 22].

Given the rarity of ocular adnexal malignancies, large-scale natural history studies or population studies of these tumors are scarce. However, the literature suggests that the risk of regional lymph node metastasis may be as high as 20–40% for conjunctival melanoma (Fig. 3.1A) [19, 20, 23, 24], 30% for eyelid melanoma [25], 10–15% for sebaceous cell carcinoma of the eyelid (Fig. 3.1B) [21], 25–60% for Merkel cell carcinoma [22], 10–30% for periocular squamous cell carcinoma [26], and 5–10% for conjunctival squamous cell carcinoma.

3.3.1 Patient Selection and Indications

Despite the fact that SLN biopsy is a minimally invasive procedure, it is best suited for lesions that have a high enough risk of metastasis to the regional lymph nodes to justify the additional surgical procedure, time, and cost. SLN biopsy has been most widely studied in cutaneous melanomas. For medium-thickness (Breslow thickness of 1.5–4.0 mm) melanomas of the skin in all locations, the overall rate of SLN positivity is approximately 15%, and this is thought to be an acceptable rate of microscopic metastasis to justify the procedure [27, 28].

The relationship between Breslow thickness and SLN positivity for cutaneous melanoma is well established. The rate of sentinel lymph node positivity is estimated to be less than 5% for lesions 0.75 mm or less in thickness and as high as 50% for lesions greater than 4 mm in thickness [16, 17, 27–31]. Similarly, thickness of conjunctival melanomas has been confirmed to be an independent predictor of regional lymph node metastasis and survival [20]. In addition to increased Breslow thickness, other high-risk features that correlate with SLN positivity in patients with cutaneous melanoma include presence of ulceration, Clark's level IV or greater, and age greater than 60 years [16].

For our ongoing trial at M.D. Anderson Cancer Center of SLN biopsy for conjunctival and eyelid tumors, we use the following indications for SLN biopsy: For conjunctival melanomas: Breslow thickness greater than 1 mm, indeterminable thickness, and large areas of diffuse conjunctival pigmentation in the background of biopsy-proven conjunctival melanoma. For eyelid-skin melanoma: Breslow thickness greater than 1 mm, Clark's level IV or higher, and indeterminable thickness. More recently, patients with sebaceous cell carcinoma and Merkel cell carcinoma of the eyelid can be considered for our trial on a case-by-case basis. There is another ongoing trial at M.D. Anderson Cancer Center that could enroll patients with squamous cell carcinoma of the head and neck skin (including eyelid) greater than 2 cm in diameter or with other high-risk features such as perineural invasion. Indications for enrollment in these trials will have to be modified as more data become available.

3.3.2 Anatomic Considerations

The eyelids and conjunctiva have a rich lymphatic drainage. Cadaver studies suggest most of the upper eyelid and the lateral half of the lower eyelid drain to the preauricular or parotid lymph nodes, whereas the medial portion of the upper eyelid and the medial half of the lower eyelid drain to the submandibular nodes by lymphatic vessels that follow the angular and facial vessels [32–35].

In a study of lymphoscintigraphy in cynomolgus monkeys, Cook et al. demonstrated drainage to the preauricular and parotid lymph nodes from the entire upper eyelid, medial canthus, and lateral lower eyelid and drainage to the submandibular lymph nodes from the medial and central lower eyelid [35]. Drainage from the central upper eyelid was to both the parotid and submandibular drainage basins in all five monkeys studied [35].

3.3.3 Technical Considerations

The mapping of SLNs begins with preoperative identification of the afferent lymphatics using radionuclide imaging [4, 13]. The lymphatic

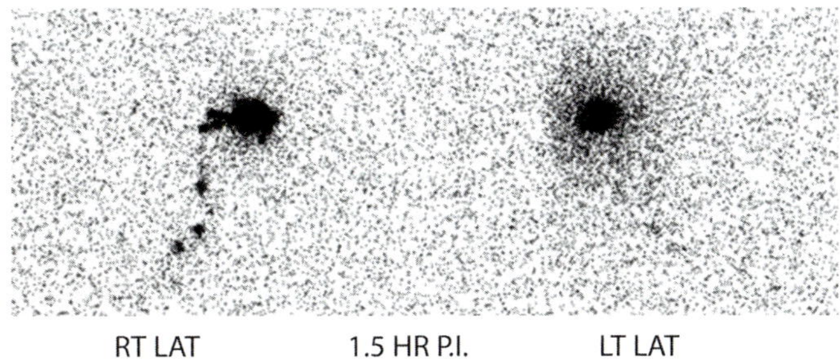

Fig. 3.2. Appearance of sentinel lymph nodes on preoperative lymphoscintigraphy in a patient with a conjunctival melanoma

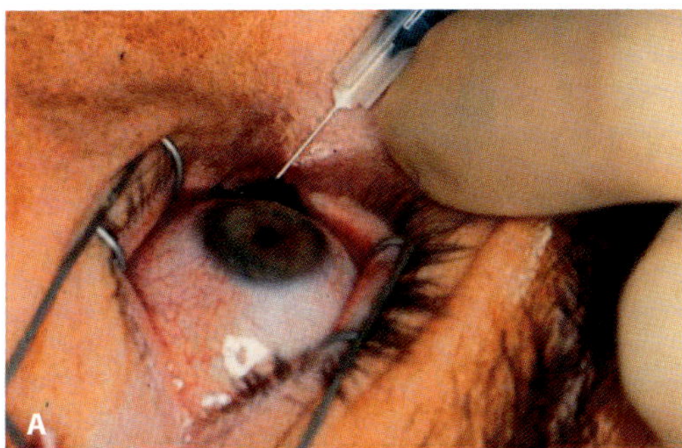

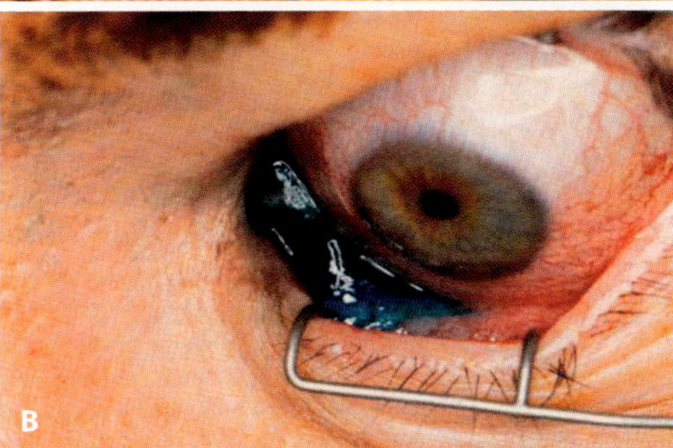

Fig. 3.3. **A** Injection of 0.2 ml of isosulfan blue dye in the subconjunctival space using a tuberculin syringe and a 30-gauge needle. **B** Appearance of blue dye immediately after injection in the inferior conjunctival fornix

drainage pattern is identified on lymphoscintigraphy. For lesions located on the eyelid or conjunctival surface, a drop of anesthetic is applied, and then 0.3 mCi of technetium-99m sulfur colloid in 0.2 ml volume is injected at two to four spots around the lesion intradermally or in the subconjunctival space. Larger volumes of injection may lead to spread of the radioactive material into the subconjunctival space and non-specific drainage from areas that might have a different pattern of lymphatic drainage than the primary tumor site.

Multiple images of the ipsilateral head and neck region are obtained in the nuclear medicine department beginning within a few minutes after radionuclide injection. The first image is obtained as soon as the first SLN is visible (Fig. 3.2). If no drainage is seen within the first 15–20 min, an attempt is made to obtain images up to 1.5 h after injection of technetium.

Intraoperatively, a combination of radiolabeled sulfur colloid and isosulfan blue dye is used to identify and biopsy the SLN(s). Several studies have shown that the rate of SLN identification is enhanced by the use of radiolabeled sulfur colloid in addition to isosulfan blue dye [36, 37]. In the first 16 patients enrolled in our trial, we used 0.2 cc of isosulfan blue dye in addition to technetium sulphur colloid (Fig. 3.3). Our experience with these patients suggests that on the ocular surface and in the periocular region, perhaps because of the very rapid transit of the blue dye, the use of isosulfan blue dye in addition to sulphur colloid is not very beneficial unless the incision over the lymphatic basin is made within a few minutes after blue dye injection. The small volume of blue dye required to avoid non-specific subconjunctival spread and the rapid transit of the blue dye in the head and neck region may be the reasons why we have not seen very many blue SLNs.

On the day of surgery, general anesthesia is induced, and 0.3 mCi of technetium-labeled sulfur colloid in 0.2 ml is once again injected at two to four spots around the lesion, either in the subconjunctival space or intradermally. A quantity of 0.2 cc of isosulfan blue dye is also injected around the lesion at this time if the surgeon chooses. After waiting the same amount of time as it took for technetium to travel to the SLN(s) on preoperative lymphoscintigraphy, the primary lesion is excised with adequate margins. Because the submandibular and parotid nodes are close to the ocular surface, it is recommended that the primary lesion be excised before intraoperative identification of the SLN(s) is attempted so that there is less background radioactivity during the search for SLNs. This ensures that the primary source of radioactivity is removed before exploration of the nodal basins with the gamma probe.

A handheld gamma probe (RIGS model 1001; Neoprobe Co., Dublin, OH) is used to transcutaneously localize SLN(s) (Fig. 3.4), which should have high radioactivity due to uptake of technetium-labeled sulfur colloid (Fig. 3.5). These should correspond to the SLN(s) identified during preoperative lymphoscintigraphy. Subtle angulation of the gamma probe away from the primary tumor site and selective use of the collimator during the search for SLN(s) reduces scatter from the primary tumor injection site and improves localization [38].

Areas of focal radioactive uptake are identified and marked on the skin. A skin incision suitable to permit exploration of the lymphatic basins at risk is made (Fig. 3.6), and these basins are explored. SLNs are defined as lymph nodes that are stained with blue dye (if dye was used) or are at least twice as radioactive as the background radioactivity. Each SLN is separated from its basin and submitted for histologic processing. The maximum ex vivo counts per second are recorded for each SLN. SLN harvest is considered to be complete when the residual radioactivity in the nodal basin is less than twice the background radioactivity. The lymphatic basins are checked again with the gamma probe after removal of the SLN(s) to confirm the lowering of radioactivity and thus confirm that no other SLNs are present.

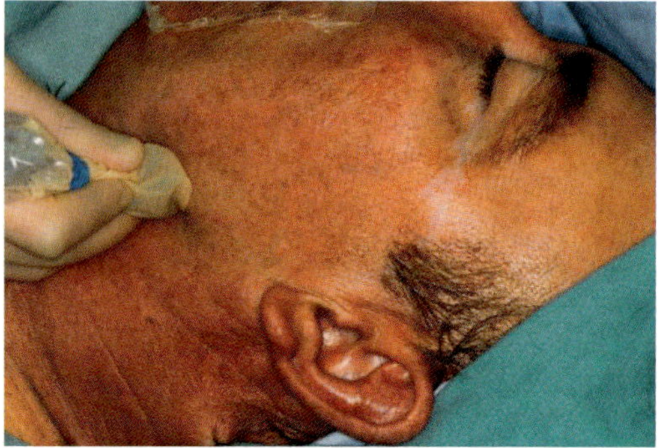

Fig. 3.4. Intraoperatively, a handheld gamma probe is used to transcutaneously localize sentinel lymph nodes intraoperatively

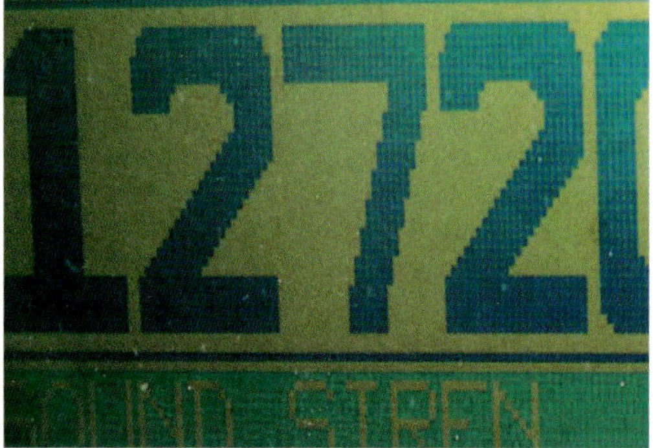

Fig. 3.5. The radioactive uptake from the sentinel nodes is recorded as an absolute number on the screen, and the signal is transmitted as a calibrated sound that increases in intensity with an increase in radioactive uptake

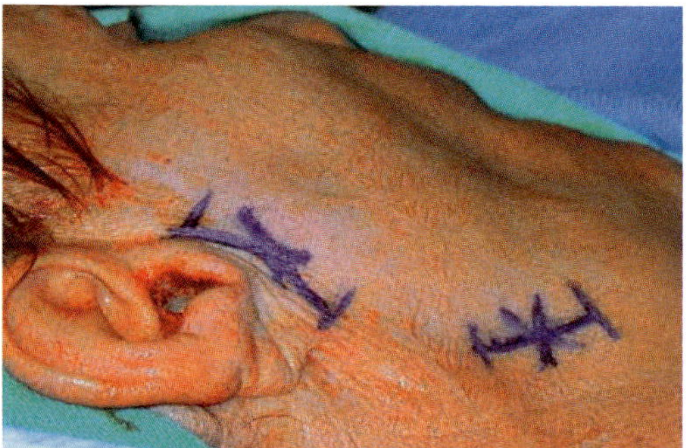

Fig. 3.6. Small (2- to 3-cm) incisions are made in the skin overlying the SLN(s). The skin incisions are planned such that they can be connected to form the incision for a possible future therapeutic neck dissection or superficial parotidectomy

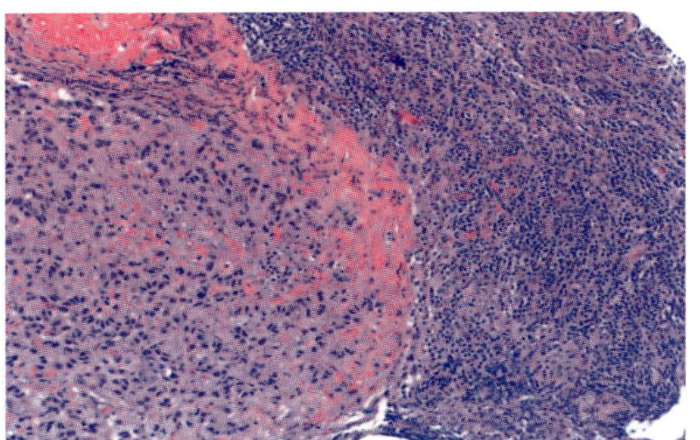

Fig. 3.7. Histologic section of a sentinel lymph node demonstrates a proliferation of cells suggesting melanoma infiltrating the lymph node parenchyma

3.3.4 Histopathologic Analysis of Sentinel Lymph Nodes

SLNs are serially sectioned ("bread-loafed") at 1-mm intervals and examined with hematoxylin and eosin (H & E) staining. If no micrometastasis is detected on the lymph node sections with H & E staining (Fig. 3.7), immunohistochemical staining is done. For melanomas, immunohistochemical staining is performed with antisera to the S-100 protein MART-1 and the melanoma antigen HMB-45. For eyelid sebaceous cell carcinoma and Merkel cell carcinoma, immunohistochemical staining is performed with antisera to cytokeratin.

Both bread-loafing, which allows for a more careful inspection of multiple thin sections, and immunohistochemical staining using appropriate antisera have increased the sensitivity of detection of micrometastasis in SLN biopsy specimens [39, 40]. The use of reverse transcriptase-polymerase chain reaction to detect mRNA for the tyrosinase gene has been reported to enhance the sensitivity of SLN biopsy in the detection of cells of melanocytic origin, but this technique remains experimental and is available only in the setting of some ongoing clinical trials [41, 42].

For conjunctival melanomas, special care is required in specimen handling and processing of the primary tumor specimen. Conjunctival melanoma specimens are friable, and the edges can curl up. In addition, most conjunctival melanoma specimens are quite small and thin compared with cutaneous melanoma specimens. These factors together frequently lead to tangential cutting of conjunctival melanoma

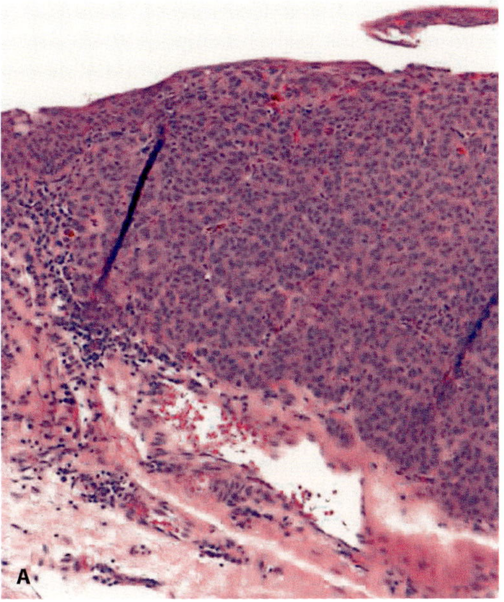

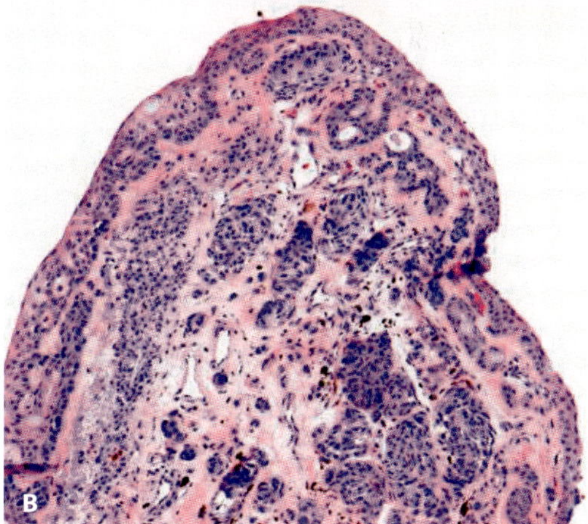

Fig. 3.8. A Histologic section of conjunctival melanoma specimen that has been cut perpendicularly. The thickness of the tumor can be measured from the surface epithelium to the furthest depth of tumor extension. **B** Histologic section of another conjunctival melanoma specimen that has been cut tangentially. The true depth of the tumor cannot be determined

specimens. Tangential cutting of the primary tumor specimen makes it impossible to determine tumor thickness (Fig. 3.8) and thus can lead to unnecessary SLN biopsy procedures. To ensure that tumor thickness can be determined, specimens must be cut perpendicularly.

3.3.5 Lymphatic Basins at Risk

The majority of patients with conjunctival or eyelid tumors who undergo SLN biopsy have more than one SLN identified. Results of our clinical trial to date indicate that the lymphatic basins that most commonly harbor SLNs are the periparotid nodes, which account for 60 % of all SLNs identified in our trial so far (parotid, 38 %; preauricular, 22 %), and the submandibular (level I) nodes, which account for 20 % of the SLNs identified. The level II nodes account for 12 % of all SLNs identified, and levels III, IV, and V each account for less than 1 % of the SLNs identified [4, 5].

3.4 Care of Patients with a Positive Sentinel Lymph Node

Identification of a micrometastasis in an SLN indicates that the patient needs to undergo a complete surgical dissection of the regional nodes (completion neck dissection) followed by external-beam radiation therapy. In the case of melanoma, the disease would be upstaged to stage III, and the patient might qualify for some of the ongoing trials of systemic adjuvant therapy in addition to completion neck dissection and superficial parotidectomy (if the parotid basin is involved) for stage III melanoma. Postoperative adjuvant radiation therapy to the regional nodes is recommended to ensure durable regional control [43, 44].

Two of the 27 patients enrolled in our M.D. Anderson trial so far have had a histologically positive SLN. Both patients had conjunctival melanoma [45]. The overall rate of SLN positivity for conjunctival melanomas in our trial is 2 of the 13 patients enrolled, or 14 %. However, the total number of patients enrolled is too small to permit definitive conclusions to be drawn about the rate of SLN positivity for any of the malignant lesions included in our trial.

The literature on SLN biopsy for cutaneous melanoma shows that patients with positive SLNs have a lower survival rate and higher rate of recurrence than patients with negative SLNs at the time of treatment of their primary cutaneous melanoma. Of the two patients in our series with conjunctival melanoma and positive SLNs, one developed distant-organ metastasis 6 months after treatment of his regional nodes, and the other had additional positive non-sentinel nodes discovered during therapeutic neck dissection and was free of distant metastasis 12 months after the SLN biopsy.

3.4.1 Potential Complications and Limitations

SLN biopsy in the parotid area requires careful delineation of the course of the facial nerve and its branches to minimize the risk of damaging the facial nerve, particularly the marginal mandibular branch. A larger incision may be required for SLN biopsy in the parotid area than for SLN biopsy in other areas to ensure safe dissection and protection of the facial nerve, particularly if an SLN is located in the deeper lobe of the parotid gland. Of the 27 patients enrolled so far in our trial of SLN biopsy for ocular adnexal tumors, only three have experienced temporary weakness of the marginal mandibular branch of the facial nerve, and this lasted only 2–3 weeks and resolved spontaneously.

The risk of blue discoloration of the eyelid skin or ocular surface remains theoretical in our experience. As shown in Fig. 3.8, the blue staining of the skin and conjunctiva resolves in 24–48 h, and in the 16 patients in whom we have used isosulfan blue dye, no tattooing of the skin or conjunctiva has been observed.

Allergic reaction to isosulfan blue dye has also previously been reported; such reactions are estimated to occur in less than 2 % of patients [46]. We have not encountered an anaphylactic reaction to the blue dye in our trial so far.

The risk of radiation damage to the eye from SLN biopsy is negligible. It is estimated that a dose of 0.3 mCi of technetium-labeled sulfur colloid emits a dose of 0.2 rad to the lens over a 6-h period even if no drainage is assumed from the subconjunctival space or the site of injection in the eyelid skin. This dose is much less than the dose associated with cataract formation or radiation retinopathy (2,000–4,000 rads) [47]. Even with two separate injections of technetium (one for preoperative lymphoscintigraphy and the other on the day of surgery for intraoperative mapping of SLNs), the dose to the eye is much less than the dose known to cause damage.

In our trial of SLN biopsy for ocular adnexal tumors, we have been able to identify the SLN(s) that correspond to the lymphoscintigraphy drainage pattern in all 27 patients enrolled. Most studies of head and neck melanomas report a rate of SLN identification greater than 90% [48–55].

The false-negative rate in our series so far is 7% – two patients with negative SLNs had clinical recurrence in their draining SLN basin. However, given the small number of patients in our study, our findings cannot be compared with those of other larger studies of SLN biopsy for head and neck melanoma. Various studies indicate that the false-negative rate of SLN biopsy for cutaneous melanomas at all locations ranges from 1.5% to 24% depending on the median length of clinical follow-up for the study [49, 50, 52, 53].

There are three major causes for false-negative findings on SLN biopsy. One is pathologic failure – i.e., because of a sampling error, the micrometastasis is not detected in the SLN specimen. Using serial sectioning and immunohistochemistry should decrease this type of error, although the technology is still not perfect. Molecular studies using reverse transcriptase-polymerase chain reaction for tyrosinase are more sensitive, but their value remains to be established. Another cause of false-negative findings on SLN biopsy is technical failure. This has to do with the method used to identify and retrieve the SLN(s). Given the limited utility of the blue dye as an adjunct to technetium in identifying the SLNs in our trial, one has to rely entirely on the gamma probe to identify the radioactive nodes, which are often located in the body of the parotid gland. The parotid gland is known to harbor a lot of background activity, making it difficult to identify SLNs in this area. The parotid nodes are also smaller and often located in a bed of fibroadipose tissue, again making their dissection more challenging. There is of course the omnipresent risk of damage to the facial nerve. But overall, several studies have corroborated our experience that SLN biopsy in the head and neck region and particularly in the parotid area is doable but is challenging and requires familiarity with the technique and the unique anatomic features of the parotid gland [48–51]. The third source of false-negative findings is biological failure. This refers to the possibility of lymphatics being obstructed by melanoma cells, which may cause rerouting of the lymph flow. As a result, the true SLN is not detected and a non-SLN is retrieved.

Another potential cause of false-negative findings on SLN biopsy that is unique to conjunctival melanoma might be an unusually high rate of local recurrence for this particular ocular malignancy. Most studies to date suggest a local recurrence rate of 20–40% for conjunctival melanomas after conservative surgical management and cryotherapy. The assumption is that each time a conjunctival melanoma recurs locally it can pose a risk to the lymphatics and the status of the regional nodes. In the case of recurrence, the lymphatic drainage pattern may be less reliable due to previous multiple surgery. The chance of local recurrence can be minimized by better handling of the specimens, more careful attention to margins, wider margins if possible, and administration of adjuvant local therapy in the form of topical chemotherapy or adjuvant radiation therapy. The utility of standard external-beam radiotherapy is limited on the ocular surface because of its toxicity to the eye, but some forms of brachytherapy or topical chemotherapy may prove to be better alternatives.

3.5 Conclusions and Future Directions

In summary, the data collected from our ongoing trial at M.D. Anderson suggest that SLN biopsy for ocular tumors is feasible and safe and can be done with a slight modification of the usual injection technique. Our data suggest that SLN biopsy can identify patients with clinically occult microscopic metastasis in their lymph nodes. The false-negative rate needs to be monitored in larger studies. Continued improvement in identification and histologic analysis of SLNs may improve the false-negative rate for SLN biopsy for ocular tumors. We are planning a phase II trial with a larger number of patients so that we can continue to evaluate the rate of positivity of SLNs, fine-tune the indications for SLN biopsy, and improve the false-negative rate. The rate of local control for conjunctival melanomas in particular would also have to be improved for the concept of regional nodal control to make sense for such tumors. Better conjunctival specimen handling, more careful attention to margins of resection, and avoidance of tangential cutting may be some preliminary steps towards this goal. Adjuvant and safe delivery of radiation therapy to the ocular surface may also be advantageous. Future efforts need to focus on the design of trials of adjuvant systemic therapy that may benefit patients who are found to have a positive SLN after they undergo completion neck dissection and regional radiation therapy. Only then can we hope to improve survival in patients with conjunctival and eyelid tumors with a definite mortality risk.

Summary for the Clinician

- **The value of sentinel lymph node (SLN) biopsy for conjunctival and eyelid cancers is currently under investigation**
- **Our experience so far suggests that SLN biopsy is technically feasible and safe to do for ocular adnexal tumors**
- **We have identified some patients who have harbored microscopic metastasis in their regional lymph nodes, thus validating the concept of utilizing SLN biopsy for these lesions**
- **Our false negative rate of 8 % may be slightly higher than in other anatomic locations; thus, there is a need for further improvement of the technique particularly when the SLNs are located in the parotid region**

References

1. Morton DL, Wen DR, Wong JH, et al. (1992) Technical details of intra-operative lymphatic mapping for early stage melanoma. Arch Surg 127: 392–399
2. Kapteijn BAE, Nieweg OE, Peterse JL, et al. (1998) Identification and biopsy of the sentinel lymph node in breast cancer. Eur J Surg Oncol 24:427–430
3. Esmaeli B (1999) Sentinel lymph node mapping for patients with cutaneous and conjunctival malignant melanoma. Ophthal Plast Reconstr Surg 16:170–172
4. Amato M, Esmaeli B, Ahmadi MA, et al. (2002) Feasibility of preoperative lymphoscintigraphy for identification of sentinel lymph nodes in patients with conjunctival and periocular skin malignancies. Ophthal Plast Reconstr Surg 19:102–106
5. Nijhawan N, Ross MI, Diba R, et al. (2004) Experience with sentinel lymph node biopsy for eyelid and conjunctival malignancies at a cancer center. Ophthal Plast Reconstr Surg 20:291–295
6. Gilchrist RK (1940) Fundamental factors governing lymphatic spread of carcinoma. Ann Surg 111:630–639
7. Zeidman I, Buss JM (1954) Experimental studies of the spread of cancer in the lymphatic system. Cancer Res 14:403–405
8. Fisher B, Fisher ER (1967) Barrier function of lymph node to tumor cells and erythrocytes. Cancer 20:1907–1913
9. Sim FH, Taylor WT, Ivins JC, et al. (1978) A prospective randomized study of the efficacy of routine elective lymphadenectomy in management of malignant melanoma. Cancer 41:948–956
10. Reintgen DS, Cruse CW, Wells KE, et al. (1994) The orderly progression of melanoma nodal metastases. Ann Surg 220:759–767
11. Vuylsteke RJ, van Leeuwen PA, Statius Muller MG, et al. (2003) Clinical outcome of stage I/II melanoma patients after selective sentinel lymph node dissection: long-term follow up results. J Clin Oncol 21:1057–1065
12. McMasters KM, Wong SL, Edwards MJ, et al. (2001) Factors that predict the presence of sentinel lymph node metastasis in patients with melanoma. Surgery 130:151–156

13. Uren R, Howman-Giles R, Thompson J, et al. (1994) Lymphoscintigraphy to identify sentinel lymph nodes in patients with melanoma. Melanoma Res 4:395–399
14. Albertini J, Cruse C, Paraparot D, et al. (1996) Intraoperative radiolymphoscintigraphy improves sentinel lymph node identification in patients with melanoma. Ann Surg 223:217–224
15. Bachter D, Michl C, Büchels H, Vogt H, Balda BR (2001) The predictive value of the sentinel lymph node in malignant melanomas. Recent Results Cancer Res 158:129–136
16. Rousseau DL, Ross MI, Johnson MM, et al. (2003) Revised American Joint Committee on Cancer staging criteria accurately predict sentinel lymph node positivity in clinically node-negative melanoma patients. Ann Surg Oncol 10:569–574
17. Gershenwald JE, Thompson W, Mansfield PF, et al. (1999) Multi-institutional melanoma lymphatic mapping experience: the prognostic value of sentinel lymph node status in 612 stage I and II melanoma patients. J Clin Oncol 17:976–983
18. Cascinelle N, Morabito A, Santinami M, et al. (1998) Immediate or delayed dissection of regional nodes in patients with melanoma of the trunk: a randomized trial – WHO Melanoma Programme. Lancet 351:793–796
19. Esmaeli B, Wang X, Youssef A, et al. (2001) Patterns of regional and distant metastasis in patients with conjunctival melanoma: experience at a cancer center over four decades. Ophthalmology 108:2101–2105
20. Tuomaala S, Kivela T (2004) Metastatic pattern and survival in disseminated conjunctival melanoma: implications for sentinel lymph node biopsy. Ophthalmology 111:816–821
21. Chao AN, Shields CL, Krema H, et al. (2001) Outcome of patients with periocular sebaceous gland carcinoma with and without conjunctival intraepithelial invasion. Ophthalmology 108:1877–1883
22. Peters GB, Meyer DR, Shields JA, et al. (2001) Management and prognosis of Merkel cell carcinoma of the eyelid. Ophthalmology 108:1575–1579
23. Seregard S, Koch E (1992) Conjunctival malignant melanoma in Sweden 1969–91. Acta Ophthalmol 70:289–296
24. Paridaens ADA, Minassian DC, McCartney ACE, Hungerford JL (1994) Prognostic factors in primary malignant melanoma of the conjunctiva: a clinicopathological study of 256 cases. Br J Ophthalmol 78:252–259
25. Esmaeli B, Wang B, Deavers M, et al. (2000) Prognostic factors for survival in malignant melanoma of the eyelid skin. Ophthal Plast Reconstr Surg 16:250–257
26. Faustina M, Diba R, Ahmadi MA, Gutstein BF, Esmaeli B (2004) Patterns of regional and distant metastasis in patients with eyelid and periocular squamous cell carcinoma. Ophthalmology 111: 1930–1932
27. Krag DN, Meijer SJ, Weaver DL, et al. (1995) Minimal access surgery for staging of malignant melanoma. Arch Surg 130:654–658
28. Chao C, Wong SL, Edwards MJ, et al. (2003) Sentinel lymph node biopsy for head and neck melanomas. Ann Surg Oncol 10:21–26
29. Joseph E, Brobeil A, Glass F, et al. (1998) Results of complete lymph node dissection in 83 melanoma patients with positive sentinel nodes. Ann Surg Oncol 5:119–125
30. Mraz-Gernhard S, Sagebiel RW, et al. (1998) Prediction of sentinel lymph node micrometastasis by histological features in primary cutaneous malignant melanoma. Arch Dermatol 134:983–987
31. Haddad FF, Stall A, Messina J, et al. (1999) The progression of melanoma nodal metastasis is dependent on tumor thickness of the primary lesion. Ann Surg Oncol 6:144–149
32. McGetrick JJ, Wilson DG, Dortzbach RK, et al. (1989) A search for the lymphatic drainage of the monkey orbit. Arch Ophthalmol 107:255–260
33. Sherman DD, Gonnering RS, Wallow IH, et al. (1993) Identification of orbital lymphatics: enzyme histochemical light microscopic and electron microscopic studies. Ophthal Plast Reconstr Surg 9:153–169
34. Gausas RE, Gonnering RS, Lemke VN, et al. (1999) Identification of human orbital lymphatics. Ophthal Plast Reconstr Surg 15:252–259
35. Cook BE Jr, Lucarelli MJ, Lemke BN, et al. (2002) Eyelid lymphatics. I: Histochemical comparisons between the monkey and human. Ophthal Plast Reconstr Surg 18:99–106
36. Gershenwald JE, Tseng C, Thompson W, et al. (1998) Improved sentinel lymph node localization in patients with primary melanoma with the use of radiolabeled colloid. Surgery 124:203–210
37. Carlson GW, Murray DR, Greenlee R, et al. (2000) Management of malignant melanoma of the head and neck using dynamic lymphoscintigraphy and gamma probe-guided sentinel lymph node biopsy. Arch Otolaryngol Head Neck Surg 126: 433–437
38. Gershenwald JE (2005) Operating room positioning: mastery of lymphatic mapping. In: Ross ME, Hunt KK (eds) Springer-Verlag, New York (in press)
39. Cochran AJ (1999) Surgical pathology remains pivotal in the evaluation of "sentinel" lymph nodes. Am J Surg Pathol 23:1169–1172

40. Yu LL, Flotte TJ, Tanabe KK, et al. (1999) Detection of microscopic melanoma metastases in sentinel lymph nodes. Cancer 86:617–627
41. Wang X, Heller R, Van Voorhies N, et al. (1994) Detection of submicroscopic lymph node metastases with polymerase chain reaction in patients with malignant melanoma. Ann Surg 220:674–678
42. McMasters KM, Noyes RD, Reintgen D, et al. (2004) Lessons learned from the Sunbelt Melanoma Trial. J Surg Oncol 86:212–223
43. Ballo MT, Bonnen MD, Garden AS, et al. (2003) Adjuvant irradiation for cervical lymph node metastases from melanoma. Cancer 97:1789–1796
44. Bonnen MD, Ballo MT, Myers JN, et al. (2004) Elective radiotherapy provides regional control for patients with cutaneous melanoma of the head and neck. Cancer 100:383–389
45. Esmaeli B, Reifler D, Prieto VG, et al. (2003) Conjunctival melanoma with a positive sentinel lymph node. Arch Ophthalmol 121:1779–1783
46. Leong SP, Donegan E, Heffernon W, et al. (2000) Adverse reactions to isosulfan blue during selective sentinel lymph node dissection in melanoma. Ann Surg Oncol 7:361–366
47. Henk JM, Whitelocke RA, Warrington AP, et al. (1993) Radiation dose to the lens and cataract formation. Int J Radiat Oncol Biol Phys 25:815–820
48. Eicher SA, Clayman GL, Myers JN, et al. (2002) A prospective study of intraoperative lymphatic mapping for head and neck cutaneous melanoma. Arch Otolaryngol Head Neck Surg 128:241–246
49. Schmalbach CE, Nussenbaum B, Rees RS, et al. (2003) Reliability of sentinel lymph node mapping with biopsy for head and neck cutaneous melanoma. Arch Otolaryngol Head Neck Surg 129:61–65
50. Wells KE, Rapaport DP, Cruse WC, et al. (1997) Sentinel lymph node biopsy in melanoma of the head and neck. Plastic Reconstr Surg 100:591–594
51. Bostick P, Essner R, Sarantou T, et al. (1997) Intraoperative lymphatic mapping for early stage melanoma of the head and neck. Am J Surg 174:356–359
52. Medina-Franco H, Beenken SW, Heslin MJ, et al. (2001) Sentinel node biopsy for cutaneous melanoma in the head and neck. Ann Surg Oncol 8:716–719
53. Chao C, Wond SL, Ross MI, et al. (2002) Patterns of early recurrence after sentinel lymph node biopsy for melanoma. Am J Surg 184:520–525
54. Carlson GW, Murray DR, Greenlee R, et al. (2000) Management of malignant melanoma of the head and neck using dynamic lymphoscintigraphy and gamma probe-guided sentinel lymph node biopsy. Arch Otolaryngol Head Neck Surg 126:433–437
55. Wagner JD, Park H-M, Coleman JJ, et al. (2000) Cervical sentinel lymph node biopsy for melanomas of the head and neck and upper thorax. Arch Otolaryngol Head and Neck Surg 126:313–321

Lacrimal Surgery

The Apparent Paradox of "Success" in Lacrimal Drainage Surgery

4

Geoffrey E. Rose

Core Messages

- The many symptoms and signs of lacrimal drainage disorders affect ocular function, ocular health and social interactions
- The highly variable size of the tear lake is dependent upon a balance between tear production and clearance from the ocular surface, the latter by evaporation or through the drainage pathways
- The lacrimal system can be considered as a three-compartment model: the tear lake being the first compartment, the lacrimal sac the second, and the nasal space the third. Two zones of poor hydraulic conductance – the canaliculi and the nasolacrimal duct – join the three compartments
- Signs and symptoms of lacrimal drainage disorders are either "flow-related" or "volume-related"
- Flow-related characteristics are due to limitations of tear conductance from the lateral canthus to the nose – but especially that due to the hydraulic resistance of the canaliculi and nasolacrimal duct. Cure of flow-related symptoms is not achievable in every patient
- Being due to fluid within – or "backwash" from – the lacrimal sac, appropriate surgery will cure volume-related characteristics in all cases
- Elimination of the second compartment (lacrimal sac) cures volume-related symptoms, this being achieved only with a large osteotomy that permits a complete opening of the sac (from the fundus to nasolacrimal duct). Primary intention healing of the mucosal union will maximise the anastomotic size and reduce fibrous contracture due to secondary intention healing – the latter typically seen after endonasal or inadequate external surgery
- During external dacryocystorhinostomy, suturing of both the anterior and posterior mucosal flaps is readily achieved if an anterior ethmoidectomy is routinely performed

4.1 Introduction

The patient with lacrimal symptoms will present when sufficiently troubled by an overfull tear lake with secondary visual impairment, by spillover of tears from the tear lake, or by either continuous or intermittent mucoid ocular discharge; all of these symptoms may be complicated by secondary bacterial infection – mucopurulent infective conjunctivitis.

It is widely assumed that an eye with watering or discharge has impairment of outflow, but the size of the tear lake is actually a fine balance between tear production (varying greatly from minimal baseline production to the copious volumes of maximal reflex lacrimation) and the loss of tears through evaporation or drainage through the lacrimal outflow passages. The complexity of this balance is manifest in two common scenarios: First, some people with complete obstruction of lacrimal outflow will be asymptomatic because their (low) rate of tear

Table 4.1. Indications for lacrimal surgery

Indications for lacrimal surgery	Cause or effect of indication
Epiphora	Cosmetic embarrassment Skin excoriation
Visual impairment (especially on downgaze)	Overfull tear-lake Mucus or pus in tear lake
Medial canthal mass	Lacrimal sac mucocoele or pyocoele Lacrimal sac pneumatocoele Lacrimal sac tumour
Ocular discharge	Chronic dacryocystitis (mucocoele or pyocoele) Chronic canaliculitis (*Actinomyces*)
Pain	Acute fluid retention in sac Acute infective dacryocystitis
Cutaneous lacrimal fistula	Congenital canalicular fistula Acquired lacrimal sac fistula
Injury	Primary repair of lacrimal drainage system Secondary repair of medial canthal injury
Tumours	Primary tumours of lacrimal drainage system Secondary involvement by orbital or sinus tumours
Intraocular surgery	Risk of endophthalmitis posed by presence of lacrimal sac muco-pyocoele

production is matched by evaporation – the latter being especially marked in hot, dry climates. Secondly, certain climatic conditions – such as cold or windy days – encourage watering due to reflex lacrimation from corneal stimulation, reduced tear evaporation with the cold, and impairment of lacrimal drainage due to nasal mucosal congestion.

There is a multitude of symptoms and signs due to abnormal lacrimal dynamics and these are, in many cases, an indication for drainage surgery – even where other factors, such as overproduction of tears, may be contributory (Table 4.1). The influence of factors other than drainage failure makes the interpretation of "success" after lacrimal drainage surgery extremely difficult: some patients will have continued symptoms despite an anatomically and physiologically patent drainage anastomosis, and others will have resolution of symptoms despite occlusion of the drainage pathway after surgery – this being an apparent "lacrimal paradox".

4.2 The "Lacrimal Paradox" and the Dichotomy of Lacrimal Characteristics

The apparent "lacrimal paradox" is well illustrated by two of the author's patients who presented with lacrimal symptoms at variance with their clinical signs.

Case 1. An elderly lady underwent open dacryocystorhinostomy for a recurrent sticky eye due to nasolacrimal duct occlusion; silicone intubation was avoided because the common canalicular opening in the lacrimal sac was noted, at surgery, to be normal. She returned to clinic a month after surgery, delighted with the postoperative result and, in her view, cured. At examination, however, there was an increased tear line on the operated side, with medial (membranous) common canalicular occlusion preventing any drainage of tears.

Table 4.2. The "volume" and "flow" characteristics or lacrimal drainage dynamics

"Volume" characteristics	"Flow" characteristics
Morning stickiness of lids and lashes especially on downgaze	Overfull tear lake causing "constant" blurred vision,
Mucoid "flooding" of tear lake, causing intermittently blurred vision	Spillover of non-mucoid tears, with "salting" of periocular skin
Strings of mucoid debris in tear-lake	Sputtering of spectacles, due to tears flicked onto lenses by wet lashes
Variable medial canthal mass, occasionally with pain of dacryocystic retention	Infrequent conjunctivitis
Expressible lacrimal sac muco-pyocoele	–
Acute infective dacryocystitis or lacrimal sac abscess	No medial canthal mass
Recurrent conjunctivitis	No dacryocystitis or pain No morning stickiness of lids or lashes

In this case we have SURGERY as an ANATOMIC FAILURE, but the PATIENT regarded the surgery as an ABSOLUTE SUCCESS.

Case 2. A middle-aged lady attended with watering eyes due to nasolacrimal duct stenosis, rather than complete occlusion, and underwent open dacryocystorhinostomy without silicone intubation. At her outpatient assessment a month after surgery, she described the operation as a "complete disaster" and threatened legal action. Although there was a somewhat increased tear lake on the affected side, spontaneous and rapid clearance of fluorescein to the nasal space was readily demonstrated and the patient was reassured that tear flow through the system would almost certainly increase over the months after surgery, as postoperative oedema resolved. A few months later she was asymptomatic.

In this case we have the PATIENT believing the surgery a FAILURE and yet the SURGICAL ANASTOMOSIS was SUCCESSFUL, both anatomically and functionally.

The enigmatic disparity between the anatomic or physiological outcome of surgery and a patient's symptoms and signs is best understood when these latter characteristics are considered in detail. Lacrimal drainage characteristics are either "*flow-related*", due to the rate of tear production (less the evaporative component) outstripping the hydraulic conductance of the outflow pathways, or "*volume-related*", due to fluid accumulation in the lacrimal sac and backwash of this debris into the tear lake (Table 4.2). A patient with volume-related difficulties will almost always have flow-related symptomatology, whereas the patient with flow-related problems will frequently *not* have any volume-related symptoms or signs.

Volume-related characteristics occur where there is free communication between an enlarged lacrimal sac, filled either with watery mucus or muco-pus, and the tear lake; they cannot, therefore, occur in the presence of complete canalicular occlusion. Symptoms are typically those of a variable mass at the inner canthus – tender or red if acute dacryocystitis is present (Fig. 4.1 A) – from which some patients will have noted that debris can be expressed into the tear lake, onto the skin (Fig. 4.1 B) or, very rarely, into the nasopharynx; the clinical signs of debris within the lacrimal sac are usually easily shown. Intermittent spontaneous drainage of the sac contents into the tear lake is associated with symptoms of "blurred vision" by strings of mucus or muco-pus and "the lids gumming closed in the morning" (Fig. 4.1 C); many patients, on waking, having to spend 5–15 min bathing their eyelids open. The presence of a significant fluid-containing "dead space" within the lacrimal sac also encourages bacterial overgrowth and predisposes to recurrent conjunctivitis (Fig. 4.1 D).

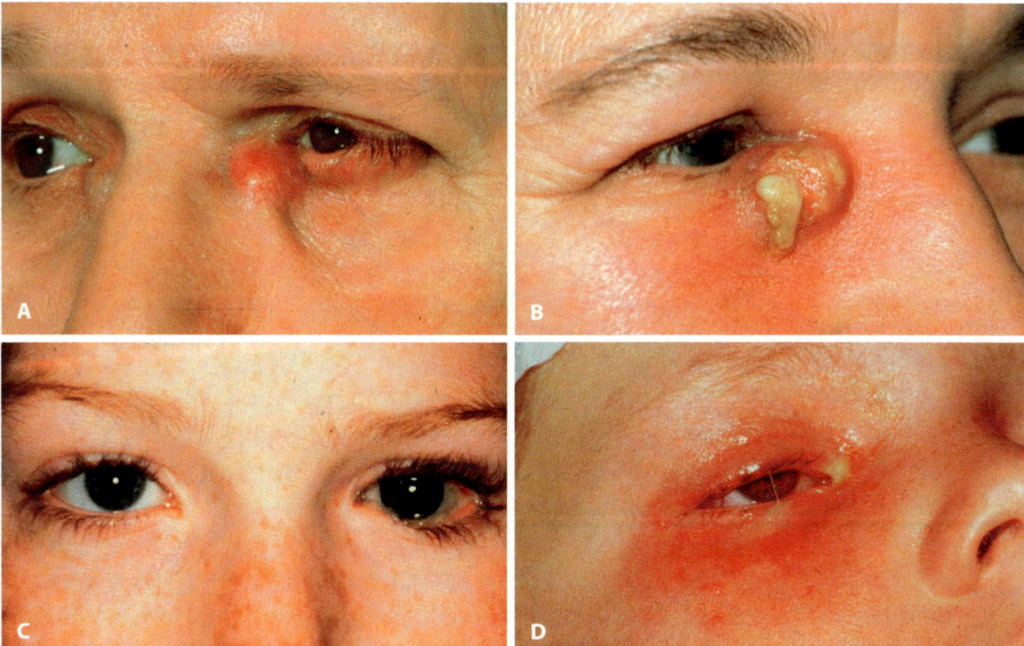

Fig. 4.1 A–D. "Volume" characteristics of lacrimal drainage: **A** Right lacrimal sac mass due to retention mucocoele and left acute infective dacryocystitis. **B** Purulent discharge from right lacrimal sac abscess. **C** Chronic mucoid discharge in left tear lake. **D** Recurrent purulent conjunctivitis and periocular skin excoriation due to occluded right lacrimal drainage

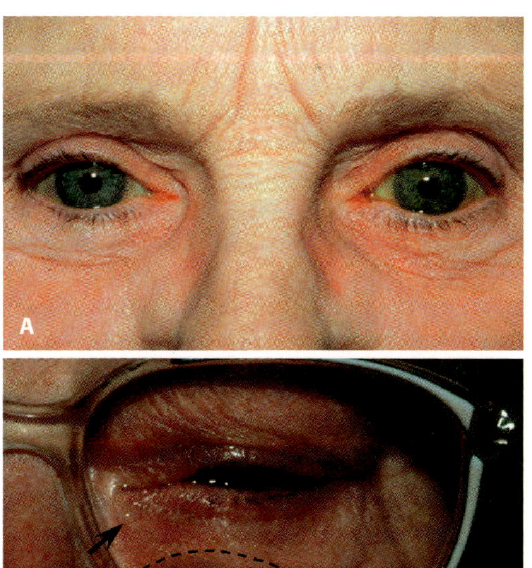

Fig. 4.2 A, B. "Flow" characteristics of lacrimal drainage: **A** Excessive tear-lake and slow clearance of fluorescein dye in both eyes, especially the left side. **B** Medial spillage of tears (*arrow*) from excessive tear lake, with pooling between spectacle lens and cheek (*outlined*)

In contrast, flow-related symptoms and signs are due to an excess of aqueous tears in the tear lake. Variable "blurred vision" due to an overfull watery (not mucoid) tear line (Fig. 4.2 A) – helped by dabbing away the tears – is probably the commonest flow-related symptom. This blurring is often worse on downgaze, such as during reading or golf, because the visual axis passes nearer to the enlarged tear meniscus on the lower lid during these pursuits and this exacerbates presbyopic symptoms. Spillage of tears – that is, true epiphora – leads to "skin soreness" and "salty deposits on the skin" and the tears, flicked from the lake by the lashes or trapped behind the spectacle lenses (Fig. 4.2 B), also lead to "repeated smearing of the glasses". Although the risk of conjunctivitis is slightly increased by slow clearance of tears, this risk is minor as compared to patients with volume-related problems and morning gumming of the lids is distinctly unusual with pure flow-related disease; likewise, dacryocystitis and dacryocystic retention are not flow-related characteristics.

Tear film dynamics can be conveniently regarded as a three-compartment hydraulic model, thus aiding understanding of volume-related and flow-related characteristics and also providing a rational explanation for the apparent "lacrimal paradox". The model also provides an understanding of the aims for lacrimal surgery, together with an unbiased and logically sound measure for "success" after lacrimal surgery.

4.3 The Three-Compartment Model of Lacrimal Drainage

Lacrimal drainage hydraulics may be considered as a three-compartment model, with the tear lake comprising the first compartment, the lacrimal sac forming the second, and the nasal space being the third compartment; the three compartments being joined by two conduits of relatively high hydraulic resistance – namely, the lacrimal canaliculi and nasolacrimal duct (Fig. 4.3).

With a freely draining nasolacrimal duct, the second compartment (the lacrimal sac) should normally contain only minimal fluid: Volume-related problems – due to fluid reflux from this second compartment into the first (tear lake) – will arise only where there is a dilated lacrimal sac, able to sequester sufficient debris to cause clinical symptoms and signs. In contrast, flow-related characteristics depend upon the hydraulic conductance of the whole drainage pathway relative to the rate of tear production, less losses by evaporation, and are largely independent of the volume of the second compartment, the lacrimal sac. Unlike volume characteristics, lacrimal flow (conductance) is also significantly affected by abnormal lower lid position and movement, by punctal apposition and function, by efficiency of the canalicular "pump", and by nasal diseases affecting drainage of the nasolacrimal duct.

The solution to the apparent "lacrimal paradox" is evident from the three-compartment model of lacrimal drainage dynamics: The first patient (with symptomatic "success", despite anatomic failure) originally had volume symptoms – with sticky eye and recurrent conjunctivitis – and these had been resolved by elimination of the lacrimal sac with open dacryocystorhinostomy; although she had an occluded common canaliculus after surgery, her tear production was insufficient to cause postoperative flow symptoms. The second patient (with symptomatic "failure", despite anatomic success) had persistent flow symptoms due to inadequate canalicular conductance probably resulting from peri-canalicular edema. As the postoperative swelling slowly resolved, so the canalicular conductance improved over several months to eventually render the patient asymptomatic.

Appreciation of the three-compartment model also allows a definition of the aims of lacrimal drainage surgery: It is a popular belief

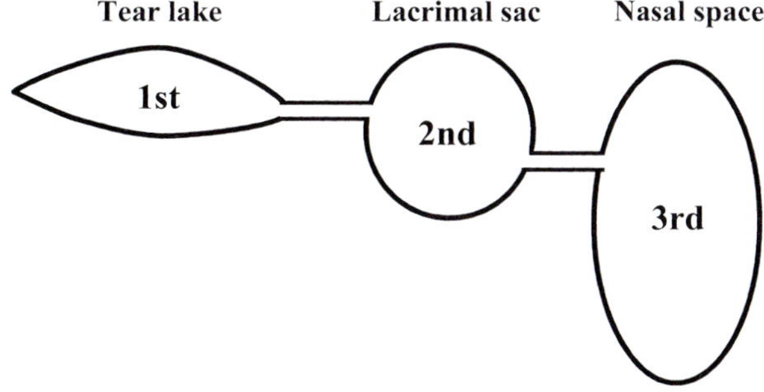

Fig. 4.3. "Three-compartment" model for lacrimal drainage dynamics, where two zones of relatively higher hydraulic resistance separate the tear lake, lacrimal sac and nasal space – namely, the canaliculi (between the first and second compartments) and the nasolacrimal duct (between the second and third compartments)

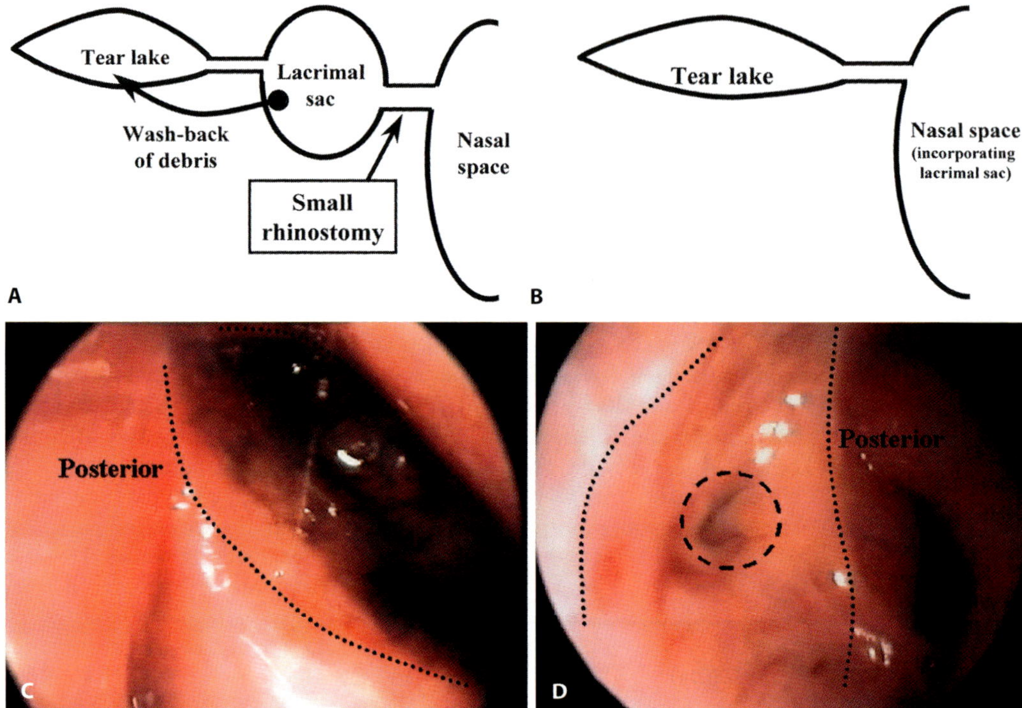

Fig. 4.4. A A small rhinostomy leads to persistent lacrimal sac (second compartment), with continued "volume" symptoms due to backwash of debris from the residual sac. **B** A correctly performed dacryocystorhinostomy eliminates the second compartment, by incorporating the lacrimal sac widely into the nasal space – thereby eliminating "volume" symptoms. **C** Intranasal endoscopic view of a widely opened left lacrimal sac after successful external dacryocystorhinostomy (*lines* indicate unions between the sac and nasal mucosae). **D** Intranasal view of right lacrimal sac after dacryocystorhinostomy, showing lines of primary intention healing of the mucosa (*dotted lines*) and the common canalicular opening (*ringed*)

that lacrimal drainage surgery creates a small anastomosis between the lacrimal sac and the nose – be this by external dacryocystorhinostomy, by the endonasal route or by reopening the nasolacrimal duct. Unfortunately, techniques based upon such ideas are liable to a relatively high failure rate (in the order of 30–50 %) due to retention of three compartments and persistent "volume" symptoms and signs (Fig. 4.4 A); persistent volume characteristics are very common in patients undergoing revisional lacrimal surgery for the "sump" syndrome [1–3]. Lacrimal drainage surgery should convert the three-compartment model into a two-compartment model, with elimination of the lacrimal sac and any possibility of "volume" symptoms (Fig. 4.4 B). The "platinum standard" for such surgery is *not* the oft-quoted "gold standard" of 95 % symptomatic cure, but rather a 100 % cure for "volume" symptoms; the patient presenting with volume symptoms should *never* get a further episode of dacryocystitis, sac retention, morning stickiness or recurrent conjunctivitis.

Flow-related symptoms are, however, dependent on a fine balance between the rate of tear production (less evaporative loss) compared with the rate of drainage – the latter being affected by several factors other than hydraulics of the drainage pathways, such as lower lid position, contour and movement. Because the resistance of the nasolacrimal duct is bypassed with an "ideal" dacryocystorhinostomy, conversion of a three-compartment system to a two-compartment one should increase the overall hydraulic conductance. Tear production in some people is, however, just too great for their canalicular conductance and these individuals will suffer persistent (albeit, probably reduced) flow symptoms. It follows, therefore, that 100% cure *cannot* be achieved for "flow" symptoms, although in most cases (where canalicular disease is absent) an outcome of over 95% is a practical reality.

A thorough understanding of the distinction between flow and volume characteristics – gained through a careful clinical history and examination – will allow an assessment of the relative proportion of symptomatology attributable to each; this judgement will, in turn, influence the informed consent for patients considering lacrimal drainage surgery. With appropriate surgery it should be possible to reassure the patient that their "volume" symptoms are totally curable, but they should be cautioned that "flow" symptoms can persist in some cases; the likelihood of continued flow symptoms will be assessed, on an individual basis, by weighing the many factors affecting tear production, evaporation and conductance.

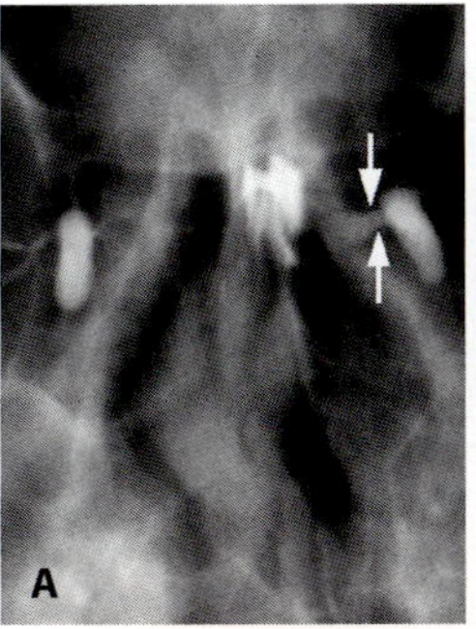

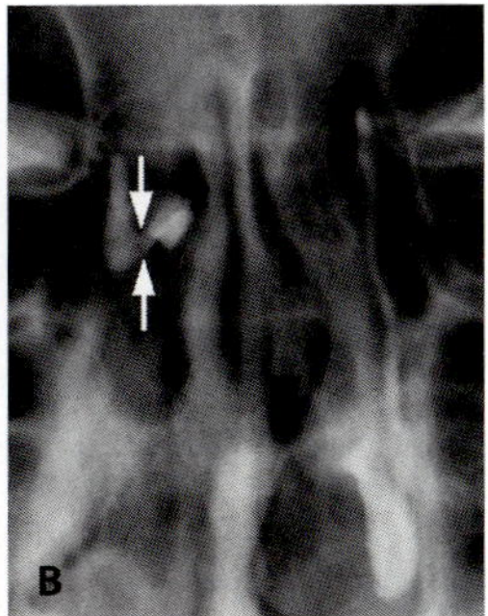

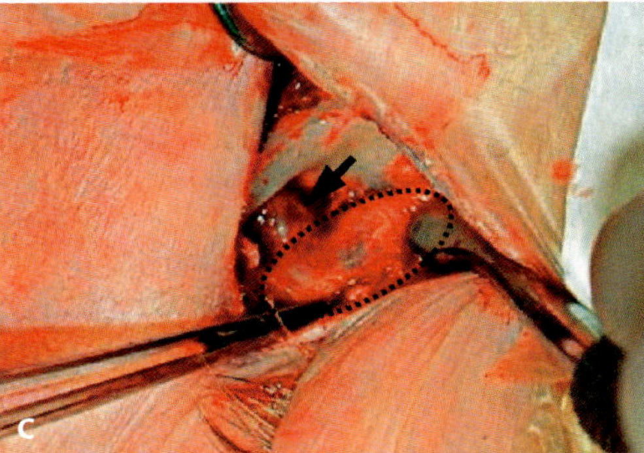

Fig. 4.5 A–C. Failure of lacrimal drainage surgery due to ring scar contracture at the site of small osteotomies (the "sump" syndrome) – with persistence of "volume" symptoms and signs in all cases: The scarred anastomosis between the residual lacrimal sac and the nose (*between arrows*) may be positioned superiorly (**A**) or, more rarely, inferiorly (**B**). **C** At the surgical revision of a failed endonasal lacrimal surgery, the small prior anastomosis is evident (*arrow*) – as is the large, unopened sac remnant (*ring*) that is giving the patient marked "volume" symptoms

4.4 Osteotomy Size and the Soft-tissue Anastomosis After Dacryocystorhinostomy

As complete cure of "volume" characteristics requires elimination of the second compartment in our hydraulic model (Fig. 4.4 B), it is *inappropriate* to regard drainage surgery as creating a small fistula between the lacrimal sac and the nose (Fig. 4.4 A): The *absolute* aim of dacryocystorhinostomy should be a wide anastomosis of the lacrimal sac into part of the lateral nasal wall (Fig. 4.4B–D), thus leaving a two-compartment model with the canaliculi as the only zone of hydraulic resistance. Unopened loculi of the lacrimal sac are a common finding at revisional lacrimal surgery [1, 2] (Fig. 4.5A–C) and these loculi can be avoided by creating a large soft-tissue anastomosis at primary dacryocystorhinostomy – ideally extending vertically from the fundus of the sac to the upper part of the nasolacrimal duct, and horizontally from nasal mucosa in front of the anterior lacrimal crest to the nasal mucosa just in front of the anterior attachment of the middle turbinate.

As would be expected due to the ring contracture of collagen maturation, most healed soft-tissue anastomoses after external DCR (with sutured mucosal flaps) are only about half of their area on the first postoperative day – this final, healed size being about 30% of the area of the original bone window [4]. An early contention that most rhinostomies contract to about 2 mm diameter after healing [5] is supported neither by ultrasonography [4] nor by endoscopic evidence (Fig. 4.4C, D), and such small anastomoses are associated with the residual second compartment of the "sump" syndrome and persistent volume characteristics (Fig. 4.5). Procedures in which only a small osteotomy is created – such as inadequate external surgery, laser dacryocystorhinostomy or balloon dacryocystoplasty – are particularly liable to having a small diameter for the final soft-tissue anastomosis. Likewise, extensive contracture of the soft-tissue anastomosis is a major problem where there is reliance on secondary intention healing with fibrosis, such as after flapless endonasal or external drainage procedures; the considerable interest in the use of anti-metabolites in lacrimal drainage surgery [6–10] tacitly acknowledging this difficulty with the fibrosis of secondary intention healing.

There is no evidence to support the belief that bone regrowth around a rhinostomy commonly leads to a reduction in the size of the osteotomy: At revisional surgery, the *original* "scalloped" edge of an osteotomy is often evident (suggesting negligible bone regrowth), and bone samples taken from the edge of such osteotomies do not show significant new bone formation – the edge of the rhinostomy being characterised mainly by a fibrous union to overlying mucosa [11]. As with other authors' experience [1, 2], most failures in this series of cases [11] were due to a small original osteotomy with a very limited soft-tissue union.

Transcanalicular procedures (laser or radiologically guided), external surgery performed without mucosal flaps, and most endonasal drainage surgeries are reliant on extensive healing by secondary intention. The body of the lacrimal sac is widely separated from nasal mucosa by about 7–10 mm of intervening anterior ethmoidal air cells, this tissue "barrier" precluding direct soft-tissue anastomosis during such procedures. This restricted access to the lacrimal sac is evident in the typical union after such "secondary intention" procedures: The soft-tissue union is narrow (due to fibrosis) and it arises from the low sac or upper duct – as the ethmoidal tissue "barrier" hampers a more direct access to the body of the sac; the anastomosis also typically passes antero-infero-medially – this being the shortest distance between the sac/duct junction and the nasal mucosa passing antero-laterally from the bulla ethmoidalis. Whilst such a limited union undoubtedly works in many cases, it leaves unopened lacrimal sac mucosa – particularly alongside the common canalicular opening – and not infrequently the persistent "second compartment" will lead these patients to seek further surgery for continued volume symptoms (Fig. 4.5 C).

Even where secondary intention healing is minimised by suturing of mucosal flaps, there is considerable contracture of the final soft-tissue anastomosis [4] and an osteotomy needs to be at least three times the area of the final union; that is, the osteotomy should be nearly twice the diameter of the anastomosis. The author routinely removes bone to about 8–10 mm in front of the anterior lacrimal crest (to create large anterior flaps), up to the level of the maxillo-frontal suture (to keep the common canalicular opening clear), inferiorly to the upper part of the lacrimal duct (to open the upper duct to the nose) and posteriorly to include an anterior ethmoidectomy. Anterior ethmoidectomy is key to optimal lacrimal surgery as it not only removes the tissue "barrier" that would otherwise prevent the wide marsupialisation of the lacrimal sac, but also allows the easy fashioning and suture of the posterior mucosal flaps.

Summary for the Clinician

- **The interpretation of lacrimal symptoms and signs should be considered in the light of a three-compartment model for lacrimal dynamics. During patient consent for any form of lacrimal intervention it is, likewise, invaluable to describe expected outcomes in terms of volume-related or flow-related symptoms**
- **Primary intention healing of a wide anastomosis between the lacrimal sac and the nose will lead to a cure of volume-related symptoms and signs in every case. Cure of flow-related symptoms is not possible in all patients**

References

1. Welham RA, Henderson PH (1973) Results of dacryocystorhinostomy – analysis of causes for failure. Trans Ophthalmol Soc UK 93:601–609
2. Welham RA, Wulc AE (1987) Management of unsuccessful lacrimal surgery. Br J Ophthalmol 71:152–157
3. Jordan JR, McDonald H (1993) Failed dacryocystorhinostomy: the sump syndrome. Ophthalmic Surg 24:692–693
4. Ezra EJ, Restori M, Mannor GE, Rose GE (1998) Ultrasonic assessment of rhinostomy size following external dacryocystorhinostomy. Br J Ophthalmol 82:786–789
5. Linberg JV, Anderson RL, Bumsted RM, Barreras R (1982) Study of intranasal ostium at external dacryocystorhinostomy. Arch Ophthalmol 100: 1758–1762
6. Zilelioglu G, Ugurbas SH, Anadolu Y, Aliner M, Akturk T (1998) Adjunctive use of mitomycin C on endoscopic lacrimal surgery. Br J Ophthalmol 82:63–66
7. Yalaz M, Firinciogullari E, Zeren H (1999) Use of mitomycin C and 5-fluorouracil in external dacryocystorhinostomy. Orbit 18:239–245
8. Liao SL, Kao SC, Tseng JH, Chen MS, Hou PK (2000) Results of intraoperative mitomycin C application in dacryocystorhinostomy. Br J Ophthalmol 84:903–906
9. Camera JG, Bengzon AU, Henson RD (2000) The safety and efficacy of mitomycin C in endonasal endoscopic laser-assisted dacryocystorhinostomy. Ophthal Plast Reconstr Surg 16:114–118
10. You YA, Fang CT (2001) Intraoperative mitomycin C in dacryocystorhinostomy. Ophthal Plast Reconstr Surg 17:115–119
11. McLean CJ, Cree I, Rose GE (1999) Rhinostomies: an open and shut case? Br J Ophthalmol 83:1300–1301

Microsurgery of the Lacrimal System: Microendoscopic Techniques

Karl-Heinz Emmerich, Hans-Werner Meyer-Rüsenberg

Core Messages

- Transcananicular endoscopy with ultrafine endoscopes has uncovered many new and previously unknown details in our understanding of lacrimal obstructions
- Combined with different tools such as the laser and drill in the simultaneous minimal invasive therapy of lacrimal obstructions, transcanicular endoscopy represents a great advance in suitable cases

5.1 Introduction

It was not possible to view the lacrimal system directly until the 1990s. In all cases of stenosis of the lacrimal system the diagnosis depended on indirect procedures. Imaging procedures such as dacryocystography with radio-opaque fluid, computer tomography, magnetic resonance tomography (MRT), high-resolution ultrasonography and radionuclide assisted procedures have been of great importance in the operative therapy of lacrimal obstructions.

In cases of mechanical obstruction of the lacrimal system, surgical therapy is almost the only way to solve the problem of permanent epiphora.

The goal of lacrimal surgery without scars led to the endonasal operation technique of internal dacryocystorhinostomy (DCR) according to West. Over the years various modifications have been developed in this field. The introduction of microscopes for endonasal surgery and flexible nasal endoscopes has considerably improved the results obtained. The combined approach of antegrade imaging and illumination of the lacrimal system with simultaneous endoscopically controlled endonasal preparation of the nasal mucosa, the bones and the lacrimal sac has achieved excellent results. To minimize the operative trauma these endonasal techniques were supplemented with the use of various lasers such as Holmium, KTP [Kalium Titanyl Phosphate] or CO_2 [1, 2, 18, 21, 22].

To be able to select a suitable operative procedure in order to eliminate lacrimal obstruction and to give an accurate prognosis, imaging is aimed at locating mechanical stenosis as precisely as possible. Operative trauma should be minimized and the benefits of the procedure can then be used optimally. The goal of being able to see pathological changes in the lacrimal passage directly led to the development of rigid and flexible endocanalicular endoscopes. The tight lumen of the canaliculi even in adults is scarcely more than 1 mm. This demands a high grade of miniaturization of the endoscopes. Thus the first endoscopes gave no satisfactory image quality and did not bring a true advance in diagnostics.

As a "spin-off" effect of the further developments in gastroduodenal endoscopes for endoscopic retrograde cholangiopancreatography (ERCP), superfine flexible endoscopes have reached a miniaturization of the diameter of down to 0.3 mm, which permits them to be used in transcanalicular diagnostics [10, 13]. The endoscopes with the smallest diameter of 0.3 mm had a possible transmission of 1,500 pixels with the resulting pictures only of fair quality. By extending the diameter up to 0.5 or 0.7 mm with a transmission of 3,000 or 6,000 pixels, a far better quality could be achieved. This was the beginning of a new phase in understanding the diseases of the lacrimal system. Direct assessment of changes of the mucosa was possible along with the detection of foreign bodies, dacryoliths and tumorous changes.

The next step was the development of miniaturized tools. Brought into the working channel as a diagnostic probe, e.g. a laser fiber, a sling or a drill could be used. In this way new procedures to eliminate lacrimal obstructions have been developed, for example, laserdacryoplasty (LDP) and microdrill dacryoplasty (MDP) [9, 12, 14, 15, 16, 17].

5.2 Dacryoendoscopy

5.2.1 Technical Equipment

5.2.1.1 Diagnostic Equipment

It was not possible to bring flexible endoscopes directly into the lacrimal system. The search to create a useful tool led to the Jünemann probe, a modified Bangerter irrigation probe with a blunt tip and a diameter of 0.8 mm. This was developed to bring a channel into the lacrimal system for intubating the system with a silicon tube. The diameter of this probe was enlarged up to 0.9 mm and a second channel for irrigation was added. The endoscope has a 70° angle view and a 0° direction view. The illumination is given by a high-power xenon cold light source connected to the camera by a TV adapter (Fig. 5.1 A).

The camera has a residual light amplification and a high shutter speed of up to 1/2,000,000 s. The endoscopically generated picture is visible on a high-performance TV monitor. During the endoscopic procedure the pictures can be recorded simultaneously through a video output and documented on an S-VHS-video recorder or more recently a DVD/CD. The quality of the documentation is, however, reduced

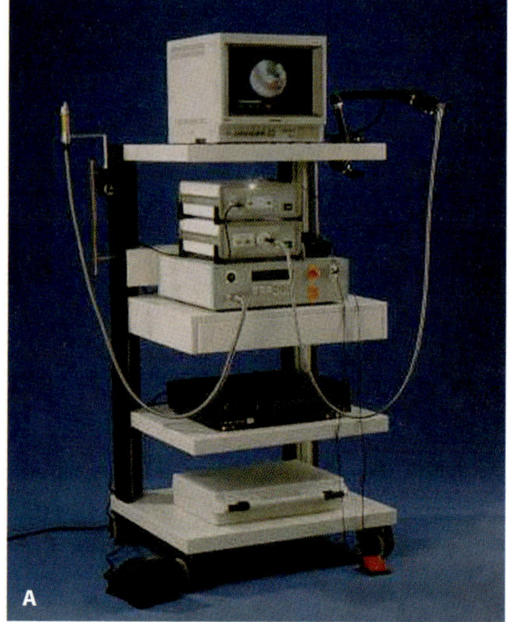

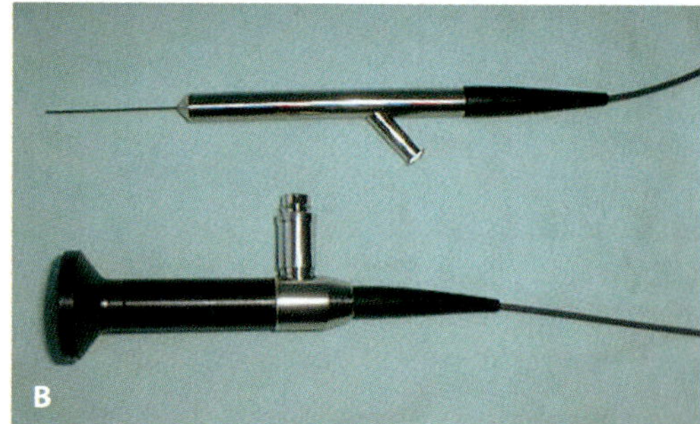

Fig. 5.1. A Endoscopic system, featuring monitor and camera, xenon light source, erbium-YAG laser and video recorder. **B** Vitroptic endoscopic system, diameter 1.0 mm

and the pictures in the text or presented by slides are of lesser quality. In spite of this, during the endoscopy the quality of the pictures is much improved.

Since the first lacrimal endoscopies, the system has had only minor changes, one change being the configuration of the endoscopes, e.g. the Vitroptic dacryoendoscope. The great advantage of this generation of endoscopes is that they (Fig. 5.1 B) do not need to be placed into the probe, for we have a fixed system. Therefore damage to the very sensitive and even expensive endoscopes can be avoided. Another step in the development of new endoscopes was the use of flexible probes as in the flexible Vitroptic dacryoendoscope. Digitalization of the picture may further improve the quality in future.

5.2.1.2
Therapeutic Equipment

First attempts at performing transcanalicular laserdacryoplasty were carried out with a holmium-YAG laser [11]. The laser probe was not connected to an endoscope. The diameter of the probe was 1.0 mm; with this laser probe a 1.0-mm cross section to the nose could be created in cases of canaliculus stenosis. The laser energy was 100 mJ and this energy was delivered by a quartz fiber.

To connect the fiber to the endoscope, the diameter of the fiber of the laser has to be very small and less than 0.4 mm. This is possible with the semiflexible fiber of a KTP laser [3]. The KTP laser is a solid body crystal laser and with an energy up to 10 W is very powerful. The released energy is sufficient for making bone holes, but the disadvantage is a certain thermal reaction with a higher scarring reaction. This technique has shown the possibility of performing transcanalicular DCR, but because of this disadvantage it has been performed only in a small number of patients and has not established itself in other lacrimal centers.

Using a modified miniaturized erbium-YAG laser developed for glaucoma surgery, a 375-μm sapphire fiber delivers the laser energy at the top of the probe up to a maximum of 50 mJ and a frequency of 1–3 Hz. The length of the used laser fiber is 10–11 cm. The erbium-YAG laser has a wavelength of 2.94 μm, a wavelength at which the maximum absorption is in water and the laser is operating photoablatively. The mucosal cells have a water content of 80 %, so the laser effect can be seen quickly. The main effect of this laser in the lacrimal passage closed by the stenosis, however, is the resulting cavitation blister and not the ablation [4]. The preparation of bone holes is not possible with the erbium-YAG laser.

The cavitation blister, which is caused by the laser impulse in the closed system, can extend over several millimeters. Punctal membranous stenosis can be opened by several impulses. The depth of penetration of the laser energy is only a few micrometers and the thermal effect is low.

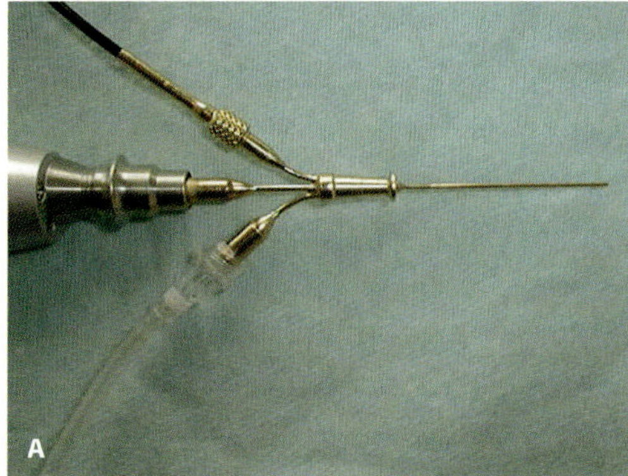

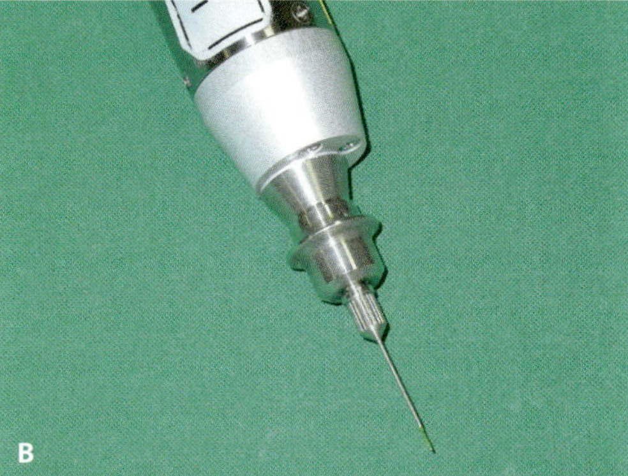

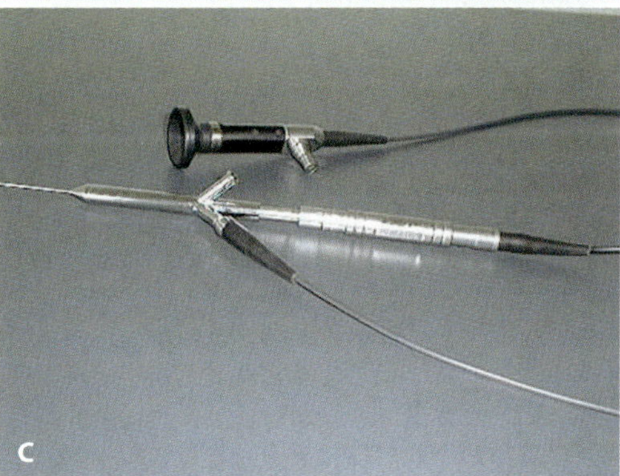

Fig. 5.2. A Three-channel probe (modified Jünemann probe), diameter 1.1 mm. **B** Four-centimeter laser probe (Sklerostom) without endoscope for treatment of canaliculus stenosis. **C** Microdrill system; three-channel probe, diameter 1.1 mm, with integrated drill

The necrosis zone is only 10–20 μm and there is no carbonization. A modification of the Jünemann probe from two to three working channels allows placement of the laser fiber (Fig. 5.2A) into the third channel and enables the laser treatment of the stenosis to be performed under endoscopic control. An additional short laser tip with a length of 4 cm has been used for the treatment of canalicular stenosis; this tip is not integrated (Fig. 5.2B) in an endoscope.

Other microendoscopic tools have been already developed, such as a sling to remove foreign bodies like dacryoliths or remains of intubation material. There is even the possibility of taking biopsies with a forceps or a brush.

5.2.2 Performing Endoscopy

In principle, performing an endoscopy in the lacrimal system is no more invasive than a deep probing of the lacrimal system. The puncta have to be dilated and it is useful to give an astringent solution some minutes before the endoscopy starts. Irrigating softly, the endoscope is inserted via the upper or lower canaliculus. The endoscope is pushed forward as far as possible, as in normal systems down to the inferior meatus, in other cases up to the point of stenosis. Unlike the endoscopies of the gastrointestinal system, the complete lacrimal passage can be judged by retracting the endoscope with simultaneous irrigation. Retracting and advancing the endoscope requires a certain amount of experience to obtain good pictures and to avoid a false passage. The learning curve is comparable to that for other endoscopic procedures such as gastroscopy, but even experienced examiners are not always able to get good pictures. In nearly every case, however, the additional information on the lacrimal system is useful.

It is possible to perform a dacryoendoscopy with anesthetizing eyedrops by irrigating the lacrimal system with 4% cocaine solution and anesthetizing the nasal city with a spray. In our experience the endoscopy is best carried out before any surgical procedure whether conventional or endoscopic. All these endoscopy procedures are performed with the patient under general anesthesia.

In children under the age of 2 years the small diameter of the lacrimal system, especially of the punctum, increases the risk of injury. Therefore, a purely diagnostic endoscopy should only be carried out in exceptional cases. Nevertheless, diseases of the lacrimal system in early childhood are mainly caused by malformations and in these cases the endoscopy cannot provide any essential additional information. Only in cases of failure following prior procedures should an endoscopy with subsequent endoscopic rechannelizing be performed to avoid a pediatric DCR [5].

5.2.2.1 Normal Findings

The endoscopic examination is concerned with observing various parts of the lacrimal system with different tissue formations such as the nasolacrimal duct, the lacrimal sac and the canaliculi. In normal findings, the canalicular mucosa appears white and smooth. The canaliculi have a narrow lumen and a homogeneous structure of the walls (Fig. 5.3A). The mucosa of the lacrimal sac is reddish, the lumen is wide and the wall is structured by flat folds (Fig. 5.3B). During endoscopy, the production of mucus can soon be seen. After touching the mucosa, a small amount of bleeding on the surface can be noted. The transition from the canaliculi to the lacrimal sac shows the Rosenmüller fold. This is like a border between different histological structures. Between the lacrimal sac and the nasolacrimal duct, the Krause fold can be seen. The lumen in the nasolacrimal duct is narrow and shows no folds. The structure of the surface is reddish as in the lacrimal sac. Polyps in the lacrimal sac can be identified (Fig. 5.4B). The nasal cavity is noticeable as an intensely red structure with a smooth surface and an enormous space (Fig. 5.3C) [20].

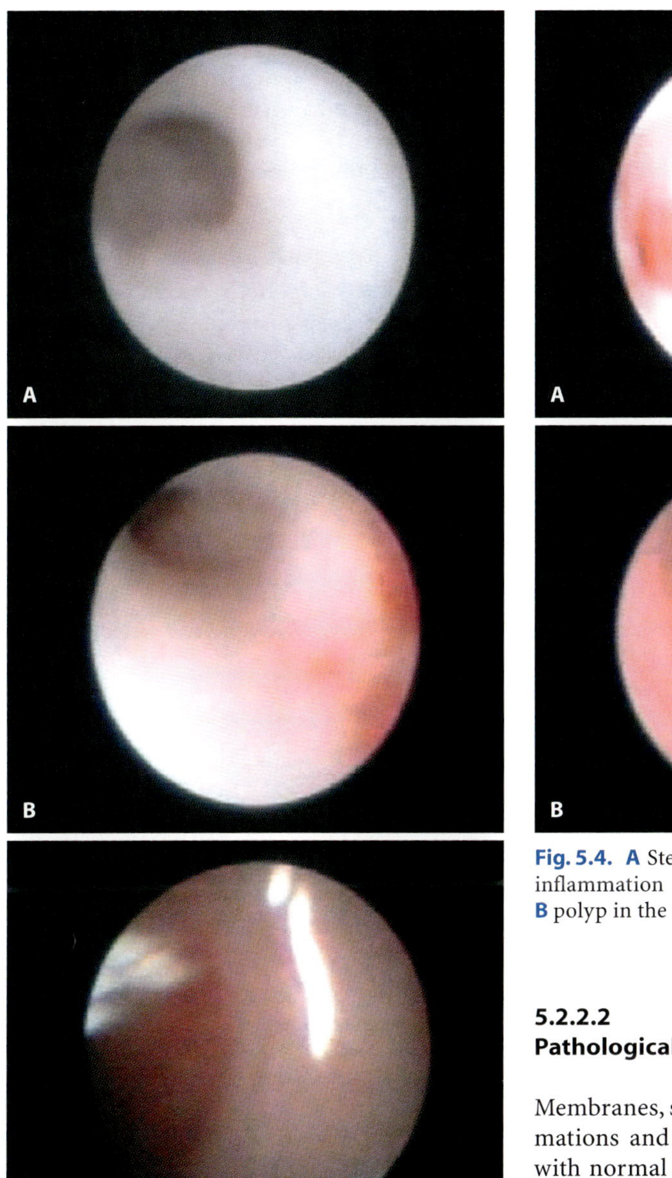

Fig. 5.3. A Normal finding of a canaliculus; **B** normal finding of a small lacrimal sac, small blendings on the surface; **C** normal finding of a nasal cavity with a red, smooth surface

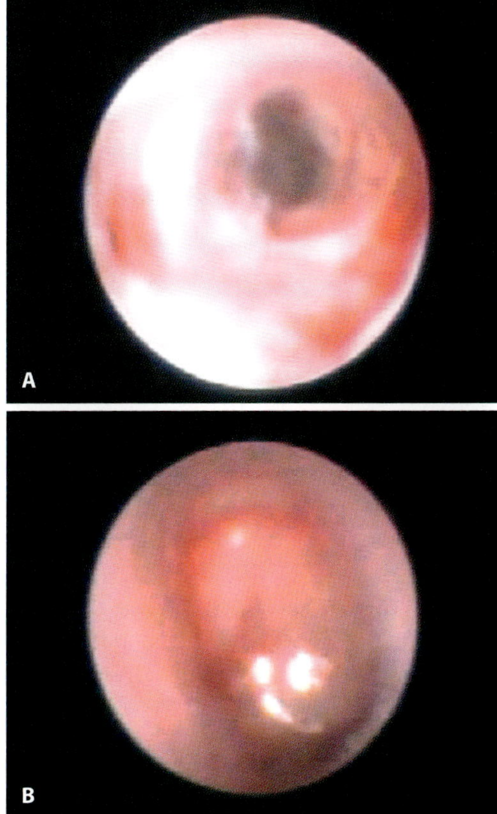

Fig. 5.4. A Stenosis of the lacrimal sac with chronic inflammation and submucosal scar formation; **B** polyp in the lacrimal sac

5.2.2.2 Pathological Findings

Membranes, surface scars, submucosal scar formations and foreign bodies can be compared with normal findings. Membranes can be seen in cases of chronic inflammations and are possible reasons for a subtotal closure of the lacrimal system, especially at the point of the preexisting valve of Rosenmüller and (Fig. 5.4 A) Krause. A submucosal scar formation is characteristic of chronic inflammations with shrinking of the lacrimal sac. Polyps in the lacrimal sac can be identified (Fig. 5.4 B). Remains of intubation material are a common reason for relapses and can easily be identified. The difference between acute and chronic mucosal inflammation can easily be seen, and depending on the findings of the endoscopy a suitable operative procedure can be selected.

5.2.3 Transcanalicular Endoscopic Procedures

The goal of lacrimal surgery without scars led to the development of internal DCR according to West a long time ago [6]. Many modifications have been developed in this field over the years [7, 19]. A great step forward was the introduction of microscopes for endonasal surgery and of flexible nasal endoscopes [8]. New possibilities resulted from the combined approach of antegrade transcanalicular illumination by cold light sources developed for pars plana vitrectomy and the endonasal endoscopic techniques. Excellent results were achieved with the preparation of nasal mucosa, the bones and the lacrimal sac. Some of these endonasal techniques were supplemented by the use of diverse lasers such as the Holmium-YAG laser, the KTP laser and the CO_2 laser [9].

With new possibilities created by the use of transcanalicular endoscopes, some groups have tried to combine the diagnostic advantages with reconstructive techniques. The concern regarding the laser was that the fiber had to be small enough to fit in the small working channel with a maximum diameter of 0.4 mm. The ideal laser should be powerful enough to create bone holes, but on the other hand the laser should not cause scarring.

With regard to the diameter of the laser fiber, the erbium-YAG laser is ideal with a fiber diameter of 375 µm. The laser has a wavelength of 2.94 µm, and as the maximum absorption is in water, the scar reaction is minimal. The only disadvantage of the erbium-YAG laser is that the maximum energy of 60 W is not able to create a bony ostium. But this energy, combined with the blister resulting in the cavitation effect, is sufficient to open membranes, which are the main cause of what clinically appears as a complete stenosis of the lacrimal system. Therefore the erbium-YAG laser made it possible to treat a high number of lacrimal stenoses by transcanalicular endoscopy [10].

5.2.3.1 Laserdacryoplasty

First attempts to rechannel a closed lacrimal system by use of a laser have been reported using a holmium-YAG laser [11]. The term “canaliculoplasty” was used for this procedure. After the introduction of transcanalicular endoscopes [12], rechannelizing of the lacrimal system was possible under endoscopic control and the term “laserdacryoplasty” was used for this procedure [14, 15].

With regard to the diameter of the laser fiber, endoscopically controlled rechannelizing by a laser system is possible. The Erbium-YAG laser has the laser energy delivered by a sapphire fiber with a diameter of 375 µm. The glass fiber of a KTP laser is similar. In our experience we first started trying to perform a transcanalicular DCR with the erbium-YAG laser but had to learn that the laser energy was not powerful enough to get through bone to the nose. Nevertheless the laser was useful enough to open closed membranes and in this way to open a blocked lacrimal system. For this procedure the term “laserdacryoplasty” was used.

Erbium-YAG Laserdacryoplasty

A modified miniaturized erbium-YAG laser developed for glaucoma surgery has been in use since 1996 and delivers the laser energy by a sapphire fiber. In different parts the laser energy depends on the width of the laser fiber and with the used sapphire fiber of 375 µm an energy of 50 mJ with 1–3 Hz can be delivered at the top of the fiber. The absorption maximum of the erbium-YAG laser is in water and the laser works photoablatively. The mucosal cells of the transitional epithelium of the lacrimal sac have a water content of nearly 80 %, so the ablation results quickly. But there is not only the ablative effect: depending on the complete closure of the lacrimal system after the introduction of the endoscopic probe, a cavitation blister results and the edges of membranes and folds, which stick together, can be opened by the laser effect. The blister can extend over several millimeters and in this way punctal membranous stenosis can be opened with just a few pulses. In many cases

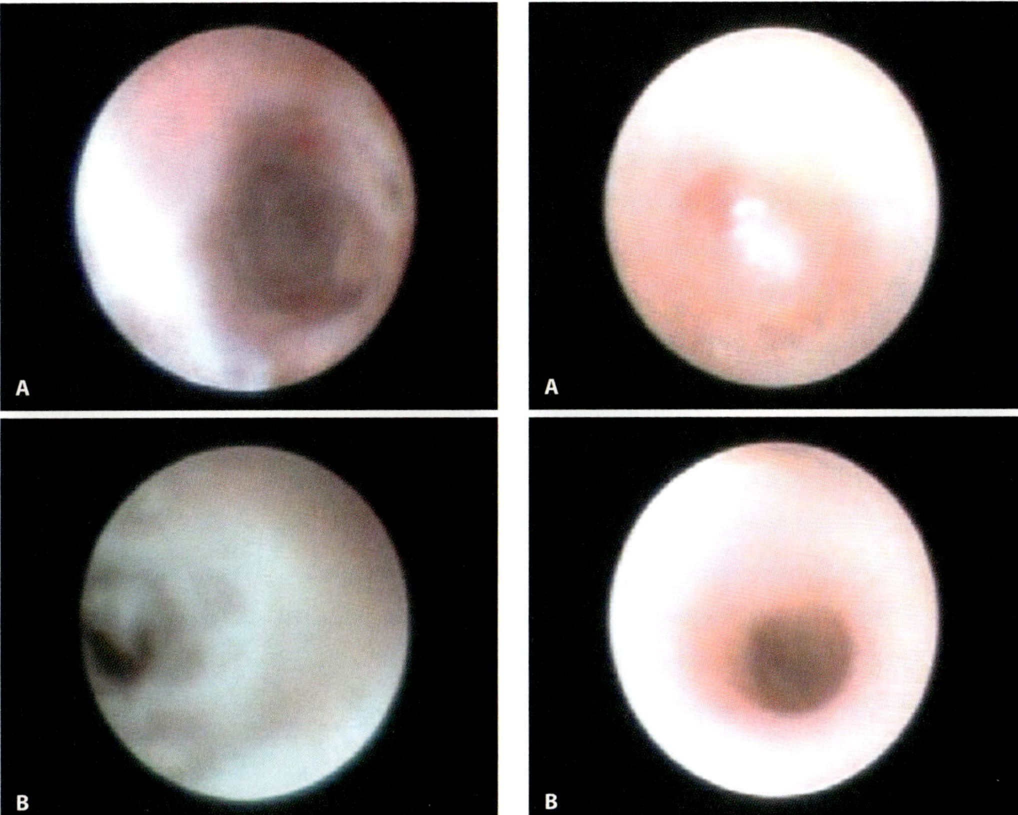

Fig. 5.5. A Complete stenosis at the end of the lacrimal sac; **B** same patient after recanalization by LDP

Fig. 5.6. A Complete stenosis of a canaliculus; **B** same patient after LDP recanalization

the energy is powerful enough to open these membranous stenoses, but not too strong to make a false passage.

Initially, a diagnostic endoscopy is performed to check the indication for surgery. With complete stenosis of the lacrimal system without a mucocele there is an indication for laser dacryoplasty. The laser fiber is brought into an endoscope with a third working channel and the laser can be applied. After several laser impulses, free irrigation can be noted. Irrigation is now possible without the former (Fig. 5.5 A, B) resistance and the endoscopic picture confirms the opening. After opening the obstruction, bicanalicular intubation using a silicon tube with a diameter of 0.64 mm is carried out to prevent postoperative adhesions of the mucosa. The tubing remains in place usually for 3 months and is removed transcanalicularly. If there is no possibility of bicanalicular intubation, then a monocanalicular stent is used according to Bernard and Fayet [23]. This Monoka intubation remains in place for at least 6 weeks. The postoperative therapy is the same as that following bicanalicular intubation, which is performed easily in the clinical setting without general anesthesia.

Using this method, the success rate of LDP related to the indicating symptom epiphora is 60–70% with a postoperative follow-up period of 20.4 months. As regards the canalicular stenosis only, the success rate is 67% and rises to 86% for isolated common canaliculus stenosis [16] (Fig. 5.6 A, B). These LDP results in treatment of canalicular stenosis are better than those following other microsurgical procedures even in the hands of experienced surgeons.

A laserdacryoplasty is possible in cases of canalicular stenosis and high or deep intrasaccal lesions. The known anatomical folds seem to be the predilection points for adhesion of the folds, causing the closure in the lacrimal system typically 10–11 mm or 18–20 mm behind the punctum. In addition, membranous occlusions following a failed DCR can be treated successfully by laserdacryoplasty. Today laserdacryoplasty is mostly performed in cases of canalicular stenosis and in saccal stenosis with only chronic and not acute inflammation with only a slightly enlarged diameter. Laserdacryoplasty is not useful in cases of acute dacryocystitis, mucoceles, or widespread adhesions following viral infections such as herpes or lacrimal stenosis caused by bone displacement after midface fractures.

5.2.3.2 Microdrill Dacryoplasty

Immediately after the introduction of transcanalicular dacryloplasty with the erbium-YAG laser, Busse had the idea of introducing another tool into the third channel of the endoscope, namely a miniaturized drill [10, 17]. The concept was to construct a microdrill for transcanalicular manipulation. The microdrill consisted of a stainless steel probe 0.3 mm in diameter which was driven by a battery-operated motor and a drill shaft. The frequency of the drill was 50 Hz. The drill was powered by a foot pedal and connected to a Vitroptic T, which is an endoscopic system where the endoscope has already been installed into the probe.

MDP Procedure

The technique of microdrill dacryoplasty is similar to that of laser dacryoplasty. Initially a diagnostic endoscopy is performed to check the indication. The drill is not powerful enough to create bone holes to perform a direct anastomo-

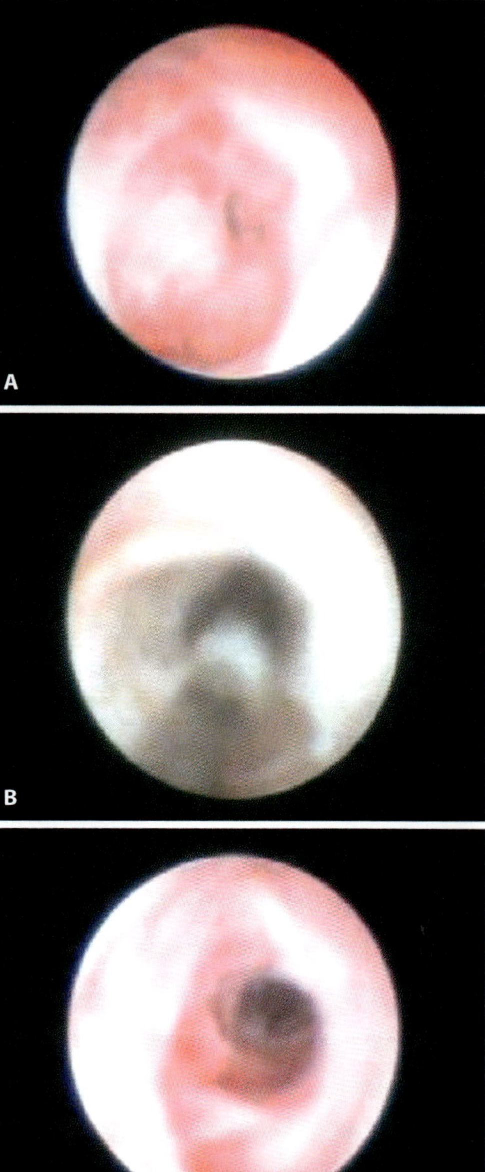

Fig. 5.7. **A** Subtotal stenosis of the lacrimal sac with a small central opening; **B** recanalization by MDP, tip of the drill from 7 to central; **C** same patient after recanalization

sis between the lacrimal system and the nasal cavity. However, in many cases a clinically completely closed system appears endoscopically not to be completely closed and shows a buttonhole like closure with a partial lumen (Fig. 5.7 A). In such cases a complete opening of the system is possible and can be performed by microdrill dacryloplasty.

The first step in performing a microdrill dacryoplasty is dilation of the upper or lower punctum in order to insert the Vitroptic T into the lacrimal system. The diameter of the system is 1.1 mm so that the procedure is possible even in children of 2 years or older. Under endoscopic control, the microdrill is brought up to the location of the stenosis and pulled forward in front of the optics (Fig. 5.7 B). A continuous irrigation is required in order to prevent lacerations and to control the success of the procedure. After removing all the obstructions, success is again assessed by irrigation under endoscopic control (Fig. 5.7 C). It is possible to compare the irrigation resistance by a special manometer. The postoperative regimen is the same as after laser dacryoplasty with bicanalicular intubation when possible and standard postoperative medical treatment.

MDP Results

According to the indications above, the success rate for microdrill dacryoplasty is even better than that for the other transcanalicular endoscopic procedures for laser dacryoplasty. Indications for performing a microdrill dacryoplasty are removal of membranes or fragmentation and removal of dacryoliths. The microdrill dacryoplasty is particularly useful in the type of stenosis which has been first described by transcanalicular endoscopic findings as the "button-hole stenosis".

Some types of lacrimal obstruction demonstrate a complete obstruction in irrigation and even a complete cessation on X-ray findings. Nevertheless, by performing endoscopy, a tight lumen at the end of the lacrimal sac located at the region of the Krause fold about 18–20 mm behind the punctum, styled like a buttonhole, can often be seen. In these cases in particular the obstruction can be removed with the microdrill performing a kind of mucosa curettage and enlarging the tight lumen. Increased resistance during initial irrigation shows an immediate decrease after a successful microdrill application. According to this model, the microdrill is not suitable for the treatment of complete stenoses, and especially for canalicular stenoses where the rotation of the drill might cause further damage in the soft tissues.

In a long term study with a minimal postoperative follow-up period of more than 12 months, the success rate is almost 78 % in reducing the symptom of epiphora.

Summary for the Clinician

- **Transcanicular endoscopy has uncovered many new and exciting details in our understanding of lacrimal obstruction**
- **Successful treatment of lacrimal obstruction with the laser or drill under endoscopic control is possible in many cases and has reduced the rate of DCR**
- **The success rate after laser dacryoplasty and microdrill dacryoplasty of about 80 % with a low rate of possible complications seems very reasonable for a first-step procedure**

5.3 Conclusions

Transcanalicular endoscopy with the new endoscopes has been useful in providing much new information about the anatomy of the lacrimal drainage pathways and the causes of lacrimal obstructions. Combining different tools for the simultaneous minimal invasive therapy of lacrimal obstructions, transcanalicular endoscopy is a great step forward in the treatment of lacrimal obstructions. It has reduced the rate of DCR which otherwise would have been necessary to be performed on our patients. Even if the success rate after laser dacryoplasty and microdrill dacryoplasty is no higher than 80 %, this rate is very reasonable for a minimally invasive first-step procedure with a low rate of possible complications.

Lacrimal endoscopy has provided new insights into the pathology of the diseases of obstruction and the morphology of the lacrimal system. With endoscopy we can see and decide at once what to do and are able to perform minimally invasive therapy with the best results for the patient. In the past only clinical impression and indirect imaging gave suggestions to what was possible, and in many cases the surgeon was surprised but not amused during surgery. Minimally invasive therapy with laser or drill is a great advance in the management of the problems of nasocrimal outflow disorders.

References

1. Bartley GB (1994) The pros and cons of laser dacrycystorhinostomy. Am J Ophthalmol 117:103–106
2. Emmerich KH, Busse H, Meyer-Rüsenberg HW, Hörstensmeyer CG (1997) External dacryocystorhinostomy: indications, method, complications and results. Orbit 16:25–29
3. Müllner K, Wolf G, Luxenberg W, Hofmann T (2001) Laser assistierte transkanalikuläre Dakryozystorhinostomie. Ophthalmologe 98:174–177
4. Mrochen M, Riedel P, Donitzky C, Seiler T (2001) Zur Entstehung von Kavitationsblasen bei der Erbium-YAG-Laser-Vitrektomie. Ophthalmologe 98:163–167
5. Emmerich KH, Meyer-Rüsenberg HW (2002) Erkrankungen der ableitenden Tränenwege im Kindesalter. Z Prakt Augenheilkd 23:19–27
6. West JM (1914) A window resection of the nasal duct in cases of stenosis. Trans Am Ophthalmol Soc 12:654
7. Berryhill BH (1982) Twenty years experience with intranasal transseptal dacryocystorhinostomy. Laryngoscopy 92:379–381
8. Lindberg JV, Anderson RL, Bumsted RM, Barreres R (1982) Study of intranasal ostium external dacryocystorhinostomy. Arch Ophthalmol 100: 1758–1762
9. Gonnering RS, Lyon DB, Fisher JC (1991) Endoscopic laser-assisted lacrimal surgery. Am J Ophthalmol 111:152–157
10. Emmerich KH, Meyer-Rüsenberg HW (2001) Endoskopische Tränenwegschirurgie. Ophthalmo loge 98:607–612
11. Dutton JJ, Holck DE (1996) Holmium laser canaliculoplasty. Ophthal Plast Reconstr Surg 12: 211–217
12. Kuchar A, Novak P, Pieh S, Fink M, Steinkogler FJ (1999) Endoscopic laser recanalisation of presaccal canalicular obstruction. Br J Ophthalmol 83:443–447
13. Kuchar A, Novak P, Ofuoglu A, Steinkogler FJ (1995) Die Endoskopie der ableitenden Tränenwege. Spektrum Augenheilkd 9:187–189
14. Emmerich KH, Lüchtenberg M, Meyer-Rüsenberg HW, Steinhauer J (1997) Dakryoendoskopie and Laserdakryoplastik: Technik und Ergebnisse. Klin Monatsbl Augenheilkd 211:375–379
15. Meyer-Rüsenberg HW, Emmerich KH, Lüchtenberg M, Steinhauer J (1999) Endoskopische Laserdakryoplastik. Methodik und Ergebnisse nach drei Monaten. Ophthalmologe 96:332–334
16. Steinhauer J, Norda A, Emmerich KH, Meyer-Rüsenberg HW (2000) Laserkanalikuloplastik. Ophthalmologe 97:692–695
17. Emmerich KH, Ungerechts R, Meyer-Rüsenberg HW (2000) Possibilities and limits of minimal invasive lacrimal surgery. Orbit 19:67–71
18. Caldwell GW (1893) A new operation for the radical cure of obstruction of the nasal duct. N Y Med J 58:476
19. Busse H, Hollwich F (1977) Kurz- und Langzeitergebnisse dacryocystorhinostomia externa nach Kaleff-Hollwich. Klin Monatsbl Augenheilkd 171: 986–989
20. Jünemann G, Schulte D (1975) Ursachen und Therapie der Stenosen der abführenden Tränenwege des Erwachsenen. In: Meyer-Schwickerath G, Ullrich (eds) Moderne Probleme der Erkrankungen der Lider und des Tränenapparates, 1st edn. Enke, Stuttgart, pp 243–264
21. Massaro BM, Gonnering RS, Harris GJ (1990) Endonasal laser dacryocystorhinostomy. A new approach to nasolacrimal obstruction. Arch Ophthalmol 108:1172–1176
22. Welham RA, Wulc AE (1987) Management of unsuccessful lacrimal surgery. Br J Ophthalmol 71: 152–157
23. Fayet B, Assouline M, Bernard JA (1998) Monocanalicular nasolacrimal duct intubation. Ophthalmology 105:1795–1796

Techniques in Endonasal Dacryocystorhinostomy

6

PETER J. DOLMAN

Core Messages

- The endonasal approach for dacryocystorhinostomy has received increasing attention over the past 20 years, with recently reported success rates rivalling or surpassing the "gold standard" external approach
- Potential advantages of the endonasal approach include reduced surgical time, no cutaneous scar or wound complications, no disruption to the medial canthal ligaments, and examination of the intranasal anatomy with each surgery
- Although early endonasal techniques used expensive technology such as lasers and video-endoscopes, excellent outcomes may be achieved using a nasal speculum and surgical loupes and simple surgical instruments
- Complications of both the external and endonasal dacryocystorhinostomy include surgical failures, epistaxis, cerebrospinal fluid leakage, and stent malfunctions. Complications more likely to occur with the endonasal approach include orbital injuries resulting from disruption to the periorbita

6.1 Introduction

The traditional procedure for acquired nasolacrimal duct obstruction is the dacryocystorhinostomy (DCR), in which an opening is created through the mucosal and bony layers separating the lacrimal sac and nasal cavity. The standard approach for the past century has been the external or transcutaneous route [1], with success rates reported between 80% and 95% [2, 3]. In the past two decades, there has been increasing interest in endonasal approaches [4, 5], with recent reports of similar success rates to the external route [6, 7]. The following chapter outlines perioperative techniques, outcomes and complications in the endonasal DCR (EN-DCR).

6.2 History

The external DCR (EX-DCR) was first described by Toti in 1904 with creation of an ostium between the lacrimal sac and nose [1]. This technique was refined by Dupuy-Dutemps and Bourguet 16 years later with the introduction of mucosal flaps to line the ostium with epithelium [8]. Although some variations have been described over the years, including changing the orientation of the incision [9], eliminating one or both mucosal flaps [10], and inserting various stents [11], the procedure has remained essentially unchanged, no doubt because of its favorable results of better than 90% success in reducing epiphora.

The idea of performing the same surgery from an endonasal route was described prior to the external route by Caldwell in 1893 [12], but fell out of favor because of difficulty using instrumentation within the nasal cavity and because of uncertainty of where the opening should be made to gain access into the lacrimal sac – a misplaced ostium could damage orbital or intracranial structures. The development of rigid nasal endoscopes and fine nasal surgical equipment for endoscopic sinus surgery in the 1970s [4], and the idea of placing a vitrectomy light pipe through the canaliculus into the lacrimal sac to act as a transillumination target in 1990 [5], resolved some of these difficulties and rekindled interest in an endonasal approach for DCRs. Over the past 20 years, there have been increasing reports in both ophthalmic and otolaryngology literature of different techniques for EN-DCRs [13–15], with recent reports of success rates rivalling the "gold standard" external approach [6, 7, 16–18]. The additional benefits for the patient of reduced surgical time [6], no cutaneous scar or wound complications, no disruption to the medial canthal ligaments and examination of the intranasal anatomy with each surgery, furthers the appeal of this approach.

6.3 Preoperative Considerations

6.3.1 Clinical Assessment of Epiphora

The standard clinical work-up for patients referred with epiphora or dacryocystitis includes a careful history, assessment of the eyelids, tear film and lacrimal drainage apparatus, and occasionally ancillary testing.

Increased lacrimation from irritative sources such as dry eyes, blepharitis, trichiasis, topical medications or exposure should be excluded. Eyelid malpositions (horizontal laxity, ectropion or entropion) and punctal abnormalities (eversion, stenosis or conjunctival overlay) can be identified and corrected surgically.

The height of the tear meniscus stained with fluorescein helps distinguish a dry eye from an excessively moist eye. The dye disappearance test with an asymmetrically high tear meniscus is particularly helpful in confirming unilateral outflow obstruction.

Anatomic testing of the lacrimal outflow tract primarily consists of irrigating through the canaliculi. Patency is confirmed by free flow of the irrigant into the nose while partial obstruction is confirmed by partial reflux of fluid through the opposite canaliculus. A complete obstruction of the nasolacrimal duct or common canaliculus is proven by complete reflux of irrigant through the opposite canaliculus. Mucus or pus may suggest acute or chronic dacryocystitis. Reflux of fluid back from the same canaliculus, often accompanied by discomfort, suggests a canalicular obstruction. The position of this obstruction along the canaliculus may be identified by measuring the point of a soft-stop on probing.

Functional testing of the lacrimal outflow tract is helpful when an anatomic blockage cannot be identified. An upper system failure may be proven by the inability of fluorescein dye instilled in the inferior cul-de-sac to reach the punctum spontaneously. A functional obstruction in the nasolacrimal duct may be suspected if dye can be seen in the punctum but cannot be detected under the inferior turbinate with a cotton tipped applicator (Jones I test).

Dacryocystography may be useful to confirm dacryoliths or diverticuli. CT scans are helpful when the clinical examination raises the possibility of neoplasms (nasal discharge, epistaxis, bloody tears or a lacrimal sac mass extending above the medial canthus) or to assess the bony and sinus anatomy in cases of previous trauma, surgery or reconstruction in the region of the lacrimal sac and duct. Dacryoscintigraphy may help support a diagnosis of functional outflow blockage when an anatomic cause for epiphora cannot be established.

6.3.2 Indications for Surgery

Indications for either external or endonasal DCRs include nasolacrimal duct and common canalicular obstructions with epiphora, dacryocystitis or symptomatic dacryoliths. Conjunctival DCRs with Jones tube placement can be performed from either the external or endonasal approach and are typically reserved for canalicular obstructions that are too extensive to be repaired with a lacrimal microtrephine or direct reconstruction, and occasionally for cases of bothersome epiphora related to facial nerve palsy refractory to lower eyelid horizontal tightening.

The external DCR should be chosen over the endonasal approach in cases of trauma with medial canthal avulsion where medial canthal reconstruction is planned or where lacerations already expose the lacrimal sac region. The external approach is preferred for suspected lacrimal sac diverticuli or lacrimal sac malignancies where biopsy or removal of the lacrimal sac or duct is planned. In my experience, patients with Down's syndrome have a very thick, flat plate of bone between the lacrimal sac and nose, often making the endonasal approach challenging, and an external route should be considered in these individuals.

6.3.3 Special Considerations in Endonasal DCRs

An assessment of the nasal cavity in the office preoperatively using a nasal speculum and headlight or endoscope may identify anatomic variations such as septal deviations or prominent middle turbinates that might require surgical correction to allow visualization or placement of instrumentation, or alternatively steer the surgeon to choose an external route [7].

Pathology such as allergic rhinitis, mucosal necrotizing vasculitis, nasal polyps or neoplasia may also be identified during this preoperative nasal inspection.

6.4 Perioperative Considerations

6.4.1 Hemostasis

A common worry of ophthalmologists regarding DCR surgery is control of bleeding. This is a particular concern for the endonasal approach where even a small amount of blood can make visualization troublesome.

A careful enquiry about anticoagulant medications allows these to be discontinued with the approval of the patient's primary care physician, cardiologist or neurologist. Coumadin should be stopped 3 days prior to surgery and prothrombin times (PT) checked on the morning of surgery. Non-steroidal anti-inflammatories, vitamin C and E, *Ginkgo biloba* and other herbal remedies with anticoagulant properties should be discontinued 1 week before surgery. Aspirin products should be discontinued 2 weeks prior to surgery if possible because of the longer duration of anti-platelet activity.

Injection of the nasal mucosa on the lateral wall anterior to the middle turbinate and injection of the anterior tip of the middle turbinate with lidocaine with 1/100,000 adrenaline significantly helps hemostasis for both external and endonasal DCRs. Cotton neuropaddies or strip gauze soaked in cocaine 4% can be placed in the middle meatus between the middle turbinate and lateral wall surgical site to decongest the nasal mucosa, inwardly displace the turbinate, and improve visualization as well as reduce bleeding.

The combination of adrenaline and cocaine should be avoided if the anesthetist feels the synergistic effect on blood pressure or heart rate might endanger the patient. The anesthetist also may help hemostasis intraoperatively by maintaining a low blood pressure [6].

During the procedure, the surgeon must avoid unnecessary trauma to the nasal mucosa distant from the site injected with adrenaline. Specifically, the instruments should not be dragged or pushed against the nasal mucosa, and the mucosa should be pulled towards the center of the ostium during its removal, rather than ripping forward, which might cause a tear into the surrounding, non-adrenalinated tissue.

6.4.2 Anesthesia

With good hemostasis, local anesthesia is possible for endonasal DCRs. This consists of infratrochlear and infraorbital blocks using lidocaine 1–2% with 1/100,000 adrenaline and monitored sedation. The lidocaine injection directly into the nasal mucosa over the planned osteotomy site and the intranasal cocaine packing provides anesthesia for the inside of the nose. For nervous patients, those for whom communication may be difficult, and for surgeons first learning the technique, general anesthesia is usually preferable.

6.4.3 Antibiotics

Oral cefazolin may be administered for patients with dacryocystitis, particularly if complicated by cellulitis. A culture of the sac contents for antibiotic sensitivities can be obtained by needle aspirate preoperatively or during the surgery. For non-infected cases of dacryostenosis, I do not advocate perioperative antibiotic coverage for endonasal DCRs. Although some surgeons have reported wound infection rates as high as 15% following external DCRs [19], I have not seen any cases of cellulitis or nasal infection following an endonasal DCR.

6.4.4 Set-up

While many surgeons may prefer a sterile set-up for endonasal DCRs, I perform these with a clean set-up, using surgical gloves, sterile instruments, and a sterile fenestrated face drape, but without prepping the skin or gowning.

6.5 Operative Techniques

6.5.1 Illumination Source

In 1990, Massaro et al. introduced the idea of threading a vitrectomy light pipe through the upper canaliculus into the lacrimal sac and viewing the transillumination target through the thin lacrimal bone within the nose [5]. Although others had described placing lacrimal probes through the sac wall to identify its location in the nose [7], the light pipe allows visualization without pushing into the nose, and provides sufficient illumination that no additional light is necessary if viewing directly with surgical loupes or an operating microscope.

Care must be taken not to injure the canalicular wall with the sharp edges of the vitrectomy light pipe – this is best achieved by pulling the eyelid laterally as the light pipe is advanced into the sac and ensuring that the tip of the pipe rests against the medial wall of the sac throughout the procedure.

The pipe may be plugged into a vitrectomy light source or into a standard headlamp light source fitted with an adaptor to fit the light pipe connector. Another possibility is to wrap sufficient surgical tape around the light pipe connector so that it fits snugly into one of the headlamp light ports.

Rarely the tip of the light pipe may be caught and crushed in the teeth of the rongeurs during bone removal – the damaged pipe can be withdrawn, the bent tip cut off with a strong pair of scissors and the light pipe repositioned within the sac.

6.5.2 Viewing Systems

Methods of visualization for the endonasal DCR include endoscopy, operating microscope or surgical loupes.

Many surgeons advocate the use of a video-endoscope, which provides a magnified view, allows video-documentation and facilitates teaching [4, 20, 21]. The 30-degree angled rigid endoscope is usually favored for endonasal DCR as it allows a view around prominent bony ridges or swollen mucosal tissues. Endoscopy is a learned skill and video-endoscopes may be unavailable in some hospitals.

The operating microscope using a 250-mm-focal-length lens provides excellent magnification but limited depth of field and relatively poor maneuverability.

Direct visualization of the osteotomy site using surgical loupes and a 5-cm-long nasal speculum provides an excellent view without any expensive equipment and with a shorter set-up time, and makes the technique considerably more affordable and portable [6]. The view is facilitated if the surgeon sits at the patient's head opposite to the side being operated on. The surgeon does not need to use a headlight as sufficient illumination is provided by the light pipe within the canaliculus.

6.5.3 Formation of the Osteotomy

The classic approach for an external DCR creates a large bony window including the lacrimal bone and the anterior lacrimal crest of the maxilla, and sutures anterior and posterior lacrimal sac and nasal mucosal flaps [8]. More recently, surgeons have reported equivalent surgical success rates even if they eliminated the posterior flaps or if they completely resected the nasal mucosa and sutured the anterior lacrimal sac flap to the periosteum at the anterior lip of the osteotomy [6]. In 1982, Linberg observed that the healed ostium was often much smaller than the original surgical passage and that even small healed ostia could have excellent functional outcomes [22].

Initially, investigators of the endonasal DCR tried a variety of lasers with different wavelengths to burn the mucosa and thin the bone, including the argon blue-green, Nd:YAG, carbon dioxide, KTP-YAG, and holmium:YAG lasers [5, 13, 23, 24]. These lasers are expensive, involve significant set-up time, and require extensive safety precautions. In addition, they are unable to remove the thicker anterior and superior bone of the internal maxillary ridge and may cause thermal damage to the delicate mucosal structures with char formation and poorer surgical outcomes [23].

Some clinicians continue to investigate an endocanalicular approach, using a Nd:YAG laser placed through the canaliculus with the laser energy directed towards the inside of the nose [25]. Advocates note a short operation time, ease of the procedure and lack of instrumentation required inside the nose, but the procedure has not gained much popularity, perhaps because of the potential for canalicular thermal damage and the small ostium size created.

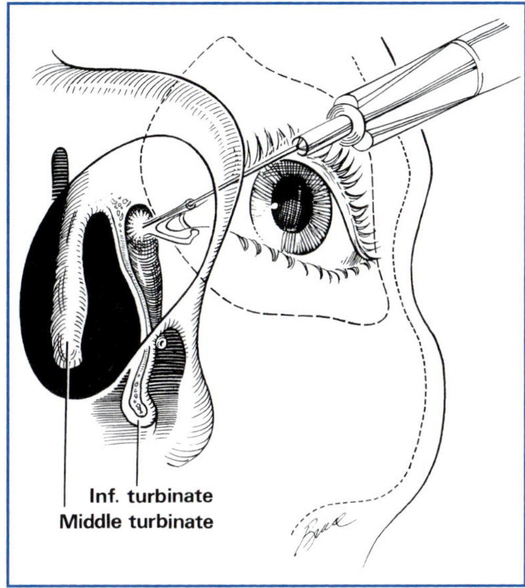

Fig. 6.1. Endonasal view during non-laser EN-DCR. The retinal light pipe is held horizontally in the upper canaliculus against the medial wall of the lacrimal sac, creating a transillumination target on the lateral wall of the nose temporal to the anterior aspect of middle turbinate. The middle turbinate has been medially displaced in this illustration and is often thicker prior to decongestion by cocaine packing. Figures 6.1–6.4 are reprinted with permission from: Dolman PJ (2003) Comparison of external dacryocystorhinostomy with non-laser endonasal dacryocystorhinostomy. *Ophthalmology* 110:78–84

A recent trend has been the use of a non-laser or mechanical approach for endonasal DCR, using simpler surgical instruments, bone microdrills or electric cautery devices, and avoiding the expensive lasers [6, 15, 26, 27].

My preferred approach uses minimal instrumentation, readily available in most operating room facilities. The 20-gauge disposable vitrectomy light pipe is placed through the upper canaliculus until it touches the bony medial wall of the lacrimal sac. The surgeon sits on the patient's side opposite to the operated side and directly views the transillumination target using surgical loupes and a nasal speculum with 5-cm blades (Fig. 6.1). A myringotomy sickle knife (or a bent disposable cataract crescent blade) is used to incise an ellipse of nasal mucosa down to bone 8–10 mm in length centered over the

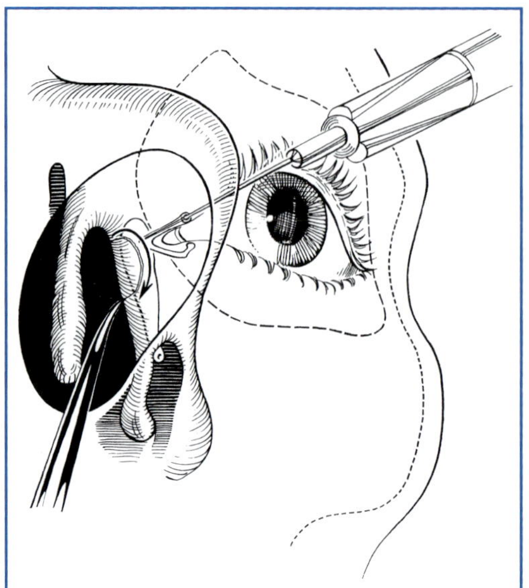

Fig. 6.2. The myringotomy knife is used to incise an ellipse of nasal mucosa overlying the transillumination target – the anterior cut is easily seen, while the posterior cut may be hidden behind the lip of the internal maxillary ridge

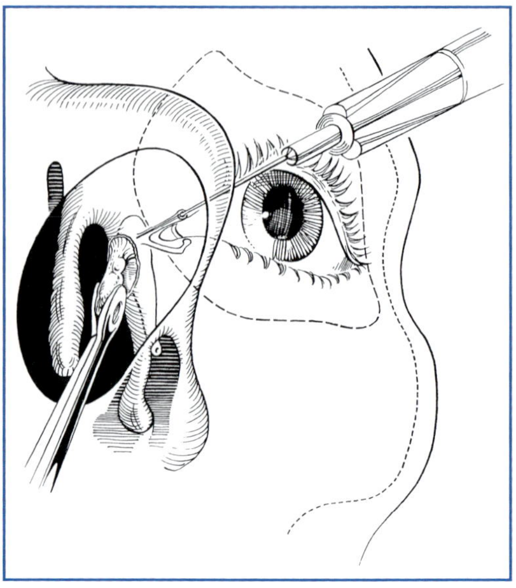

Fig. 6.3. Ethmoid forceps are used to peel away the nasal mucosa from the underlying bone

transillumination target. This is typically centered over the maxillary ridge, which extends above the base of the inferior turbinate, lateral to the anterior lip of the middle turbinate (Fig. 6.2). A Cottle periosteal elevator can be employed to strip the mucosa towards the center of the ellipse from the underlying bone. The mucosa is then peeled free using a straight Weil-Blakesley ethmoid forceps (Fig. 6.3).

The underlying bone at the osteotomy site usually has a vertical ridge with a posterior lip – the internal portion of the frontal process of the maxilla. The tip of a 3-mm right-angled up-biting Ruggles-Kerrison rongeur is slipped behind this ridge of bone, outfracturing the thin bone overlying the posterior portion of the lacrimal sac. The bone is nibbled away anteriorly through the thicker maxillary bone and then superiorly (Fig. 6.4). The bone widens superiorly as it curves horizontally onto the base of the middle turbinate, making removal increasingly difficult. However, an attempt is made to rongeur sufficient bone superiorly to allow the end of the light pipe to indent the lacrimal sac mucosa when held horizontally within the superior canaliculus. Sufficient bone is removed to visualize easily the entire width and most of the length of the lacrimal sac and duct (Fig. 6.4, insert). Tearing the underlying lacrimal sac and duct with either the rongeur or the light pipe is avoided.

Several adjunctive bone removal procedures may be considered to improve exposure of the lacrimal sac. Bruno Fayet has described excising the uncinate process, the mucosal-lined bony plate lying directly behind the lacrimal bone, to augment a posterior access to the lacrimal sac [28]. Tsirbas et al. have described using a curved 15-degree diamond burr on a powered microdebrider to remove bone superiorly above the attachment of the middle turbinate to expose the fundus of the lacrimal sac [27]. While this may improve the chances of directly connecting the internal common punctum to the nasal cavity, care must be taken to avoid creating a cerebrospinal fluid leak. Excision of the head of the middle turbinate may be considered to improve visualization and access of instruments to the

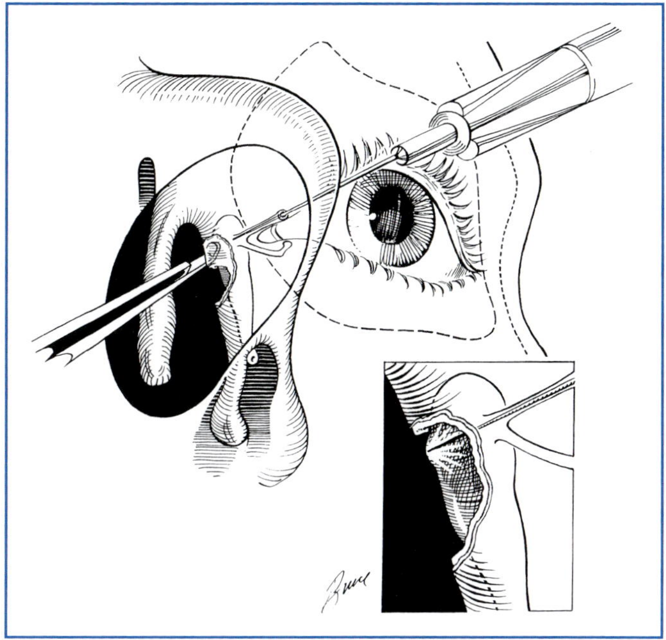

Fig. 6.4. The 3-mm up-biting Kerrison rongeur is slid posterior to the ridge of bone formed by the internal portion of the frontal process of the maxilla and is used to nibble away the bone anteriorly and superiorly. *Inset* shows the light pipe tenting the underlying lacrimal sac mucosa nasally through the bony opening. A myringotomy knife or cataract crescent knife is then used to incise the mucosa at the anterior margins allowing the flap to fold posteriorly

osteotomy site and also to lessen the risk of adhesions between the osteotomy and turbinate. In most cases, I have not found it necessary to perform these adjunctive measures.

6.5.4 Fenestrating the Lacrimal Sac

Marsupializing the lacrimal sac into the nasal cavity is one of the more technically difficult stages of the endonasal DCR, and one of the more likely causes of surgical failure.

Some proponents of the external DCR argue that suturing of anterior and posterior lacrimal sac and nasal mucosal flaps are crucial for the success of the procedure. However, other surgeons have modified the external DCR technique by eliminating posterior flaps, or by excising the nasal mucosa entirely, and suturing the anterior lacrimal flap to the periosteum at the anterior lip of the osteotomy, with good outcomes [6].

From an endonasal approach, the objectives are to create a large window within the medial wall of the lacrimal sac, avoiding any trauma to the lateral wall and common internal punctum [29, 30]. Ideally, the opening should be superior enough that the internal punctum is well visualized by the endoscope or surgical loupes, and sufficiently inferior to avoid a "sump syndrome" with pooling of tears or mucus below the opening [7]. The cut edges of the lacrimal sac should also be placed as far from each other as possible to prevent them from sealing shut again. Lastly, care should be taken to avoid traumatizing the delicate mucosa on the middle turbinate or nasal septum in order to limit adhesions forming between the lacrimal sac and these structures.

The medial wall of the lacrimal sac is tented with the retinal light pipe or probe with one hand while incising the mucosa with the other, avoiding damage to the lateral wall and orbital structures. Some authors have proposed injecting viscoelastics or vinyl polysiloxane into the sac to protect the sac and the common internal punctum [31]. In cases of mucocele or acute dacryocystitis, the distended sac is easier to incise safely than with scarred, shrunken sacs typical with chronic recurrent dacryocystitis [30].

The sac may be incised with a sickle knife, electrocautery, radiofrequency unit or laser. I prefer to create a large posteriorly based lacrimal sac flap, hinging it backwards to separate it widely from the cut anterior border. Care must be taken to avoid making a simple slit in the sac as the cut ends will readily seal. The flap may be removed for biopsy purposes with an ethmoid or micropituitary forceps, but care should be taken to avoid extending the mucosal tear beyond the sac into the orbit. If residual anterior mucosal flap remains, the light pipe or probe can be used to tent it towards the nasal cavity to facilitate additional trimming.

6.5.5 Mitomycin-C

This is an alkylating agent that inhibits fibroblast proliferation and has been promoted to help improve success rates in both external and endonasal DCRs. Most surgeons suggest placing a cotton-tipped applicator soaked with 0.3–0.5 mg/ml MMC over the osteotomy site for 3 min postoperatively, but surgeons have disagreed about its efficacy in improving surgical outcomes [32, 33]. A recent prospective study of patients undergoing EN-DCR with or without adjunctive MMC found no apparent benefit for surgical success [34].

6.5.6 Stenting

Bicanalicular silicone stents may be placed to keep the cut edges of the lacrimal mucosal flaps apart and help prevent osteotomy closure. Some surgeons have suggested enhancing the effect by using double stents, red-rubber catheters or Gelfoam in the osteotomy site [35, 36]. Silicone stents may prolapse into the eye if tied too loosely, or cause cheese-wiring of the canaliculi if tied too tightly. In rare cases, they may induce pyogenic granuloma formation on the conjunctival or nasal mucosal side. For this reason, removal at 2–3 months postoperatively is recommended.

6.6 Postoperative Care

On discharge, the patient is advised to avoid exertion and nose-blowing for 1 week and shown how to manage nosebleeds. In the rare instance where a nasal pack is required following EN-DCR, it should be removed in the recovery room or in the office the following day.

The patient is prescribed a steroid-antibiotic drop for 2 weeks and either a saline or steroid nasal spray once daily for 2 weeks. Systemic antibiotics can be prescribed for acute dacryocystitis alone, although some clinicians recommend prophylactic use.

Follow-up visits are arranged for 2 and 8 weeks postoperatively at which time irrigation of the canaliculi and inspection of the ostium can be performed. If a laser is used, more frequent follow-up examinations may be necessary to debride char from the ostium site [23].

The silicone stents are usually removed between 2 and 3 months postoperatively, but may be removed earlier if they are too tight or loose.

6.7 EN-DCR for Specific Conditions

6.7.1 Pediatric EN-DCR

Over 95% of cases of congenital nasolacrimal duct obstruction resolve spontaneously by the first year. Persistent obstruction can usually be cured with probing and/or silicone stenting. Dacryocystorhinostomy in childhood is reserved for those rare cases of congenital obstruction that persist in spite of probing and stenting, or for cases of acquired dacryostenosis or canalicular agenesis. EN-DCR in the pediatric population has been described in several series with excellent outcomes [37, 38]. Visualization remains excellent and the same instrumentation as in adult cases may be used in spite of the relatively small space within the child's nose [6].

6.7.2 EN-DCR with Canalicular Stenosis

Discrete canalicular scars, particularly those located along the distal canaliculus near the lacrimal sac, may be cured by the lacrimal microtrephine and silicone stents. Those symptomatic cases in which the canalicular stenosis is too broad to treat by trephination are best approached with a conjunctivo-dacryocystorhinostomy with a Jones Pyrex tube. The endonasal approach is well suited for this procedure, which bypasses the lacrimal system but which requires careful placement of the tube away from nasal obstructions. My preferred technique is to angle the retinal light pipe inferiorly in the medial canthus behind the lower eyelid insertion. The surgical site can be viewed using the loupes with the surgeon sitting on the opposite side of the patient's head. The mucosa and bone are resected as described previously although less bone removal is necessary superiorly. Local anesthetic with adrenaline is then injected in the conjunctiva medially for hemostasis. A 20-gauge needle is then threaded through the conjunctiva where the light pipe was aimed, passed through the osteotomy, and the tip viewed from within the nose. The needle is positioned so that it can be seen within the nasal cavity but not so deep that it might impinge medial structures such as the middle turbinate or nasal septum. A middle turbinectomy may be necessary. A hemostat is then placed on the shaft of the needle on the conjunctival side close to the conjunctival entry site. This allows selection of the appropriate Jones Pyrex tube length. The passage is bluntly widened with a lacrimal dilator or the gold dilators provided with the Pyrex tube set. The 20-gauge needle can be placed through the Pyrex tube and used to push it into position through the opening into the nose. The nasal end should be carefully examined to be sure it is well within the nasal cavity but not abutting any medial nasal structures. Water irrigated onto the surface of the eye should pass freely into the nose.

6.8 Complications

The most common complications from both external and endonasal DCRs include surgical failures, epistaxis, CSF leaks and stent malfunctions.

Surgical failures most commonly arise in the first 3 months following surgery. The leading causes noted by endonasal inspection are bridging scars between the ostium site and the middle turbinate or septum, insufficient exposure of the lacrimal sac superiorly from inadequate bone removal, and scar formation over the lacrimal sac opening or over the common internal punctum [6]. Adhesions are best avoided by minimizing abrasions to the middle turbinate mucosa and by excising the head of the middle turbinate if it lies too close to the ostium site. The lacrimal and maxillary bone should be rongeured or drilled sufficiently superiorly that the common internal punctum can be visualized when the lacrimal sac is opened. Opening the lacrimal sac with a large posteriorly based flap and hinging this backwards helps prevent the two cut ends of the sac scarring together.

Postoperative epistaxis can usually be controlled with external nostril compression, cold compresses on the nasal bridge, and sitting upright. Epistaxis sufficient to require nasal packs (Vaseline gauze or Gelfoam) is equally rare from either the external or endonasal approach. CSF leaks may occur from disruption of the cribriform plate, particularly from torsion of the middle turbinate with rongeurs [7].

Silicone stent complications include displacement and canalicular cheese-wiring as well as pyogenic granuloma formation [39]. Early removal is indicated for any of these complications. Jones Pyrex tubes may also cause granulomas and may migrate towards the nose or be extruded. A number of different tubes have been devised to try to prevent migration; my preference is a tube with a suture fixation hole in the collar.

Orbital injuries resulting from disruption to the periorbita are more likely in EN-DCR. These include orbital fat protruding into the nasal cavity and potentially obstructing the ostium, medial rectus trauma, orbital hemorrhage, and orbital emphysema (from nose-blowing).

Wound complications that may rarely occur in EX-DCR, such as webbing, medial canthal disinsertion or infection, do not occur in EN-DCR.

6.9 Comparison of EN-DCR and EX-DCR

Controversy persists in the ophthalmologic and otolaryngology literature over which approach is preferable for dacryocystorhinostomy [2, 3, 6, 17, 18, 40, 41].

Those favoring an external route argue that it has been performed for many years with an excellent success rate, with high patient satisfaction and that it remains the gold standard for lacrimal surgery. They note that the endonasal approach uses expensive equipment (lasers and video-endoscopes) and has had poorer success rates reported in the literature.

In many early series of EN-DCR, particularly when lasers were used, the success rates *were* lower in EN-DCR, ranging from 60% to 90% [16, 42], compared to the reported rates for the EX-DCR of between 75% and 95% [2, 3]. However, surgeons increasingly have refined the EN-DCR technique, using rongeurs and drills to remove even the thick superior bone of the maxillary ridge, and emphasizing opening the lacrimal sac with flaps hinged backwards to limit adhesions and scarring. The technique I have described even eliminates the need for video-endoscopes and maintains an overall success rate better than 90% [6].

Using these refined techniques, expensive instrumentation can be eliminated for the endonasal approach, and in the last 5 years success rates reported for EN-DCR have improved to the 75–99% range [17]. A report by the American Academy of Ophthalmology on endonasal DCR found that it was difficult to make a definite conclusion about the relative efficacy of the external versus endonasal route [17].

There are several advantages to the EN-DCR over the EX-DCR. Wound complications such as oedema, haematomas, infection, discomfort or scarring are eliminated. Although the scar is usually minimal from the external approach, I have found that the patients who have undergone both an external and endonasal DCR have all preferred the latter approach [6].

Underlying nasal pathology is directly viewed and can be addressed at the time of the EN-DCR. The operative time is shortened: my retrospective review of both EN-DCR and EX-DCR found the average operative time for the endonasal (18.5 min) was little over half that of the external route (34.3 min) [6].

6.10 Transition to EN-DCR

Surgeons wishing to try the endonasal DCR may choose a graded transition, similar to a cataract surgeon first learning phacoemulsification surgery. A first stage is to become familiar with the nasal anatomy by viewing the light pipe within the lacrimal sac before performing an external DCR and then viewing the osteotomy at the end. Revision surgery in cases of failed EX-DCR is a good second step, practising removal of scar tissue without requiring much bone removal. When primary cases are first tried, the surgeon may always switch to an external approach when difficulties are encountered.

Observing and performing several EN-DCR surgeries under the guidance of another surgeon experienced with this approach is recommended. Unfamiliarity with nasal anatomy could lead to violation of the orbital or cranial barriers, leading to trauma to the orbital fat or medial rectus muscle or CSF leak.

While there are a variety of expensive instruments proposed by many authors for viewing the surgical site and for creating the osteotomy and mucosal flaps, my experience has been that good outcomes can be achieved using a nasal speculum and surgical loupes, and simple surgical instruments such as the Kerrison rongeur, Blakesley ethmoid forceps and myringotomy sickle knife.

Summary for the Clinician

- The clinical work-up for patients with tearing or dacryocystitis includes a directed history, assessment of the eyelids, tear film and lacrimal drainage apparatus, and occasionally ancillary testing including dacryoscintigraphy, dacryocystography or CT scan
- Advantages of the endonasal approach include a reduced surgical time, no wound complications, no disruption of the medial canthal ligaments, and an examination of the intranasal anatomy with each surgery
- The external approach may be favored in cases of trauma with medial canthal avulsion or with wounds exposing the lacrimal sac, for suspected lacrimal sac diverticuli or malignancies, and in cases of Down's syndrome
- The most common endonasal DCR operative technique involves placing an illumination source within the canaliculus acting as a transillumination target. The surgical site may be viewed with operating loupes, microscope or endoscopy. The ostium may be created with lasers or mechanically with drills or surgical instruments such as ethmoid forceps, myringotomy blades and Kerrison bone rongeurs. Excellent success rates have been reported with a rapid, inexpensive method using a nasal speculum and surgical loupes and simple surgical instruments
- Recently reported success rates for the endonasal dacryocystorhinostomy rival or surpass those of the external approach
- Complications for both the endonasal and external DCR include surgical failures, epistaxis and stent malformations. Orbital injuries such as medial rectus trauma, orbital fat herniation, or orbital hemorrhage are rare, but are more likely to occur from the endonasal approach from disruption to the periorbita
- Surgeons wishing to try the endonasal DCR are recommended to observe and perform initial surgeries under the guidance of another surgeon experienced with this approach

References

1. Toti A (1904) Nuovo metodo conservatore di cura radicale delle suppurazioni croniche del sacco lacrimale (dacriocistorinostomia). Clin Mod Firenze 10:385–387
2. Tarbet KJ, Custer PL (1995) External dacryocystorhinostomy: surgical success, patient satisfaction, and economic cost. Ophthalmology 102: 1065–1070
3. Hartikainen J, Grenman R, Puukka P, Seppa H (1998) Prospective randomized comparison of external dacryocystorhinostomy and endonasal laser dacryocystorhinostomy. Ophthalmology 105: 1106–1113
4. McDonogh M, Meiring JH (1989) Endoscopic transnasal dacryocystorhinostomy. J Laryngol Otol 103:585–587
5. Massaro BM, Gonnering RS, Harris GJ (1990) Endonasal laser dacryocystorhinostomy: a new approach to nasolacrimal duct obstruction. Arch Ophthalmol 108:1172–1176
6. Dolman PJ (2003) Comparison of external dacryocystorhinostomy with nonlaser endonasal dacryocystorhinostomy. Ophthalmology 110:78–84
7. Watkins LM, Janfaza P, Rubin PAD (2003) The evolution of endonasal dacryocystorhinostomy. Surv Ophthalmol 48:73–84
8. Dupuy-Dutemps MM, Bourget ET (1920) Note preliminaire sur un proded de dacryocystorhinostomie. Ann D'Ocul (Paris) 157:1445–1447
9. Harris GJ, Sakol PJ, Beatty RL (1989) Relaxed skin tension line incision for dacryocystorhinostomy. Am J Ophthalmol 108:742–743
10. Becker BB (1988) Dacryocystorhinostomy without flaps. Ophthalmic Surg 19:419–427
11. Hurwitz JJ (1989) Teflon tubes for stenting and bypassing the lacrimal drainage pathways. Ophthalmic Surg 20:855–859
12. Caldwell GW (1893) Two new operations for obstruction of the nasal duct with preservation of the canaliculi and an incidental description of a new lacrymal probe. N Y Med J 57:581–582
13. Gonnering RS, Lyon DB, Fisher JC (1991) Endoscopic laser-assisted lacrimal surgery. Am J Ophthalmol 111:152–157
14. Montynen J, Yishitsuga M, Rautiainen M (1997) Results of dacryocystorhinostomy in 96 patients. Acta Otolaryngol Suppl 529:187–189
15. Javate RM, Campomanes BS, Co ND et al. (1995) The endoscope and the radiofrequency unit in DCR surgery. Ophthalmic Plastic Reconstr Surg 11:54–58

16. Boush GA, Lemke BN, Dortzbach RK (1994) Results of endonasal laser-assisted dacryocystorhinostomy. Ophthalmology 101:955–959
17. Woog JJ, Kennedy RH, Custer PL et al. (2001) Endonasal dacryocystorhinostomy. A report by the American Academy of Ophthalmology. Ophthalmology 108:2369–2377
18. Bartley GB (1994) The pros and cons of laser dacryocystorhinostomy. Am J Ophthalmol 117: 103–106
19. Hanna IT, Powrie S, Rose GE (1998) Open lacrimal surgery: a comparison of admission outcome and complications after planned day case or inpatient management. Br J Ophthalmol 82:392–396
20. Fayet B, Racy E, Halhal M et al. (2000) Forage osseux protégé lors des dacryocystorhinostomies par voie endo-nasale. J Fr Ophtalmol 23:321–326
21. Whittet HB, Shun-Shin GA, Awdry P (1993) Functional endoscopic transnasal dacryocystorhinostomy. Eye 7:545–549
22. Linberg JV, Anderson RL et al. (1982) Study of intranasal ostium external dacryocystorhinostomy. Arch Ophthalmol 100:1758–1762
23. Woog JJ, Metson R, Puliafito CA (1993) Holmium:YAG endonasal laser dacryocystorhinostomy. Am J Ophthalmol 116:1–10
24. Seppa H, Grenman R, Hartikainen J (1994) Endonasal CO_2–Nd: YAG laser dacryocystorhinostomy. Acta Ophthalmol 72:703–706
25. Pearlman SJ, Michalos P et al. (1997) Translacrimal transnasal laser-assisted dacryocystorhinostomy. Laryngoscope 107:1362–1365
26. Fayet B, Racy E, Halhal M et al. (2000) Endonasal dacryocystorhinostomy (DCR) with protected drill. J Fr Ophtalmol 23:321–326
27. Tsirbas A, Wormald PJ (2003) Mechanical endonasal dacryocystorhinostomy with mucosal flaps. Br J Ophthalmol 87:43–47
28. Fayet B, Racy E, Assouline M (2004) Complications of standardized endonasal dacryocystorhinostomy with unciformectomy. Ophthalmology 111:837–845
29. Olver J (2003) The success rates for endonasal dacryocystorhinostomy. Br J Ophthalmol 87:1431
30. Goldberg RA (2004) Endonasal dacryocystorhinostomy. Is it really less successful? Arch Ophthalmol 122:108–110
31. Goldberg RA, Beizai P, Kim J, McCann JD (2002) Use of vinyl polysiloxane impression material to protect and identify the nasolacrimal sac in endonasal dacryocystorhinostomy. Ophthal Plast Reconstr Surg 18:205–210
32. Camara JG, Bengzon AU, Henson RD (2000) The safety and efficacy of mitomycin C in endonasal endoscopic laser-assisted dacryocystorhinostomy. Ophthal Plastic Reconstr Surg 16:114–118
33. Liao SL, Kao SCS, Tseng JHS et al. (2000) Results of intraoperative mitomycin C application in dacryocystorhinostomy. Br J Ophthalmol 84:903–906
34. Dolman PJ, Alas E (2004) Prospective comparison of adjunctive mitomycin-C for endonasal DCR [abstract]. Presented at the American Society of Ophthalmic Plastic and Reconstructive Surgeons, 2004, Los Angeles, CA
35. Hurwitz JJ, Archer KF et al. (1988) Double stent intubations in difficult post-traumatic dacryocystorhinostomy. Ophthalmic Surg 19:33–36
36. Leone CR (1982) Gelfoam-thrombin dacryocystorhinostomy stent. Am J Ophthalmol 94:412–413
37. Cunningham MJ, Woog JJ (1998) Endonasal endoscopic dacryocystorhinostomy in children. Arch Otolaryngol Head Neck Surg 124:328–333
38. Wong JF, Woog JJ et al. (1999) A multidisciplinary approach to atypical lacrimal obstruction in childhood. Ophthal Plast Reconstr Surg 15:293–298
39. Allen K, Berlin AJ (1989) Dacryocystorhinostomy failure: association with nasolacrimal silicone intubation. Ophthalmic Surg 20:486–489
40. Szubin L, Papageorge A, Sacks E (1999) Endonasal laser-assisted dacryocystorhinostomy. Am J Rhinol 13:371–374
41. Tsirbas A, Davis F, Wormald PJ (2004) Mechanical endonasal dacryocystorhinostomy versus external dacryocystorhinostomy. Ophthal Plast Reconstr Surg 20:50–56
42. Sadiq SA, Ohrlich S, Jones NS, Downes RN (1997) Endonasal laser dacryocystorhinostomy – medium term results. Br J Ophthalmol 81:1089–1092

Monocanalicular Lacrimal Pathway Intubation with a Stable Punctal Attachment

7

Bruno Fayet, Jean-Marc Ruban

Core Messages

- Monocanalicular intubation has been made effective by the manufacture of a device combining a punctal plug device and a connecting silicone tube or rod (the Mono-Ka® device)
- The results for congenital dacryostenosis are similar to those seen with bicanalicular intubation
- The Mono-Ka® device is particularly useful for cases of punctal atresia of a single channel with associated nasolacrimal duct obstruction
- The Mini-Mono-Ka® is a modified device with a punctal plug and a Silastic rod useful for the repair of canalicular lacerations
- Complications with these devices are infrequent but include early extrusion, damage to the punctum or burying of the device

7.1 Introduction

Monocanalicular intubation has been used for many years but primarily for lacrimal trauma. Most of the time this intubation required the surgeon's ingenuity in order to modify a medical device originally made for other purposes (e.g. angiocath silicone guide, embolectomy catheter). The surgeon had to fit together a silicone rod and a probe in order to enable lacrimal intubation to be performed. The device had to be taped or sutured to the eyelid or inferior fornix or otherwise secured with tape to the skin in the punctal area.

Preparing a useful device was time consuming for the surgeon. Moreover, all of these devices lacked a safe method for punctal fixation, thus requiring exteriorization of the device as described above. Improvement was achieved by a manufactured coupling of a punctal plug (as popularized by Freeman) and a silicone rod used for lacrimal intubation (Long, Fayet).

7.2 Description and Fitting for Monocanalicular Stenting: The Mono-Ka® Device

This device consists of three components:

1. A silicone rod, which is a hollow tube 0.64 mm in external diameter and 27 cm long
2. A superior fixation device (SFD), which allows for a secure seating of the punctal plug part of the device in the ampulla
3. A seating instrument, which can either be a metallic or a plastic probe point to push the plug securely into the punctum

7.2.1 Description of the Superior Fixation Device (SFD)

In cutout view the SFD looks like an onion or an ace of spades. The collarette, which is wider than the lacrimal meatus, prevents the burying or migration of the Mono-Ka® into the canaliculus. It is the only part of the device which is visible once the Mono-Ka® has been properly placed in the lacrimal duct. It permits postoperative evaluation and simple removal of the

Mono-Ka® when appropriate. Three sizes of collarettes are available. These are fused to a bulb, which forms the inferior part of the SFD.

When the Mono-Ka® is in place, the bulb is securely fixed in the ampulla. Its bulbous shape prevents the spontaneous extrusion of the SFD. Yet its size is not so wide that it would prevent simple removal when desired. The silicone tubing is fused together with the bulb, forming a right angle.

7.2.2 Monocanalicular Intubation: Technique for Insertion

Intubation of the silicone tube can be achieved by utilizing a system described by Fayet [1]. The stability of the Mono-Ka® in the punctum is linked to its SFD. The setting of the SFD in the punctum can be achieved with the specific device described earlier as used to secure punctal plugs. Once the silicone tube has been introduced into the lacrimal pathways and retrieved from the nostril, the end is trimmed with scissors. Care should be taken not to pull the tube too tightly while cutting it so that the end does not retract past the valve of Hasner at the distal end of the nasolacrimal duct. The end of the silicone tube should remain free under the inferior meatus without any fixation device or knot.

7.2.3 Limitations of the Mono-Ka® Device

As in the other types of silicone intubation, the "active" part of the device is the free part of the silicone tube, which prevents the development of scarring in the nasolacrimal duct. Moreover, the SFD also allows for enlargement of the punctal meatus in order to reduce the occurrence of punctal stenosis. However, the lack of an intermeatal silicone loop, as seen with bicanalicular intubation, reduces the possibilities of curing caruncular or semilunar fold disease as well as any associated punctal position abnormalities.

7.2.4 Indications and Contraindications for the Mono-Ka®

The indications for monocanalicular stenting are fewer than those for bicanalicular intubation. The best indication is the treatment of nasolacrimal duct impatency associated with canalicular agenesis. In the treatment of congenital tearing from lacrimal duct impatency, Mono-Ka® and Bi-Ka® have the same success rate. The choice between one or the other device depends more on the surgeon's preference. The main indication for Mini-Mono-Ka® is for canalicular injury in the distal or medial third of the canaliculus and, for some surgeons, for the treatment of canaliculitis.

7.2.5 Caution

The meatal tolerance of the Mono-Ka® device decreases as time goes by. Mono-Ka® intubations should not be used when an extended canalicular intubation is required. The effectiveness of Mono-Ka® intubation in common canalicular stenosis is less than that for bicanalicular intubation. It is not recommended to place two Mono-Ka® devices on the same side in order to cure lacrimal pathway stenosis (risk of increased epiphora during duration of intubation). Cure of epiphora can occur after withdrawal of a Mono-Ka® device in many cases because a single canaliculus is sometimes sufficient in lacrimal drainage obstruction. Conjunctival tolerance to Bi-Ka® silicone loop is better for conjunctival diseases such as pterygium or pinguecula as compared to conjunctival contact with the Mono-Ka® SFD.

7.3 The Mini-Mono-Ka® Device

This device does not utilize any probe to insert tubing into the nasolacrimal duct. It is a solid silicone rod. The SFD allows the Mini-Mono-Ka® to remain stable in the canaliculus. Its use is specifically for canalicular injuries. Placement of this device requires gentle punctal dilation of the meatus. The proximal part of the punctum and canaliculus is intubated with the free silicone rod part of the device, which is brought out via the wound. Then a smooth pulling of the free silicone part of the Mini-Mono-Ka® allows the SFD to set into the punctum. The punctal plug seating delivery device may sometimes be needed. The end of the rod is then shortened sufficiently to pass into the distal canalicular wound and only slightly into the lacrimal sac. Sutures are carefully placed to close the canalicular wound and to reconstruct the canthal tendon by standard techniques. The average duration of intubation is 2 months.

7.4 Supervision and Removal of the Mono-Ka® Device

The Mono-Ka® device once placed in the lacrimal drainage system is almost invisible. The collarette lies flat on the lid margin, and the functional tolerance of the SFD is usually very good. Removal of the Mono-Ka® device is achieved with an atraumatic forceps by pulling the collarette, thus permitting the Mono-Ka® to be pulled from the lacrimal drainage apparatus.

Summary for the Clinician

- **The Mono-Ka® stent is useful for congenital dacryostenosis and some cases of punctal agenesis**
- **The device consists of a punctal plug and silicone tube**
- **The tubing is introduced into the system and then seated with a special device**
- **A Mini-Mono-Ka® device with a solid rod attached to the punctal plug is useful for the repair of canalicular trauma**

7.5 Complications

The complications of the Mono-Ka® device are similar to those noted with punctal plugs and to complications with bicanalicular intubation.

7.5.1 Complications Related to the Insertion of the Mono-Ka® Device

7.5.1.1 Meatal Ring Rupture

This is usually the consequence of inadequate dilation of the punctal meatus and is not due to a complication of the Mono-Ka® device itself. Some authors describe a meatal ring rupture as a stricturotomy. This is really a specific complication only of bicanalicular intubation and is not appropriate as this really refers to slitting of the canaliculus. Indeed, the axis of the canalicular laceration is always orientated according to the main axis of the eyelid, which can be very important in stricturotomies. On the contrary, the axis of the meatal ring rupture with plug insertion is variable with respect to the main axis of the eyelid. It does not occur postoperatively following proper surgical insertion of the device, and it will always remain localized. Should this complication occur during insertion, however, then use of the Mono-Ka® will be contraindicated as the punctal plug (SFD) will not remain in position. Stricturotomy, in the true sense, does not result from the Mono-Ka® device, and this fact represents one of its main advantages.

7.5.1.2 Burying of the Mono-Ka® During Seating

This complication can occur in two main situations:

1. Excessive pressure with SFD insertion in the meatus using the punctal plug seating device (PPSD) improperly
2. Excessive pulling of the free silicone rod in the nose

In these two instances, the SFD is pulled beyond the meatal ring.

Prevention of burying of the Mono-Ka® can be achieved by careful insertion and seating technique. The SFD should be gently pushed into the meatus and should never be inserted into the meatus by pulling on the nasal free end of the silicone rod alone. On the contrary, the

SFD should be gently inserted with the punctal plug setting device only after a gentle dilation of the former has been done. Scissors can be used to sever the free silicone tubing under visual control beneath the inferior turbinate without any pulling on the silicone. One should not at any time suture the silicone tubing in the nose or fix it on the lid with an adhesive strip.

One should never neglect a buried Mono-Ka® that occurs with insertion. Repositioning of the SFD is easy to perform. The collar of the SFD is catheterized with the PPSD. Then a 45° bending of this latter device is performed in an anteroposterior plane (and not in a frontal plane, which increases the risk of worsening the complication) so as to withdraw the SFD by causing a reverse motion. If this is not sufficient, the SFD can be withdrawn by using a small toothed forceps. Canaliculotomy is rarely necessary in order to remove a buried SFD but may be required if the plug is passed into the horizontal part of the canaliculus.

7.6 Undesirable Side Effects of the Mono-Ka® After Placement in the Lacrimal Pathways

7.6.1 Dyeing of the Silicone

Acquired dyeing of the SFD is often a consequence of the instillation of methylene blue solution. The dyeing does not have any consequence on the anatomic tolerance of the Mono-Ka® and should not be a cause for early withdrawal of the silicone. We have not encountered any dyeing of the silicone with the use of fluorescein, rifamycin (orange dye), rose bengal (red dye) or indocyanine green (green dye).

Late yellow coloring of the silicone rod beyond the SFD is quite frequent, but we have never noticed any yellowing of the SFD itself, even with long duration intubation (>6 months). One should be aware that some amount of discharge can accumulate in the lumen of the collar and represent an infection spot. Intraocular surgery should not be performed until the Mono-Ka® is removed.

7.6.2 Itching

Itching can occur secondary to rubbing of the SFD against the medial part of the conjunctiva, especially during reading. This side effect is increased when the inner part of the bulbar conjunctiva is scarred or edematous (pinguecula, pterygium, loose conjunctiva, etc.). Dye tests (rose bengal, indocyanine green) can confirm the possibility of anatomic sequelae to the conjunctiva. If the conjunctival dye tests are immediately positive (conjunctival dye staining), removal of the Mono-Ka® is still not required because this side effect is common during the first days after insertion of the Mono-Ka® and will gradually disappear as time goes by. In any case of corneal erosion confirmed by dye testing, however, the Mono-Ka® should be removed. This complication is more frequent with the wide collarette Mono-Ka® (4 mm) compared with the standard collarette Mono-Ka® (3 mm) now most commonly used.

7.6.3 Impermeability

The Mono-Ka® device is impervious to tear flow because of its design as a punctal plug for dry eyes. This is not a problem in most cases because a single canaliculus is usually sufficient to achieve tear drainage in indoor basic conditions. This has been confirmed by several papers comparing the Mono-Ka® and Bi-Ka® devices in the treatment of congenital lacrimal impatency [3, 5, 6]. These papers have also confirmed that the rate of cure is similar between bicanalicular and monocanalicular intubation. On the other hand, one should not automatically seek an early secondary procedure if epiphora persists while the Mono-Ka® is in place. The silicone tubing fills the nasolacrimal duct and may cause epiphora unless the surrounding space is sufficiently large for tears to drain around the tube. Following removal, there may still be some edema that causes epiphora. We, therefore, recommend waiting at least 3 months following tube removal before performing further lacrimal surgery.

7.7 Late Complications of the Mono-Ka® After Insertion in the Lacrimal Drainage Pathway

7.7.1 Externalization or Extrusion

In some cases, extrusion or loss of the tube is obvious when the patient brings back the Mono-Ka® device to the surgeon's office. In other cases, it can be suspected by observing the absence of the SFD while inspecting the punctal area. In such cases, probing can be helpful in confirming an open lacrimal pathway in adults. In children, however, this can only be an assumption, which will require a general anesthetic and further lacrimal surgery if symptoms persist. Externalization of the Mono-Ka® device is less frequent than the irreversible Bi-Ka® externalizations. Its mechanism is linked to a direct pull on the SFD. Inadequate seating of the SFD into the punctal ampulla facilitates its externalization. Therefore, it is important, as one should do after a punctal plug seating procedure, to check for the correct positioning of the collarette on the lid margin. There is no difference between the rate of wide collarette SFD extrusion and that of the medium collarette nor does it matter whether the SFD has been secured in the inferior punctum compared to the superior punctum.

7.7.2 Intracanalicular Migration

In some cases, it is obvious when the patient returns postoperatively that the Mono-Ka® is not visible. This can mean that it has either come out or has migrated into the canaliculus. In the intracanalicular migration situation, the SFD is inside the lumen of the canaliculus, and probing the lacrimal pathway is then impossible.

Intracanalicular migration can occur in two main circumstances: (1) migration during the seating of the Mono-Ka®, and (2) later during the postoperative period, which is very rare.

Once a migration of the Mono-Ka® has occurred, two possibilities can be encountered:

1. Good tolerance with no symptoms:
   Observation of the patient is then the rule except when the migration is a complication secondary to placement of the SFD. The medium and larger size collarette have been well tolerated with few examples of migration.
2. Tearing and canaliculitis:
   If these problems persist, the surgeon has to remove the Mono-Ka®. It is not advisable to try to push the Mono-Ka® device further into the lacrimal pathway because no sight control is possible using this technique. If the surgeon can feel the SFD with his fingers, a posterior (conjunctival approach) canaliculotomy will permit the extraction of the Mono-Ka®. If the surgeon cannot feel the SFD in the eyelid but can see the distal free silicone rod under the inferior turbinate, pulling the silicone gently is often sufficient to remove a small collarette Mono-Ka® (2 mm wide). With larger collarettes, however, this maneuver is not advisable. We have tested the resistance of the silicone plug to inferior pulling and never noticed any rupture between the SFD device and the proximal silicone part of the Mono-Ka®. However, as nothing can ever be excluded in daily medical practice, this problem may yet be observed.

7.8 Prevention of Intracanalicular Migration of the Mono-Ka®

This depends on:

1. Gentle dilation of the meatal ring
2. Careful seating of the SFD into the punctum

An alteration of the SFD design (J.M. Ruban) may also prevent this type of migration.

7.9 Complications of the Mini-Mono-Ka® Device

The complications described with the Mono-Ka® device can also occur with the Mini-Mono-Ka® device. Only one is specific to the Mini-Mono-Ka®, however, namely, wound dehiscence. The indication for use of the Mini-Mono-Ka® is as a stent for repair of canalicular lacerations. It is of great importance to adjust the length of the silicone rod in the distal portion of the wound. There should be enough length to intubate the distal canalicular part for a distance of at least 2 mm. Shortening the distal silicone rod has to be performed after the SFD is settled in the meatus. The distal free end of the rod should never reach the lacrimal sac. If this situation happens, the risk of wound rupture increases with eventual disunion of the canalicular mucosa and subsequently the eyelid tissues (orbicularis and skin). The only way to avoid this situation is to reseat the Mini-Mono-Ka® properly. There must be no resistance from an excess length of tubing. The distal length of the tubing must be shortened or the silicone device removed.

Summary for the Clinician

- **Complications of the Mono-Ka® include extrusion and migration or burying of the punctal plug early**
- **Extrusion often still results in cure if the tube has remained in place for at least several weeks**
- **Migration or burying of the tube is infrequent if properly placed. It may require a canaliculotomy on the inner tarsal surface**
- **If the plug causes corneal staining, then the device should be removed**
- **The Mini-Mono-Ka® device is particularly useful as a stent for canalicular laceration repair**

References

1. Fayet B, Bernard JA (1990) Une sonde monocanaliculaire à fixation méatique autostable dans la chirugie des voies lacrymales d'excrétion. Ophtalmologie 4:351–357
2. Fayet B, Bernard JA, Pouliquen Y (1989) Repair of recent canalicular wounds using a monocanalicular stent (in French). Bull Soc Ophtalmol Fr 89: 819–825
3. Fayet B, Bernard JA, Assouline M, Benabderrazik S, Pouliquen Y (1993) Bi-canalicular versus mono-canalicular silicone intubation for naso-lacrimal duct impatency in children. Orbit 12: 149–156
4. Goldstein SM, Goldstein JB, Katowitz JA (2004) Comparison of monocanalicular stenting and balloon dacryoplasty in secondary treatment of congenital nasolacrimal duct obstruction after failed primary probing. Ophthal Plast Reconstr Surg 20:352–357
5. Ruban JM, Boyrivent V (1994) Intérêt de l'intubation mono-canaliculo-nasale de courte durée dans le traitement de l'imperméabilité des voies lacrymales d'excrétion du nourrisson. Ophtalmologie 8:296–298
6. Ruban JM, Guigon P, Boyrivent V (1995) Analyse de l'efficacité de la sonde d'intubation mono-canaliculo-nasale grande collerette dans le traitement par obstruction congénitale des voies lacrymales d'excrétion du nourrisson. J Fr Ophtalmol 18:377–383

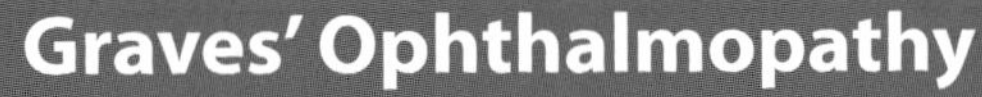
Graves' Ophthalmopathy

The Role of Orbital Radiotherapy in the Management of Thyroid Related Orbitopathy

Michael Kazim

8

Core Messages

- The treatment protocol for orbital radiotherapy published in 1973 by Donaldson et al. has been adopted by all radiation oncology centers worldwide
- Patients are presently exposed to a total of 20 Gy delivered in ten fractional sessions with the beam directed at the retro-ocular tissues, posteriorly at 5°, to avoid excessive exposure to the retina and lens
- While there is no clear understanding of the mechanism by which low-dose radiation modulates the local inflammatory response in the orbit, a number of in vitro studies provide evidence to suggest multiple mechanisms by which the currently held model for thyroid associated orbitopathy may be modified to blunt the downstream consequences of fibroblast activation
- The majority of patients suffering with Graves' orbitopathy are not candidates for radiotherapy
- Patients with mild disease or stable phase disease will not benefit from the treatment when compared to the natural history of the disease
- In more severely affected patients, reversal of optic neuropathy, improvement in extraocular motility and decrease in congestive signs and symptoms can be anticipated after treatment with 20 Gy

8.1 Introduction: Historical Background

The use of radiotherapy to treat exophthalmos resulting from Graves' disease dates to 1936 [1]. The early reports detail external beam radiation directed at the pituitary gland, which at the time was believed to be the cause of the exophthalmos, resulting in regression of proptosis. It would appear, in retrospect, that the radiation field fortuitously included the orbital tissues thereby producing the observed effects in the orbit. Subsequently, small case series provided further support for the use of orbital radiotherapy [2–7]. A significant change in the treatment protocol occurred after the 1973 publication by Donaldson et al. from Stanford University [8]. The protocol has subsequently been adopted by all radiation oncology centers worldwide. The most critical improvement was the conversion from cobalt to linear accelerator electron beam as the radiation source. This produced a finer edge to the isodose curves and thereby reduced the collateral injury associated with the cobalt sources. Patients are presently exposed to a total of 20 Gy delivered in ten fractional sessions with the beam directed at the retro-ocular tissues, posteriorly at 5°, to avoid excessive exposure to the retina and lens.

Over the subsequent 20 years, as the treatment protocol was universally adopted by centers dedicated to the treatment of thyroid related orbitopathy, a series of retrospective studies published that further supported the efficacy of the treatment [9–11]. In the retrospective study published in 1991, Donaldson's group reported a

20-year experience of the treatment of 311 patients [12]. Radiotherapy in their study arrested the progression of the ophthalmic manifestations of the disease in 95% of cases. There was no difference in clinical response noted in the groups treated with 20 Gy or 30 Gy. Seventy-six percent of patients were able to discontinue steroids after radiotherapy treatment. The study suffered from the lack of clinical classification of disease by an orbital specialist. Moreover, all non-prospective, controlled studies suffered from the lack of comparative natural history data.

Kazim and Trokel reported results of the treatment of 84 patients suffering with acute phase thyroid related orbitopathy comparing corticosteroid to radiation therapy [13]. Patients treated with radiotherapy were more likely to have improvement in both subjective and objective signs of orbital congestion than patients treated with steroids alone. Moreover, of the 29 patients who received radiotherapy to treat compressive optic neuropathy, only one (6%) failed to respond and required surgical decompression. Conversely, among the 16 patients with optic neuropathy who were treated with oral corticosteroids, 6 (37%) required surgical decompression, the indication of treatment failure.

Lloyd and Leone reported results for 36 patients who were treated with oral corticosteroids initially for thyroid related orbitopathy and ultimately became intolerant to the medications [14]. After receiving 20 Gy of orbital radiotherapy, 33 patients no longer required steroid treatment. The three failures were treated with alternate forms of immunosuppression.

More recently there have been two studies conducted in a prospective randomized fashion, both with clinical parameters defined and measured by orbital specialists in an attempt to address the limitations of the preceding studies. In a study from Utrecht, Mourits et al. constructed a randomized double-blind trial in which 30 patients suffering with moderately severe orbitopathy were assigned to one of two groups [15]. The first received 20 Gy radiotherapy and the second was sham irradiated. The treatment outcome was measured qualitatively. Improvements in the treated group were significant when assessing a decrease in diplopia, improved elevation of the globes and improved field of binocular vision. There was no significant improvement in proptosis or eyelid swelling. As a consequence, 25% of patients treated with radiotherapy were spared the need for strabismus surgery.

In a follow-up study published in 2004, the Dutch group performed a randomized double-blind study of 88 patients suffering mild orbital disease [16]. Forty-four were treated with 20 Gy and the others sham treated, in an attempt to determine if the treatment would prevent disease progression at a rate greater than the natural history of the disease. Their findings supported the earlier report with the respect to the improvement in eye muscle function and a decrease in diplopia; however, overall radiotherapy failed to prevent progression of disease. Therefore among mildly affected cases radiotherapy, they felt, was no better than the "wait and see" natural history of the disease.

The study that has to date produced the greatest controversy is one first reported in 2001 from the Mayo Clinic with subsequent follow-up reported in 2002 and 2003 [17–19]. The clinic conducted a double-blind study to eliminate some of the confounding variables that plagued even the prospective Dutch studies. Fifty-three patients with moderate thyroid related orbitopathy were enrolled in the study. One eye was treated with a novel radiotherapeutic protocol to limit exposure to the contralateral eye, which was simultaneously sham treated. The clinical parameters of disease were monitored over a period of 6 months, at which time the contralateral orbit was treated and the initially treated orbit, sham treated. The results showed no significant difference in clinical measurements between the two orbits at either 6 months or 1 year. The authors concluded that the results proved that radiotherapy had no significant benefit in the treatment of thyroid associated orbitopathy. The study was limited by several factors. First, the average length of orbital disease in the enrolled group was 18 months. Consequency the patients enrolled in the study were on average in the stable phase of the orbitopathy and thereby not expected to respond to an immunomodulator. Secondly, over the course of the first 6 months there was no progression of disease in the sham-treated orbit. This observation lends further support to the conclusion that the patients enrolled were in the stable phase of the disease. If active, one would anticipate the disease parameters would worsen in the 6-month time interval. Third, the novel protocol for radiotherapy, which constructed a treatment field that limited the contralateral orbital dose, is a significant departure from the accepted protocol. This variance from the accepted treatment protocol may produce a significant therapeutic variation. Finally, the protocol necessitated the exclusion of patients with compressive optic neuropathy. Patients with compressive optic neuropathy are among the most severely affected. In many centers the presence of optic neuropathy is the primary indication for treatment with orbital radiotherapy. This study has not addressed this group of patients or those with rapidly progressive orbitopathy. Therefore it would be reasonable to conclude from the Mayo study that the course of mild or stable phase thyroid related orbitopathy is not significantly improved compared to the natural history of the disease when treatment is delivered according to the protocol that was constructed. The debate over the study was chronicled in a series of editorials both accompanying the initial paper and three further publications in the *Ophthalmic Plastic and Reconstructive Surgery Journal* [20–22].

8.2 Biological Effects of Radiotherapy

While there is no clear understanding of the mechanism by which low-dose radiation modulates the local inflammatory response in the orbit, a number of in vitro studies provide evidence to suggest multiple mechanisms by which the currently held model for thyroid associated orbitopathy may be modified to blunt the downstream consequences of fibroblast activation [23].

Lymphocytes are generally highly radiosensitive; however, activated lymphocytes are, on the contrary, relatively radio-resistant to low doses of radiation. In either case, the singular sterilization of the orbit of lymphocytes by the treatment with ten sessions of 2 Gy is inadequate to explain the more long lasting effects appreciated clinically. It would be anticipated that soon after conclusion of treatments the orbits would become repopulated with bone marrow derived lymphocytes directed to the orbit.

It has been shown that radiation induces terminal differentiation in progenitor fibroblasts over a 2- to 3-week interval in response to doses of radiation as low as 1 Gy. This mechanism would argue for treatment with oral corticosteroids for some interval of time after completing the radiotherapy to allow for the full effect of the radiation treatment to be appreciated on a cellular level.

The orbital fibroblast has been recently identified as the target of the immune system within the orbit. In response to cytokines, induction of glycosaminoglycan production occurs. This effect is site specific, affecting the orbit as expected and to a lesser extent the pretibial region. These fibroblasts can actively participate in the immune response, and promote further movement of lymphocytes to the orbit. In addition, a subset of fibroblasts has been shown in vitro to differentiate into fat cells and may account for the clinically observed expansion of the orbital fat compartment resulting in proptosis in patients younger than 40 years.

If radiotherapy were to act by inducing terminal differentiation among orbital fibroblasts, it may explain the cessation of glycosaminoglycan deposition, preadipocyte differentiation into fat cells, and lymphocyte accumulation in the orbit.

Radiotherapy in low doses has been shown to decrease the adhesion of blood-borne lymphocytes to activated endothelial cells. This effect may blunt the local effect of such activated lymphocytes in the orbit. Furthermore, mounting evidence suggests that, unlike high dose radiotherapy, low dose radiotherapy may blunt the secretion of proinflammatory cytokines from activated macrophages.

8.3 Safety

The safety of orbital radiotherapy has been investigated by a number of longitudinal studies.

The risk of carcinogenesis has been examined by four studies [24–27]. The theoretical rate of cancer induction from the typical treatment protocol has been calculated to be between 0.7% and 1.2%; however, long-term longitudinal studies have failed to identify an increased rate of development of tumors or tumor associated death when patients were followed postradiation for between 5 and 30 years. However, most centers will limit the age of radiotherapy treatment to approximately 30 years to decrease the theoretical risks of the treatment. Fortunately, this is not an age group that typically requires this intervention. Furthermore, the studies have shown no increased risk in the development of cataract as compared to an age-matched control [28].

The risk of radiation-induced retinopathy has been demonstrated to be higher among patients with insulin dependent diabetes or pre-existing retinopathy (both diabetic and hypertensive) when treated with radiotherapy. In a 3-year follow-up to the Mayo study, among the 42 patients treated with radiotherapy, patients with pre-existing microvascular changes, uveitis, hypertension, and borderline elevated blood glucose levels were more likely to have evidence of the development and/or progression of retinal macular and vascular abnormalities [19].

Taken together these considerations have led to the recommendation to withhold radiotherapy in the younger patient and those at risk of retinal vascular injury.

8.4 Pre-treatment Analysis

To determine which patients would be most likely to benefit from orbital radiotherapy, a number of diagnostic maneuver have been employed. Most widely utilized is the steroid trial of oral prednisone at doses of 1 mg/kg for 2–4 weeks. A therapeutic response during the trial defines acute phase disease and the reversible nature of the orbitopathy. Although not studied in a prospective fashion, response to the steroid trial should be mirrored by treatment with radiotherapy.

As an alternative, there have been a number of studies examining the predictive value of MRI (contrast enhanced T1, and T2 relaxation time) [19, 29–32] and octreotide scans [30, 33]. Overall, the data are no more compelling than clinical assessment of disease activity.

8.4.1 10- vs. 20-Gy Dose Treatment

Studies of higher versus lower dose orbital radiotherapy (20 Gy vs. 10 Gy [34] and 2.4 Gy vs. 16 Gy [35]) have failed to prove that lower dose treatment has any advantage or is even as effective as the higher dose. Although 20-Gy protocols have been utilized for 30 years with reasonable success and without significant incidence of adverse affect, their efficacy at this time still remains in question. It would be advisable, however, to conduct efficacy trials of treatment at the 20-Gy level before attempting to modify the current treatment protocol.

8.5 Recommendations and Future Developments

At present the following recommendations regarding the use of orbital radiotherapy to treat thyroid related orbitopathy are supported by the available data.

The majority of patients suffering with Graves' orbitopathy are not candidates for radiotherapy. Patients with mild disease or stable phase disease will not benefit from the treatment when compared to the natural history of the disease. The definition of mild disease may be debated, as severity or activity scores are typically flawed in their construct; however, it would generally be agreed that the presence of compressive optic neuropathy or rapidly progressive orbitopathy over the first 1–3 months after presentation constitutes the more severely affected group. In this more severely affected group, reversal of optic neuropathy, improvement in extraocular motility and decrease in congestive signs and symptoms can be anticipated after treatment with 20 Gy. A positive response to oral corticosteroids typically anticipates response to orbital radiotherapy.

The lack of response to steroids, or the lack of change in signs and symptoms of the orbitopathy over a 6-month interval, are likely evidence of stable phase disease that is unlikely to respond to orbital radiotherapy. In the future, we anticipate that large multicenter natural history studies and treatment trials will provide a clearer understanding of the role of radiotherapy in the management of thyroid related orbitopathy.

Summary for the Clinician

- **Safety considerations have led to the recommendation to withhold radiotherapy in the younger patient and those at risk of retinal vascular injury**
- **The most widely utilized diagnostic maneuver to determine which patients are most likely to benefit from orbital radiotherapy is the steroid trial of oral prednisone at doses of 1 mg/kg for 2–4 weeks. A therapeutic response during the trial defines acute phase disease and the reversible nature of the orbitopathy. Although not studied in a prospective fashion, response to the steroid trial should be mirrored by treatment with radiotherapy**
- **Studies of higher versus lower dose orbital radiotherapy (20 Gy vs. 10 Gy [34] and 2.4 Gy vs. 16 Gy [35]) have failed to prove that lower dose treatment has any advantage or is even as effective as the higher dose**
- **Patients with mild disease or stable phase disease will not benefit from the treatment when compared to the natural history of the disease**
- **It would generally be agreed that the presence of compressive optic neuropathy or rapidly progressive orbitopathy over the first 1–3 months after presentation constitutes the more severely affected group of patients. In these patients, reversal of optic neuropathy, improvement in extraocular motility and decrease in congestive signs and symptoms can be anticipated after treatment with 20 Gy**

References

1. Thomas HM Jr, Woods AC (1936) Progressive exophthalmos following thyroidectomy. Bull Hopkins Hosp 59:99–113
2. Jones A (1951) Orbital X-ray therapy of progressive exophthalmos. Br J Radiol 24:637–646
3. Beiewaltes WH (1951) Irradiation of the pituitary in the treatment of malignant exophthalmos. J Clin Endocrinal Metab 11:512–530
4. Beierwaltes WH (1953) X-ray treatment of malignant exophthalmos: a report on 28 patients. J Clin Endocrinol Metab 13:1090–1100
5. Gedda PO, Lindgren M (1954) Pituitary and orbital roentgen therapy in the hyperophthalmopathic type of Graves' disease. Acta Radiol 42:211–220
6. Wijndbladh HJ, Mossberg H, Liungman S (1954) On exophthalmos and its treatment. Acta Endocrinol 17:442–451
7. Hermann K (1972) Pituitary exophthalmos: an assessment of methods of treatment. Br J Ophthalmol 36:1–19
8. Donaldson SS, Bagshaw MA, Kriss JP (1973) Supervoltage orbital radiotherapy for Graves' ophthalmopathy. J Clin Endocrinol Metab 37:276–285
9. Marcocci C, Bartalena L, Bogazzi F, Bruno-Bossio G, Lepri A, Pinchera A (1991) Orbital radiotherapy combined with high dose systemic glucocorticoids for Graves' ophthalmopathy is more effective than radiotherapy alone: results of a prospective randomized study. J Endocrinol Invest 14: 853–860
10. Marcocci C, Bartalena L, Bogazzi F, Bruno-Bossio G, Pinchera A (1991) Role of orbital radiotherapy in the treatment of Graves' ophthalmopathy. Exp Clin Endocrinol 97:332–337
11. Kao SC, Kendler DL, Nugent RA, Adler JS, Rootman J (1993) Radiotherapy in the management of thyroid orbitopathy. Computed tomography and clinical outcomes. Arch Ophthalmol 111:819–823
12. Petersen IA, Kriss JP, McDougall IR, Donaldson SS (1990) Prognostic factors in the radiotherapy of Graves' ophthalmopathy. Int J Radiat Oncol Biol Phys 19:259–264
13. Kazim M, Trokel S, Moore S (1991) Treatment of acute Graves orbitopathy. Ophthalmology 98: 1443–1448

14. Lloyd WC 3rd, Leone CR Jr (1992) Supervoltage orbital radiotherapy in 36 cases of Graves' disease. Am J Ophthalmol 113:374–380
15. Mourits MP, van Kempen-Harteveld ML, Garcia MB, Koppeschaar HP, Tick L, Terwee CB (2000) Radiotherapy for Graves' orbitopathy: randomised placebo-controlled study. Lancet 355:1505–1509
16. Prummel MF, Terwee CB, Gerding MN, et al. (2004) A randomized controlled trial of orbital radiotherapy versus sham irradiation in patients with mild Graves' ophthalmopathy. J Clin Endocrinol Metab 89:15–20
17. Gorman CA, Garrity JA, Fatourechi V, et al. (2001) A prospective, randomized, double-blind, placebo-controlled study of orbital radiotherapy for Graves' ophthalmopathy. Ophthalmology 108:1523–1534
18. Gorman CA, Garrity JA, Fatourechi V, et al. (2002) The aftermath of orbital radiotherapy for Graves' ophthalmopathy. Ophthalmology 109:2100–2107
19. Robertson DM, Buettner H, Gorman CA, et al. (2003) Retinal microvascular abnormalities in patients treated with external radiation for Graves ophthalmopathy. Arch Ophthalmol 121: 652–657
20. Wiersinga WM (2002) Perspective – part III: retrobulbar irradiation in Graves orbitopathy: the Dutch experience. Ophthal Plast Reconstr Surg 18:175–176
21. Kazim M (2002) Perspective – part II: radiotherapy for Graves orbitopathy: the Columbia University experience. Ophthal Plast Reconstr Surg 18: 173–174
22. Bartley GB, Gorman CA (2002) Perspective – part I: the Mayo orbital radiotherapy for Graves ophthalmopathy (ORGO) study: lessons learned. Ophthal Plast Reconstr Surg 18:170–172
23. Trott KR, Kamprad F (1999) Radiobiological mechanisms of anti-inflammatory radiotherapy. Radiother Oncol 51:197–203
24. Marcocci C, Bartalena L, Rocchi R, et al. (2003) Long-term safety of orbital radiotherapy for Graves' ophthalmopathy. J Clin Endocrinol Metab 88:3561–3566
25. Akmansu M, Dirican B, Bora H, Gurel O (2003) The risk of radiation-induced carcinogenesis after external beam radiotherapy of Graves' orbitopathy. Ophthalmic Res 35:150–153
26. Snijders-Keilholz A, De Keizer RJ, Goslings BM, Van Dam EW, Jansen JT, Broerse JJ (1996) Probable risk of tumour induction after retro-orbital irradiation for Graves' ophthalmopathy. Radiother Oncol 38:69–71
27. Schaefer U, Hesselmann S, Micke O, et al. (2002) A long-term follow-up study after retro-orbital irradiation for Graves' ophthalmopathy. Int J Radiat Oncol Biol Phys 52:192–197
28. Wakelkamp IM, Tan H, Saeed P, et al. (2004) Orbital irradiation for Graves' ophthalmopathy: Is it safe? A long-term follow-up study. Ophthalmology 111:1557–1562
29. Just M, Kahaly G, Higer HP, et al. (1991) Graves ophthalmopathy: role of MR imaging in radiation therapy. Radiology 179:187–190
30. Gerding MN, van der Zant FM, van Royen EA, et al. (1999) Octreotide scintigraphy is a disease-activity parameter in Graves' ophthalmopathy. Clin Endocrinol (Oxf) 50:373–379
31. Ott M, Breiter N, Albrecht CF, Pradier O, Hess CF, Schmidberger H (2002) Can contrast enhanced MRI predict the response of Graves' ophthalmopathy to orbital radiotherapy? Br J Radiol 75: 514–517
32. Prummel MF, Gerding MN, Zonneveld FW, Wiersinga WM (2001) The usefulness of quantitative orbital magnetic resonance imaging in Graves' ophthalmopathy. Clin Endocrinol (Oxf) 54:205–209
33. Terwee CB, Prummel MF, Gerding MN, Kahaly GJ, Dekker FW, Wiersinga WM (2005) Measuring disease activity to predict therapeutic outcome in Graves' ophthalmopathy. Clin Endocrinol (Oxf) 62:145–155
34. Kahaly GJ, Rosler HP, Pitz S, Hommel G (2000) Low- versus high-dose radiotherapy for Graves' ophthalmopathy: a randomized, single blind trial. J Clin Endocrinol Metab 85:102–108
35. Gerling J, Kommerell G, Henne K, Laubenberger J, Schulte-Monting J, Fells P (2003) Retrobulbar irradiation for thyroid-associated orbitopathy: double-blind comparison between 2.4 and 16 Gy. Int J Radiat Oncol Biol Phys 55:182–189

Bony Orbital Decompression Techniques

9

K.E. Morgenstern, Paul Proffer, Jill A. Foster

Core Messages

- Inflammation of the orbital soft tissues in Graves' orbitopathy, which is characterized by infiltration of the extraocular muscles, orbital fat, and lacrimal gland, may necessitate surgical intervention to preserve vision
- The resulting discrepancy between the closed bony space of the orbit and the expanding inflamed soft tissue volume within may be managed by performing boney orbital decompression surgery
- Indications for bone decompression include patients who fail medical therapy, suffer from globe subluxation or pain from a "tight" orbit, have documented ocular hypertension, or who may have significant cosmetic concerns
- Different types of incisions may be used to gain access to the walls of the orbit and include the lateral canthal, transconjunctival, transcaruncular, transcutaneous, antral and endoscopic approaches
- Multiple surgical techniques exist to decompress the lateral wall, orbital floor, and medial walls of the orbit
- The incision and bone decompression technique chosen is dependent upon the clinical situation, the surgeon's experience, and the patient's expectations

9.1 Introduction

The soft tissue compartment of the orbit undergoes pathologic expansion in Graves' orbitopathy. The resulting discrepancy between space and volume may result in the need to surgically enlarge the boundaries of the bony orbit. Alteration of the orbital soft tissues is characterized by infiltration of the extraocular muscles, orbital fat, and lacrimal gland by inflammatory cells such as lymphocytes [1]. Activation of orbital fibroblasts and deposition of glycosaminoglycans are typical of the inflammatory phase of the disease. During this acute or inflammatory phase, the patient may complain of deep orbital discomfort, tearing, photophobia, visual changes and diplopia. The clinician may observe exophthalmos, corneal exposure from lid retraction or proptosis, congestive changes in the conjunctiva, and motility disturbances. In severe cases, optic neuropathy may develop secondary to an orbital compartment syndrome with increased orbital pressure. In such cases, the patient may present with or develop decreased vision. Clinical assessment may reveal an afferent pupil defect, dyschromatopsia, and/or visual field defects [2, 3].

Mild acute orbitopathy may be managed conservatively but more severe cases may require steroids, orbital radiotherapy, or surgical decompression in order to protect vision. The role of orbital decompression surgery in Graves' orbitopathy, its history, indications, techniques, and complications will be the focus of this chapter.

9.2 History of Bony Decompression

Dollinger was the first to perform a bony orbital decompression in 1911. His technique, modeled after Kronlein's lateral approach to the orbit for tumors, involved removing the lateral wall and decompressing the orbital contents into the temporalis fossa [4–7]. This technique resulted in minimal orbital volume expansion. In 1931, Naffziger described an approach through the orbital roof to decompress both orbital apices simultaneously in cases of bilateral optic neuropathy [8]. Unfortunately, this exposed the patient to risk of meningitis and transmission of cerebral pulsations to the eye [1]. It did not provide significant volume augmentation of the orbit. Sewall's decompression described in 1936 involved ethmoidectomy while Hirsch in 1950 was the first to describe an inferior orbitotomy [1]. The Walsh and Ogura technique reported in 1957 involved a transantral Caldwell-Luc decompression of the medial and inferior orbital walls avoiding an external incision [1]. This was often complicated by postoperative diplopia and infraorbital hypoesthesia. Preservation of the anterior periorbita has been suggested by Seiff et al. in order to reduce these postoperative motility disturbances [9]. In the early 1990s, endoscopic technology improved endonasal orbital decompression techniques as described by Kennedy and others [10]. Absence of an external incision scar and diminished surgical force on the already compressed structures of the tight orbit were advocated as advantages of this technique as well as better access for removal of the ethmoid air cells and medial orbital floor. Shortly thereafter, Olivari described a technique for removal of orbital fat to diminish orbital volume in Graves' orbitopathy [11]. Kazim and Trokel modified the technique of fat decompression to treat optic neuropathy in patients where computed tomography (CT) preoperatively identified a relative increase in the volume of the intraorbital fat [6]. Transconjunctival approaches to the medial orbital wall and orbital floor have also proven valuable in minimizing postoperative scar [12], and have proven to be efficacious for the treatment of compressive optic neuropathy [13].

Techniques for orbital decompression continue to evolve. Terms such as "balanced orbital decompression" and "graded orbital decompression" indicate that today's approach to surgical enlargement of the orbital space relies on combinations of these techniques. The surgical approach, incision and the extent of bony wall removal should be tailored to the individual patient's needs and the surgeon's experience. Advancements made in this field have led to a broader range of indications for performing orbital decompression surgery.

9.3 Indications

Nonsurgical management of the inflammatory phase of Graves' orbitopathy includes protective lubrication, systemic steroids and external beam radiation. Patients who fail to respond and are developing progressive optic neuropathy or visually threatening exophthalmos such as globe subluxation or corneal exposure can be considered for bony decompression. Patients with thyroid eye disease may also have a "tight orbit", which can result in significant orbital pain. Orbital decompression surgery has been shown to provide pain relief in some of these patients [14]. Ocular hypertension is also associated with Graves' orbitopathy. This may be the result of several factors, and decompression may help to lower intraocular pressure [15].

Those with longstanding stable disease can also be considered for orbital expansion surgery to improve aesthetically objectionable exophthalmos. These cosmetic indications have more recently been accepted as legitimate criteria for orbital decompression because of the social and psychological implications of proptosis. Lyons and Rootman described a case series of 65 transantral orbital decompression procedures for 34 patients who had surgery for this reason. Inclusion criteria for cosmetic decompression included Hertel measurements of 23 mm or more in men and 20 mm or more in women. Occupational history and old photographs were also taken into consideration [16].

Goldberg et al. performed a series of decompressions for six cases of non-Graves-associated proptosis. Inclusion criteria included congenitally shallow orbits, enlarged globes secondary to high myopia, and hypoplastic malar eminences with scleral show [17]. Together these studies have helped to establish these new indications.

9.4 Characterizing Decompressive Surgery

Perhaps the easiest way to characterize bony orbital decompression surgery is by the surfaces that are removed. There are three walls in the orbit that are available for surgical decompression. The first is the medial wall, which overlies the ethmoid air cells. Removing the medial wall from the posterior lacrimal crest back to the anterior face of the sphenoid sinus is particularly effective in treating compressive optic neuropathy and in modestly increasing orbital volume. The second surface is the floor of the orbit overlying the maxillary sinus. The surgical orbital floor has two areas for bone reduction. It is divided into the medial and lateral floor by the infraorbital groove and nerve. The medial floor extends from the medial orbital strut to the infraorbital nerve, and the lateral surgical floor is bounded by the path of the infraorbital nerve nasally and the inferior orbital fissure laterally. The third surface for decompression includes both the anterior aspect of the lateral wall adjacent to the temporalis muscle and the deep lateral wall of the orbit consisting of the greater and lesser wings of the sphenoid between the superior and inferior orbital fissures. Decompression in the anterior lateral wall is limited by the temporalis muscle and posteriorly by the dura of the anterior and middle cranial fossa [14].

In contrast to bony decompression to create volume expansion and thus diminish soft tissue compression, orbital fat decompression works by reducing the total intraorbital volume. This technique relies on removal of intraconal orbital fat and can be used in conjunction with bony decompression or as an isolated procedure.

9.5 Surgical Approach

There are several incisions that may be used to gain access to the walls of the orbit. The approach chosen is dependent upon the clinical situation, the surgeon's experience, and the patient's expectations. For example, the medial wall can be approached through an external Lynch incision (Fig. 9.1), a transcaruncular incision, or an endoscopic endonasal approach. The Lynch incision made in the skin between the medial junction of the upper and lower eyelids and the bridge of the nose provides excellent exposure to the medial wall, but leaves a skin scar. The transcaruncular incision has a somewhat more limited view, but leaves no visible skin scar. Endoscopic endonasal techniques also leave no external scar, but have more technically challenging variability in anatomy, and more difficulty in leaving the medial strut intact while removing the medial wall. The orbital floor may be approached with an external subciliary incision, a transconjunctival incision, or a transantral approach with a buccal gingival sulcus incision. As with the endoscopic endonasal approach, the transantral approach creates some technical difficulty in reaching the inferomedial wall without removing the medial orbital strut. The lateral orbit can be approached from upper eyelid crease incisions, an extended lateral canthal incision, a lateral orbital rim incision, or a coronal incision. When the lateral orbital surface and the orbital floor are simultaneously needed for access, the most direct approach is through a lateral canthal "swinging eyelid" flap with release of the lateral canthal tendon and a transconjunctival incision to reach the floor. This same incision may also be extended up through the caruncle to better reach the medial orbital wall.

There are numerous techniques that may be used and a combination of orbital walls that may be altered to successfully decompress the orbit. The plan of approach should therefore be tailored to the surgeon's experience as well as to the specific patient's needs. For example, if control of compressive optic neuropathy is the primary goal, then the surgeon should choose a

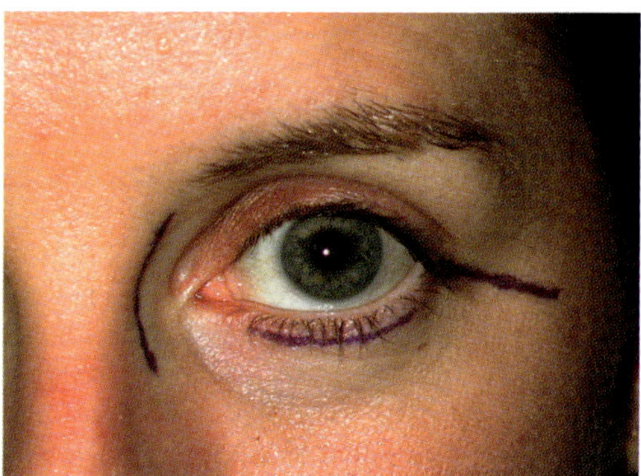

Fig. 9.1. The Lynch incision made in the skin between the medial junction of the upper and lower eyelids and the bridge of the nose provides excellent exposure to the medial wall. The orbital floor may be approached through an external subciliary incision as shown as well as a transconjunctival incision. An extended lateral canthal incision may be used to gain wide exposure to the lateral bony rim

procedure with proven efficacy while minimizing complications. In this case altering any of the three walls in the orbit or removing orbital fat would be appropriate since each has been shown to be beneficial in treating optic neuropathy.

It is recognized that postoperative diplopia is seen more frequently with inferomedial decompression, asymmetric decompression, and removal of the medial orbital strut. Since our first goal is preservation of vision, these considerations may become less important when an urgent decompression is needed. Postoperative motility disturbance may also be influenced by features unrelated to surgical technique such as degree of orbital inflammation at the time of surgery, the presence of optic neuropathy, and preoperative radiotherapy [18].

In contrast to compressive optic neuropathy, if the primary purpose of the surgery is to reposition the orbital contents, certain axioms may then be applied; the more walls removed, the greater the potential space is created, and the more walls removed, the longer the surgery time. As a rule of thumb, each wall provides 2–3 mm of reduction in proptosis. Fat decompression will add an additional 2–4 mm. Lateral wall advancement or orbital rim augmentation can change the relationship of the lateral canthus to the corneal surface by 2–3 mm in Hertel measurements. It is therefore necessary to document the extent of the preoperative exophthalmos and the relative protrusion compared to the fellow eye. The three-dimensional position of the globe relative to the contralateral eye also becomes crucial in selecting the surgical approach when repositioning the eye. If the only eye to be operated on is vertically level with the unoperated side, then a maximal floor decompression with removal of the nasal floor and drilling out the floor lateral to the groove will likely result in vertical globe dystopia, and may not be the first surgical choice. If, however, the side planned for surgery shows several millimeters of hyperglobus, the surgeon may choose to do a thorough removal of the bony floor.

9.6 Bony Decompression Techniques

9.6.1 Anterior and Posterior Lateral Wall

In a 1998 editorial, Goldberg advocated that the lateral wall should be the first wall to decompress [14]. He supported this premise with data from his and other studies showing that in contrast to the medial and floor decompression, the lateral decompression has less chance of causing diplopia because the muscle cone is not shifted inferomedially [19]. Up to 5 cm^3 of bony volume and 6 mm of retro-globe placement can be achieved through this approach [14]. An upper eyelid crease incision or a lateral canthal incision and inferior conjunctival incision are the most direct approaches to the lateral orbital wall. A coronal flap has been described and does allow access to the posterior aspect of the lateral wall but is typically reserved for severe proptosis requiring maximal decompression or in the patient adamant about avoiding visible surgical scars. The lateral wall may be removed and anteriorly replaced [20] or it may be left in position and sculpted using a drill and burr.

The authors of this chapter approach maximal decompression of the lateral orbital wall using a lateral canthal incision made with a #15 Bard Parker blade (Fig. 9.2). The incision is car-

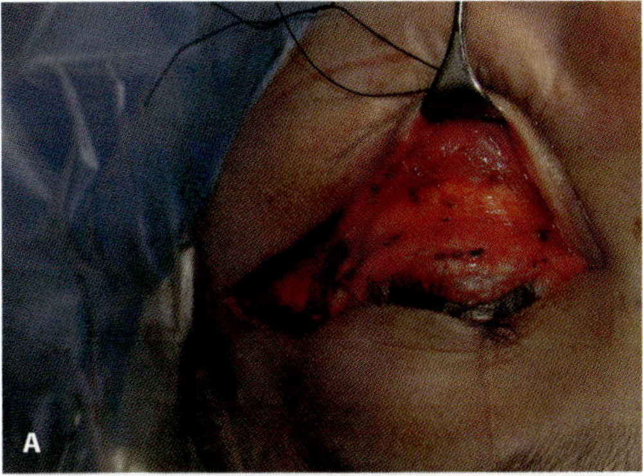

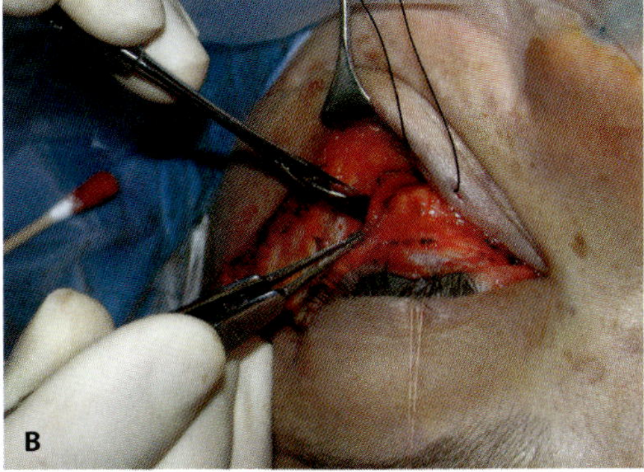

Fig. 9.2. A When performing a lateral orbital wall decompression a lateral canthal incision is made using a #15 Bard Parker blade. The incision is carried down 2 cm lateral to the lateral orbital rim. A lateral cantholysis is then fashioned to release the lower eyelid. **B** Additional inferior exposure is obtained with a transconjunctival incision across the lower eyelid. The periosteum is then scored with the monopolar cautery and elevated off the anterior bony rim and laterally off the backside of the zygomatic and frontal bone portions of the lateral orbital rim

ried down 2 cm lateral to the lateral orbital rim. A lateral cantholysis is then fashioned to release the lower eyelid. Additional inferior exposure may be obtained with a transconjunctival incision across the lower eyelid. The deep temporalis fascia and underlying muscle below the horizontal incision are incised. The periosteum is then scored with the monopolar cautery and elevated off the anterior bony rim and laterally off the backside of the zygomatic and frontal bone portions of the lateral orbital rim. The periosteum is then elevated off the internal orbital lateral bony wall. Care is taken to leave the periosteum of the orbit as intact as possible to facilitate exposure. The periosteum is most adherent along the arcus marginalis, and thin in the lacrimal gland fossa. The assistant holds Sewell retractors or ribbon retractors to retract the orbital contents once the periosteum has been partially released. The surgeon uses the suction in one hand and a periosteal elevator in the other. A headlight becomes essential for illumination once the deeper orbit is reached. The inferior orbital fissure provides a landmark for the junction between the "surgical" lateral orbital wall and the floor. For maximal volumetric decompression, the technique described includes removal of the lateral wall with anteroplacement of the lateral orbital rim. In order to achieve this, an oscillating saw is used to deeply score the lateral rim in two places: the lateral wall at the zygomatic-frontal suture line superiorly and just above the zygomatic arch inferiorly. While operating the saw, ribbon retractors are used to protect the soft tissues of the orbit, and Desmarres retractors used to pull back the soft tissue along the rim. Two large Kocher clamps are placed on the bony rim, and the rim is outfractured. Remaining fragments of the thin lateral rim are removed with rongeurs. The inner table of the bone that is too thick to remove or inaccessible with rongeurs is then sculpted with a 3-mm burr down to the level of the marrow (Fig. 9.3 A). Bleeding indicates this level has been reached. The bleeding may then be treated with cautery, bone wax or switching to a diamond burr. An incision of the orbital periosteum above and below the lateral rectus muscle may then allow the orbital contents to shift more easily to take up the additional space that has been created by the bone removal.

When the desired amount of bone has been removed posteriorly, the rim can then be replaced either at its original position, or may be advanced 2–3 mm anterior to its original location, and fixed into place using titanium plates [20] (Fig. 9.3 B). The periosteum is then reapproximated and the temporalis muscle is sutured together using interrupted Vicryl sutures. The incision is closed in a layered fashion and the lateral canthus is reconstructed.

A variation of this technique has been described by Goldberg et al. In this method, the wall is not removed, but the inner aspect is sculpted using the burr with lateral rim intact.

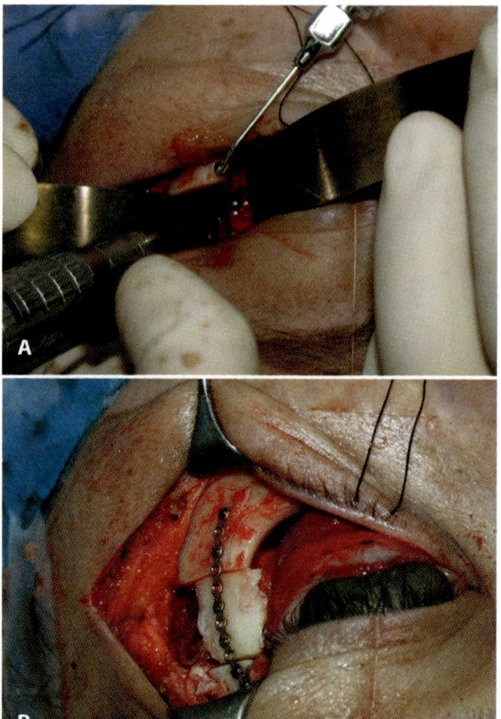

Fig. 9.3. A The inner table of the bone that is too thick to remove or inaccessible with rongeurs is then sculpted with a 3-mm burr down to the level of the marrow. B When the desired amount of bone has been removed posteriorly, the rim can then be replaced advancing the repositioned bone 2–3 mm anterior to its original location, and then fixing the bone into place using titanium plates

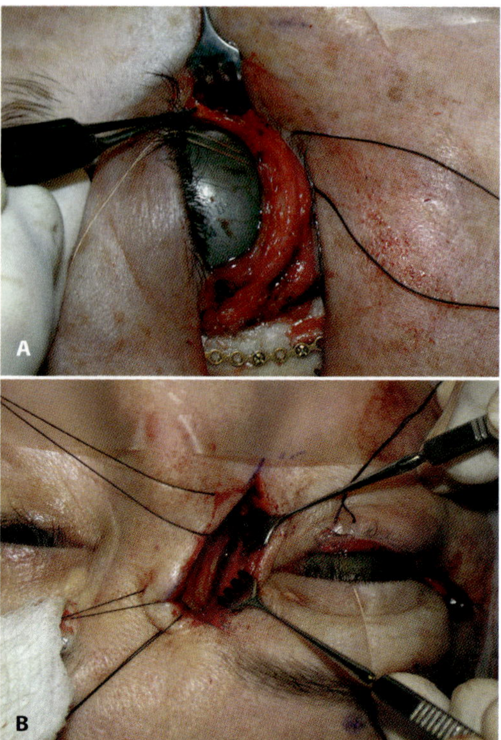

Fig. 9.4. A In approaching the medial wall a transcaruncular approach is quick and allows visualization to the optic canal ring. It leaves no cutaneous scarring and requires no special equipment setup. It has the benefit of being used alone or as an extension of an inferior fornix incision commonly used to access the orbital floor. B In cases of extreme orbital swelling, however, visualization may be difficult and the Lynch incision may be used. Visualization is often better but an unsightly scar may develop

In place of the anterior movement of the actual bone, onlay grafts may be added to anteriorly displace the attachments of the lateral canthal tendon and eyelids [17].

9.6.2 Medial Wall

The medial wall decompression may be performed as an isolated single wall alteration, or as an adjunct to other types of bony orbital expansion. In addressing the medial wall, a transcaruncular (Fig. 9.4A) approach may be used to avoid a cutaneous incision, while providing excellent exposure. The transcaruncular incision has the flexibility of being used alone or as an extension of a transconjunctival incision, which is commonly used to access the orbital floor. In cases of extreme orbital swelling and exophthalmos, visualization may be difficult and the Lynch incision (Fig. 9.4B) may be used. Visualization is often better, but scarring in the medial canthal region is unpredictable. An endoscopic transnasal approach has also been described [21] and can allow for simultaneous medial wall and floor decompression without leaving an external incision. In the inflamed orbit, the transnasal approach may avoid the need to retract or manipulate inflamed and friable orbital tissues. Finally, a coronal approach has been described but offers no significant advantages [22].

Patients are induced with general anesthesia and local anesthetic is injected in the areas of the incisions. Supraorbital and infraorbital nerves should also be anesthetized for postoperative comfort. The nose may be packed with 4% cocaine, Neosynephrine, or oxymetazoline soaked neuro paddies. Patients are given a dose of intravenous antibiotic as a successful decompression results in sinus communication with the orbit. A standard prep and drape is then performed. In the transcaruncular approach a Westcott scissor is used to incise the caruncle. A 6–0 Vicryl suture is used to mark the edges of the caruncle for ease of alignment and closure at the end of the case. A Steven's scissor can then be placed through the incision at a posterior medial angle. The tips are then spread vertically, enlarging the incision. Skin hooks or lacrimal rakes are employed by the assistant to improve exposure. The periosteum is visualized along the medial wall and can be incised vertically using the sharp edge of a periosteal elevator. Blunt dissection releases the medial orbital periosteum from the bone. Care should be taken to avoid uncontrolled disruption of the anterior and posterior ethmoid arteries. Gentle pressure can then be applied to the medial wall infracturing the bone into the ethmoid sinuses. Using the ethmoid arteries as a guide to the most superior aspect of the decompression will help avoid unintentional entry of the cribriform plate and anterior cranial fossa. Takahashi forceps are helpful if the mucosa of the air cells needs to be removed. Thick bone may be removed with the drill, but is not usually necessary for an adequate medial decompression of the orbit. Incisions are made in the periosteum above and below the medial rectus muscle to allow egress of the orbital fat through the periosteal openings into the space created by the destruction of the sinuses.

9.6.3 Floor

A floor decompression with preservation of the maxillary strut is often used in combination with the medial wall decompression. It can be approached through an inferior conjunctival fornix incision, transantral incision, or endoscopic transnasal approach. Unfortunately, using the latter two of these incisions makes it slightly more difficult to spare the maxillary strut, which can be a significant source of postoperative diplopia. That said, a orbital decompression that leaves the ethmoid-maxillary strut intact may still result in diplopia and globe displacement. By decompressing the floor and medial wall, the maxillary and ethmoid sinuses respectively are violated and chronic sinusitis can result. The dura above the fovea ethmoidalis is not typically visualized during this type of decompression and inadvertent laceration can result in intracranial bleeding or even chronic cerebrospinal fluid leaks [14].

The inferior fornix incision is made approximately 3 mm below the inferior edge of the lower lid tarsus and is the most commonly used approach among oculoplastic surgeons (Fig. 9.5 A). In combining this incision with a transcaruncular approach to the medial wall, one should be aware of the inferior oblique muscle which originates from the anterior medial aspect of the inferior rim. The dissection plane is anterior to the septum and carried down to the orbital rim. The periosteum is scored and elevated off the floor of the orbit using a periosteal elevator. The inferior orbital canal is usually easily identifiable and is used as the lateral aspect of the floor decompression (Fig. 9.5 B). The bone along the medial aspect of the floor is relatively thin and can usually be easily removed using a Kerrison punch or bone rongeur. Using this direct approach to the floor makes it relatively easy to preserve the maxillary strut medially. The posterior limit of decompression is the back wall of the maxillary sinus and can usually be detected as the bone in this area becomes thicker and more difficult to remove. Once bone removal has been completed, the periosteum is scored and the intraconal

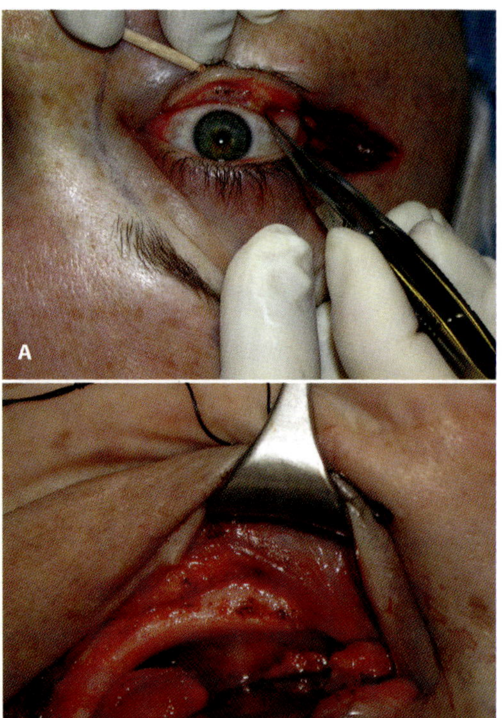

Fig. 9.5 A–B. The inferior fornix incision is made approximately 3 mm below the inferior edge of the lower lid tarsus and is the most commonly used approach among oculoplastic surgeons. This approach allows excellent exposure to the orbital floor and medial maxillary strut

fat is teased out along the radial incisions. Care should be taken when making these incisions in the periosteum to avoid injuring the rectus muscles, which are often enlarged in thyroid eye disease. Although less satisfying in the amount of volume augmentation that it provides, there is a triangle of bone between the infraorbital canal and the inferior orbital fissure that may also be debulked. Removal of this bone will require the use of the drill. Occasionally there will be access to the maxillary sinus through this space; other times one drills until soft tissue is encountered. The floor decompression technique may also be used in concert with a lateral wall decompression or with removal of intraconal orbital fat.

Removal of the inferior and medial walls together has been associated with risks of strabismus, infraorbital anesthesia, CSF rhinorrhea, nasolacrimal duct obstruction, oroantral fistula, and blindness [23]. Recent attention to the preservation of the maxillary strut and the bone overlying the infraorbital nerve has been more successful in protecting the nerve and reduces the risk of hypoglobus [24].

9.6.4 Roof

A decompression of the orbital roof as opposed to the deep lateral wall (sphenoid wing) was first described as a neurosurgical procedure. This approach to Graves' orbitopathy proved more effective than the original lateral decompression but had a significant morbidity associated with it. These patients had longer hospital stays, frontal lobe signs such as confusion or disorientation, rhinorrhea, pulsating globes, and risks of meningitis [22, 25]. Proptosis was reported to have decreased anywhere from 1 to 7 mm. Gorman et al. compared the results of lateral and frontal decompression with transantral decompression and found them to be equally effective. While the morbidity was lower in the latter, the incidence of diplopia was higher [26]. Practically speaking, the superior orbital roof would be the last wall considered for orbital decompression.

9.7 Alternative Approaches to Orbital Decompression

9.7.1 Transantral

The transantral approach (Caldwell-Luc) is an effective way of decompressing the orbit into the maxillary and ethmoid sinuses. Ogura first reported on a large series of patients treated with transantral decompression by removing a portion of the orbital floor and medial wall [27]. Most patients had improvement of their visual symptoms; however, four of them actually had a decrease in their measured acuity. While overall results of the transantral approach have been good, there have been significant complications reported [2, 28–30].

This technique is approached through the canine fossa. This area of mucoperiosteum superior to the teeth on the face of the maxilla is infiltrated with local anesthetic and adrenaline. An incision is made and carried down to the bone. The tissue is elevated superiorly off the maxillary face until the maxillary nerve (infraorbital nerve), which exits the infraorbital foramen in the midpupillary line, is identified. Care is taken not to injure this nerve. The face of the maxillary sinus is then opened using a chisel to create an entry point and then Kerrison rongeurs to enlarge the opening. The orbital floor is now visualized and can be removed using rongeurs. Leaving bone intact around the infraorbital nerve will help prevent postoperative hypoesthesia. The periosteum is then incised and the orbital fat allowed to prolapse into the sinuses. Exenteration of the ethmoid air cells may also be achieved through this approach, allowing the surgeon to perform both a medial wall and orbital floor decompression. Finally, an inferior nasal antrostomy is performed for drainage.

9.7.2 Endoscopic

Two major advantages of the intranasal approach are that there is no cutaneous scarring and it provides the ability to directly visualize the apical area of the orbit. The contraindications for endoscopic decompression include sinusitis, nasal polyps, contracted maxillary antrum, and thick orbital floor. Because of these issues, CT scanning of the orbit preoperatively is imperative. This approach is limited in the amount of anterior orbital floor that can be removed.

The floor and medial wall may also be approached using an endoscopic transnasal technique. The patient is placed supine and the nose is packed using 4% cocaine, Neo-synephrine or oxymetazoline. The whole face is then prepped into the surgical field and submucosal injection of local anesthetic is placed in the lateral nasal wall and middle turbinates. This is usually done under direct endoscopic visualization. The middle turbinate is infractured, displaced medially, or resected when necessary for access. A surgical incision is then created in the uncinate process. The incision is just posterior to the maxillary line on a bony eminence that extends from the anterior attachment of the middle turbinate to the root of the inferior turbinate. The bone of the uncinate process is then removed. The maxillary ostium should then be enlarged to provide optimal exposure of the orbital floor. The medial wall may be downfractured with a curette. Bone is then removed in a posterior direction stopping at the back of the maxillary sinus. Anterior removal stops at the thick bone of the frontal process of the maxilla, which protects the nasolacrimal duct. The ostium is enlarged superiorly to the level of the orbital floor and inferiorly to the root of the inferior turbinate. A 30-degree endoscope may be used to enter the maxillary sinus and to identify the infraorbital nerve along the roof of the sinus. The medial wall is removed by performing an ethmoidectomy under direct visualization. The anterior and posterior ethmoid arteries can be identified during this procedure avoiding unnecessary bleeding. The bones of the lamina papyracea are excised. The thick bone encountered approximately 2 mm anterior to the sphenoid face represents the annulus of Zinn and should not be removed. Attention is then directed back to the orbital floor where remaining bone medial to the infraorbital nerve can be removed. The nerve will mark the lateral limits of the orbital floor decompression.

After bony removal the periosteum can then be scored using a sickle knife and the orbital fat teased out into the ethmoid and maxillary sinuses. In cases of acute inflammatory thyroid eye disease, the fat may prolapse easily. If extensive fibrosis has occurred, then gentle teasing of the fat may be necessary. It is important to remember when making this incision that the rectus muscles lie immediately deep to this tissue plane and may be enlarged secondary to thyroid disease.

Like other techniques of bony decompression, the endoscopic approach may also be coupled with lateral wall decompression or orbital fat removal [21].

9.7.3 Orbital Fat Decompression

Decompression of the intraorbital fat content, termed fat removal orbital decompression (FROD), has been mentioned intermittently through this chapter. Although it does not involve actual bone removal it has been reported to reduce proptosis with less morbidity than that of bony decompression [6, 15]. It is becoming more common to include this technique at least as an adjunct to bony orbital expansion.

A retrospective review of 41 FROD surgeries performed by transseptal excision of extra- and intraconal fat demonstrates adequate proptosis reduction with fewer side effects. Mean reduction of proptosis by 4.7 mm was achieved by excising 7.31±1.9 ml of orbital fat. Using this technique one must be careful of the lacrimal gland laterally, the superior oblique and medial rectus medially, and the superior orbital nerve superiorly. There is a lower rate of motility disturbances after FROD when compared with the traditional bony decompression techniques. In these studies, it was attributed to balanced fat removal around the eye as apposed to selective removal of one or several bony walls.

In Trokel's series of 158 fat decompressions performed there was an average reduction of 1.8 mm with the greatest reduction of 3.3 mm achieved in those with proptosis >25 mm. Gockel et al. found an improvement in visual field, motility, and IOP in five patients who received a fat decompression with microsurgical liposuction using a lateral canthotomy [31].

Historically, fat decompression had been limited in its clinical indication to reducing exophthalmos, eliminating orbital pain, and reducing congestion. More recently it has been used to treat optic nerve compression in patients who have failed medical management and whose CT or MRI scans demonstrate enlargement of the orbital fat compartment. This may be identified by direct measurements of the orbital fat volume.

Surgically, patients receive preoperative steroids and antibiotics. A lid crease incision is made in the medial half of the upper lid. A subciliary incision is made in the lower lid. The orbital septum is opened and prolapsing orbital fat removed using blunt surgical dissection and cautery. The use of ribbon retractors enables dissection deep into the orbit. Traction on the anterior orbital fat may be used to gain access to the intraconal fat. It is important not to transect the pedicle of fat until the final depth of the dissection is reached. The fat retracts and is difficult to relocate. On average, 3–6 ml of fat may be removed from the lower compartment and 2 ml through the superior compartment. After inspecting for bleeding, the incisions are closed. Patients should be observed for 24 h to monitor for postoperative bleeding [6, 32].

9.7.4 Potential Complications

Complications associated with orbital decompression surgery range from transient diplopia to visual loss or CSF leaks and death. The risk of the complications often differs based on the surgical approach taken. For example, Hochberg et al. showed that with a low frontal approach, the frontal branch of cranial nerve VII can be damaged. Goldberg et al. looked at the incidence of medial entropion after orbital decompression. In their series of 69 patients, they found that 20 % had postoperative medial entropion – with 6 % requiring further surgery. They found a strong correlation between these complications and the transantral approach, when it was compared with transconjunctival surgery.

Postoperative bleeding can be severe enough to damage the optic nerve and lead to central retinal vein occlusion. The anterior and posterior ethmoidal arteries are common sources, especially when working on the medial wall during an orbital or endoscopic approach. Medial bone removal should be below the ethmoidal suture line and posterior to the lacrimal sac fossa [33]. The anterior and posterior ethmoidal arteries exit just superior to the ethmoidal suture line.

Diplopia remains one of the most problematic effects of this surgery. Although it may be present prior to surgery, the procedure may amplify the amount of diplopia. This is often the result of more extensive decompressions, for example, those involving three walls. In addition, when these extensive decompressions involve the ethmoid sinus and the floor, a medial strut should be maintained. Without preservation of this strut, ocular dystopia with inferomedial displacement of the globe can result. This is caused by displacement of the muscle cone along with its orbital connections into the maxillary or ethmoid sinuses.

Other complications consist of hypoesthesia if the infraorbital nerve is damaged during orbital floor decompressions, and postoperative scarring if a skin approach is employed. Sinusitis may occur. An entropion may also occur if contraction of the conjunctiva occurs. CSF leaks may also occur if a decompression is carried above the frontal ethmoid suture line or too far posteriorly.

9.8 Conclusion

Both bony and soft tissue orbital decompression can reverse optic neuropathy, elevated IOP, exposure keratitis, extreme exophthalmos and some of the cosmetic changes produced by Graves' orbitopathy. Preoperative planning based on informed discussions with the patient, detailed clinical exam, and careful analysis of computed tomography, magnetic resonance imaging, and old photographs will help the surgeon choose the most appropriate procedure. Modern surgical techniques offer a variety of approaches that produce predictable results and lower rates of complications.

Summary for the Clinician

- **Graves' orbitopathy is an inflammatory condition that may cause the muscles and adipose tissues of the orbit to expand within the confines of the rigid orbital walls**
- **An orbital bone decompression may be performed to expand orbital volume and decrease pain, preserve vision, or improve cosmesis**
- **The lateral wall may be approached using a lateral canthal incision. The anterior aspect of the wall may be removed, burred down, and then replaced slightly anteriorly. Simultaneously, the posterior aspect of the lateral wall may be removed using rongeurs or alternatively with a 3-mm burr**
- **The orbital floor may be duly approached through the conjunctiva, endoscopically, or with a transantral incision. The bone is removed medial to the infraorbital nerve leaving the maxillary strut intact to minimize postoperative diplopia**
- **The medial wall decompression may be approached through a transcaruncular or Lynch incision and is completed by infracturing the medial wall into the ethmoid air cells**
- **Fat decompression surgery provides an alternative or adjunctive approach to boney decompression surgery**
- **Using modern techniques, and the tailoring of surgery to the specific patient needs, improves surgical outcomes and minimizes complications postoperatively**

References

1. Rizk SS, Papageorge A, Liberatore LA, et al. (2000) Bilateral simultaneous orbital decompression for Graves' orbitopathy with a combined endoscopic and Caldwell-Luc approach. Otolaryngol Head Neck Surg 122:216–221
2. Carter RD, Frueh BR, Hessburg TP, et al. (1991) Long term efficacy of orbital decompression for compressive optic neuropathy of Graves' disease. Ophthalmology 98:1435–1442
3. Kazim M, Goldberg RA, Smith TJ (2002) Insights into the pathogenesis of thyroid associated orbitopathy. Arch Ophthalmol 120:380–384
4. Dollinger J (1911) Die Druckentlastung der Augenhoehle durch Entfernung der Aeusseren Orbitalwand bei hochgradigem Exophthalmus (Morbus Basedoweii) und konsecutiver Hornhauterkrankung. Dtsch Med Wochenschr 37:1888
5. Kronlein RU (1913–1914) Die Traumatische Meningitis. In: Handbuch der praktischen Chirugie, vol 4
6. Trokel S, Kazim M, Moore S (1993) Orbital fat removal: decompression for Graves' orbitopathy. Ophthalmology 100:674–682
7. Weisman RA, Osguthorpe JD (1994) Orbital decompression in Graves' disease. Arch Otolaryngol Head Neck Surg 120:831–834
8. Lund VJ, Larkin G, Fells P, et al. (1997) Orbital decompression for thyroid eye disease. J Laryngol Otol 111:1051–1055

9. Seiff SR, Tovilla JL, Carter SR, et al. (2000) Modified transantral orbital decompression for dysthyroid orbitopathy. Ophthalmic Plast Reconstr Surg 16:62–66
10. Kennedy DW, Goodstein JL, Miller NR, Zinreich SJ (1990) Endoscopic transantral orbital decompression. Arch Otolaryngol Head Neck Surg 116: 275–282
11. Olivari N (1991) Transpalpebral decompression of endocrine ophthalmopathy (Graves' disease) by removal of intraorbital fat: experience with 147 operations over 5 years. Plast Reconst Surg 87: 627–643
12. Garcia GH, Goldberg RA, Shorr N (1998) The transcaruncular approach in repair of orbital fractures: a retrospective study. J Craniomaxillofac Trauma 4:7–12
13. Perry JD, Kadakia A, Foster JA (2003) Transcaruncular orbital decompression for dysthyroid optic neuropathy. Ophthalmic Plast Reconstr Surg 19: 353–358
14. Goldberg RA (1998) The evolving paradigm of orbital decompression surgery. Arch Ophthalmol 116:95–96
15. Adenis JP, Robert PY, Lasudry JG, et al. (1998) Treatment of proptosis with fat removal orbital decompression in Graves' ophthalmopathy. Eur J Ophthalmol 8:246–252
16. Lyons CJ, Rootman J (1994) Orbital decompression for disfiguring exophthalmos in thyroid orbitopathy. Ophthalmology 101:223–230
17. Goldberg RA, Hwang MM, Garbutt MV, et al. (1995) Orbital decompression for non-Graves' orbitopathy: a consideration of extended indications for decompression. Ophthalmic Plast Reconstr Surg 11:245–252
18. George JL, Tercero ME, Maalof T, et al. (2001) Clinical course and prognosis of diplopias after orbital bony wall decompression for thyroid related orbitopathy. J Fr Ophtalmologie 24:245–252
19. Hurwitz JJ, Birt D (1985) An individualized approach to orbital decompression in Graves' orbitopathy. Arch Ophthalmol 103:660
20. Wulc AE, Popp JC, Bartlett SP (1990) Lateral wall advancement in orbital decompression. Ophthalmology 97:1358
21. Metson R, Dallow R, Shore JW (1994) Endoscopic orbital decompression. Laryngoscope 104:950–957
22. Naffziger HC (1948) Exophthalmos: some surgical principles of surgical management from the neurosurgical aspect. Am J Surg 75:25–41
23. Van der Waal KG, de Visscher JG, Boukes RJ, et al. (2001) Surgical treatment of Graves' orbitopathy: a modified balanced technique. Int J Oral Maxillofac Surg 30:254–258
24. Paridaeins DA, Verhoeff K, Bouwens D, et al. (2000) Transconjunctival orbital decompression in Graves' ophthalmopathy: lateral wall approach ab interno. Br J Ophthalmol 84:775–781
25. Poppen JL (1950) The surgical treatment of progressive exophthalmos. J Clin Endocrinol 10:1231
26. Gorman CA, DeSanto LW, MacCarty CS, Riley FC (1974) Optic neuropathy of Graves' disease. Treatment by transantral or transfrontal orbital decompression. N Engl J Med 290:70
27. Ogura JH, Walsh TE (1962) The transantral orbital decompression operation for progressive exophthalmos. Laryngoscope 72:1078
28. Warren JD, Spector JG, Burde R (1989) Long term follow up and recent observation of 305 cases of orbital decompression for dysthyroid orbitopathy. Laryngoscope 99:35
29. Sessions RB, Wilkings RB, Weycer JS (1972) Endocrine exophthalmos. Arch Otolaryngol 95:46
30. Stell PM (1969) Transmaxillary orbital decompression for malignant exophthalmos. Proc R Soc Med 62:23
31. Gockel R, Winter R, Sistani F, et al. (2000) Minimal invasive decompression of the orbit in Graves' orbitopathy. Strabismus 8:251–259
32. Kazim M, Trokel SL, Acaroglu G, Eliott A (2000) Reversal of dysthyroid optic neuropathy following orbital fat decompression. Br J Ophthalmol 84:600–605
33. Colvard DM, Waller RR, Neault RW, DeSanto LW (1979) Nasolacrimal duct obstruction following transantral ethmoidal orbital decompression ophthalmus. Ophthalmic Surg 10:25

Orbital Decompression Using Fat Removal Orbital Decompression

10

Jean-Paul Adenis, Pierre-Yves Robert

Core Messages

- Orbital decompression can be achieved successfully by fat removal orbital decompression (FROD) or bone removal orbital decompression (BROD) in Graves' ophthalmopathy
- FROD leaves the possibility of concomitant palpebral and/or oculomotor surgery
- FROD or BROD, or combined surgery, may be performed initially, depending on the severity of clinical presentation, radiologic findings and previous treatments
- FROD is probably better indicated in patients with large bony orbital volume, large orbital fat volumes and stretched muscles, or cosmetic "grotesque" disability
- BROD is probably better indicated in patients with small bony orbital volume, small orbital fat volumes and enlarged muscles and/or with compressive optic neuropathy

10.1 Introduction

Dysthyroid orbitopathy (or Graves' ophthalmopathy) can cause increased orbital pressure, optic neuropathy, palpebral retraction, lagophthalmos and corneal exposure. For many patients their appearance is grotesque and esthetically unacceptable. Conservative treatment may involve systemic steroids or retrobulbar radiation therapy and a slow return to a normal thyroid status with the help of the endocrinologist. However, although effective in the treatment of the inflammatory component of the disease, these methods show little efficacy in the treatment of proptosis. Classical bone removal orbital decompression (BROD) has potential side effects, including infraorbital anesthesia, aggravation of ocular motility, globe displacement, and blindness.

In 1988, Olivari [1, 2] demonstrated that significant reduction of proptosis can be achieved by fat removal orbital decompression (FROD) alone. Thereafter, Trokel [3] published a series of 158 FROD procedures in 81 patients. Various types of surgical decompression combining FROD and BROD have been performed over the years: Hecht [4] described a two-wall decompression where the orbital medial wall and floor were removed, and resection of orbital fat was added through several incisions of the periorbita. Roncevic [5, 6] described a three-wall decompression (floor, lateral and medial wall) where defatting was added with removal of small lobules of fat. Liu [7] performed FROD alone in two children, with few complications. Morax [8] recently published 69 BROD procedures in which 57 were associated with fat removal. Moreiras [9] described a combined FROD-BROD technique through a small upper eyelid crease incision of 15–20 mm and his experience has extended to more than 1,000 cases. In the present article we describe the technique of FROD, report our experience and try to evaluate the advantages and drawbacks compared with BROD or with combined procedures

Therefore the challenge for the orbital surgeon for orbital decompression in the past was to choose between various techniques removing bone. More recently the choice is more complex between BROD, FROD, or both.

Summary for the Clinician

- **Graves' ophthalmopathy may induce proptosis, compressive optic neuropathy, palpebral retraction, lagophthalmos and corneal exposure**
- **Orbital decompression is required after failure of medical treatments (steroids, radiotherapy)**
- **FROD has developed since 1988 as an alternative to BROD. At present the choice and/or the association between both techniques is under discussion**

10.2 Description

The operation is performed with the patient under general anesthesia using an operating microscope (a 275-mm lens) and the help of two assistants [9].

10.2.1 The Upper Eyelid (Figs. 10.1–10.7)

After placement of a 4–0 Prolene suture, in the upper tarsus border near the eyelashes downward traction is applied to the upper eyelid. The incision is then made along the superior palpebral crease (as a blepharoplasty incision).

After dissecting off the orbicularis oculi muscle from the tarsus and the septum with the electric knife, the aponeurosis of the levator palpebrae superioris muscle and then the orbital septum are identified.

1. The dissection begins with the superomedian fat pad, while carefully avoiding injury to branches of the frontal nerve. Incision of the septum reveals the intraorbital fat, which bulges through the opening, and the lacrimal gland laterally. Whitnall's ligament can be visualized after the fat is retracted using a Desmarres' retractor. The resection begins at this point. The fat lobules are carefully resected after dissection with Vannas' long scissors, or directly with bipolar diathermy. This dissection can be hampered by bleeding (value of using bipolar diathermy) or especially fibro-

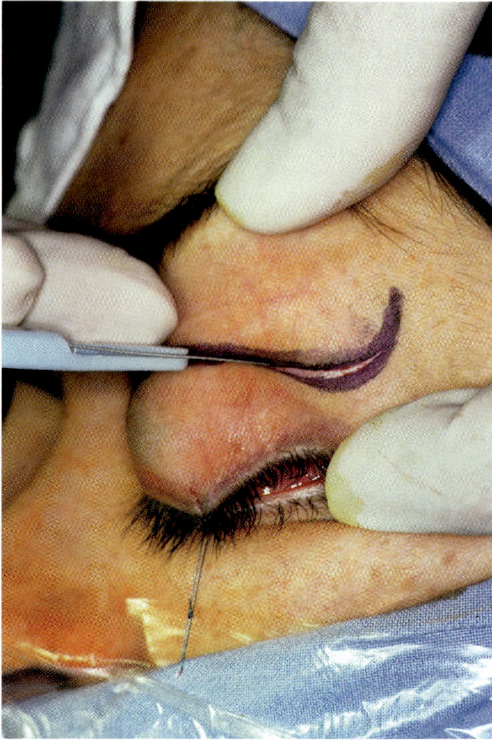

Fig. 10.1. Incision line in the upper eyelid skin crease

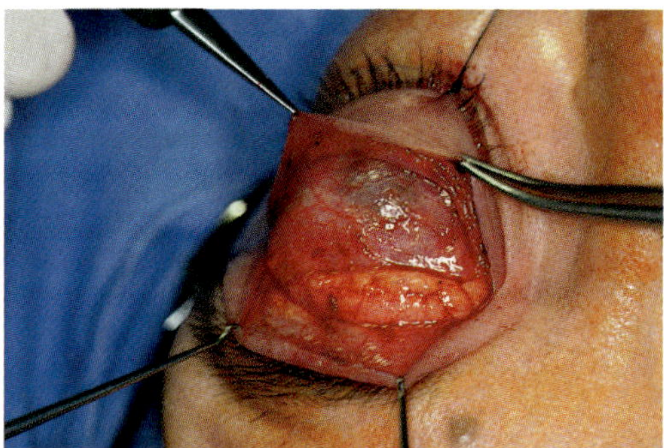

Fig. 10.2. Prolapse of the median fat pad behind the septum

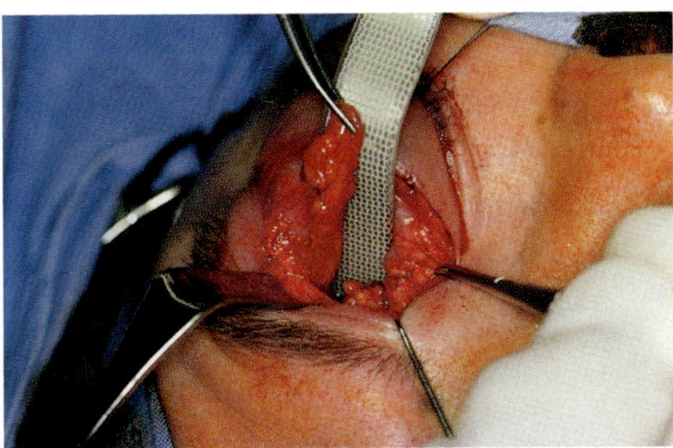

Fig. 10.3. Fat removal of the superior median fat pad after incision of the medial orbital septum

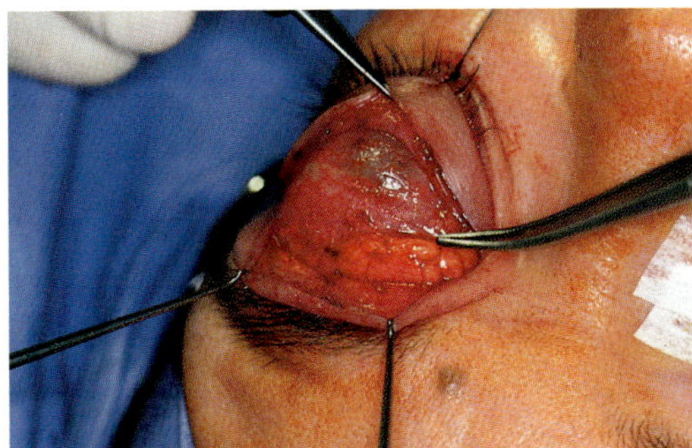

Fig. 10.4. Prolapse of the medial fat pad

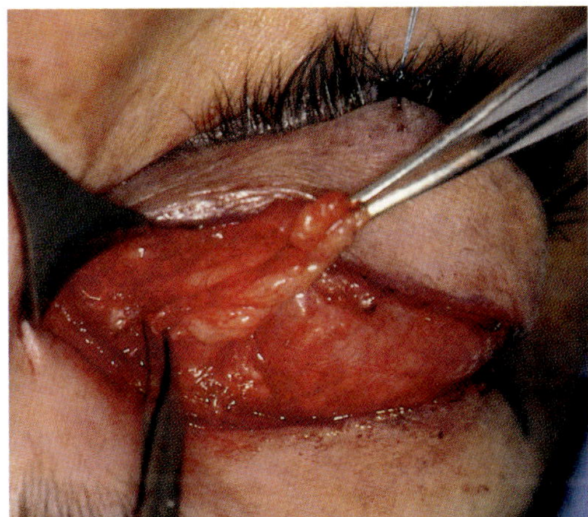

Fig. 10.5. Fat removal of the superior medial fat with retractors on the superior oblique and on the medial rectus muscle

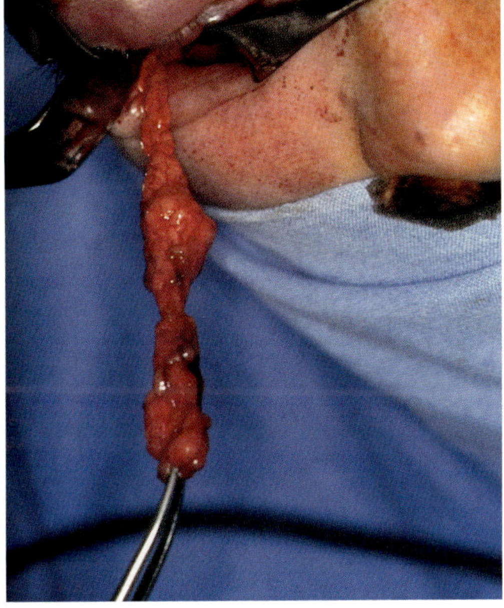

Fig. 10.6. Large volume of fat removed on a profile view

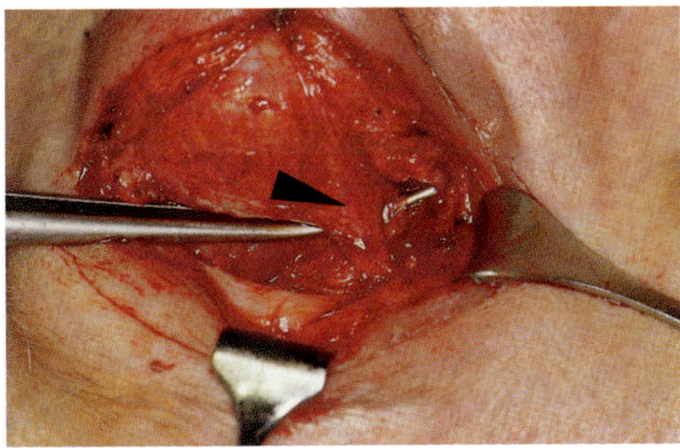

Fig. 10.7. Indirect portion, trochlea and direct portion of the superior oblique after fat removal

sis of the orbital septa, in particular if the patient has previously undergone radiotherapy. In this case, the fat lobules can tightly adhere to the extraocular muscles fascia and the veins are dilated. The dissection is then continued deeper by exerting gentle traction on the adipose tissue. It is thus possible to resect the extraconical and intraconical orbital fat. Adequate hemostasis is essential to avoid the complication of retro-orbital hematoma.
2. The second step addresses the superomedial fat pad. During this part of the dissection, it is necessary to avoid injury to the supraorbital nerve, the superior oblique muscle, and further below, the medial rectus muscle. A second assistant is helpful at this time to retract the muscular structures and provide better access to the deep orbital fat.

10.2.2 The Lower Eyelid (Figs. 10.8–10.10)

The lower eyelid is then dissected after performing an anterior lamella incision 2 mm below the eyelid margin.

The orbicularis oculi muscle is retracted, allowing visualization of the septum, which in turn is incised at a distance from the inferior border of the tarsus.

1. The dissection begins with the inferolateral fat pad, which is by far the largest, and does not involve risk to the adjacent anatomical structures.
2. Once inside the inferomedial fat pad, the dissection must carefully avoid injury to the inferior rectus muscle. Lastly, very deep inside, after retracting the orbicularis oculi muscle with a Desmarres' retractor, the inferior oblique muscle on the outside and the medial rectus muscle above, the inferior medial fat pad is removed.
3. The inferior median fat pad surrounds the inferior rectus muscle and is removed by pieces around this muscle. Fat below the muscle is not totally removed to maintain the bumper effect of fat at this level. If necessary FROD can be combined with lower eyelid lengthening with ear cartilage grafting (Figs. 10.11, 10.12). The skin is then sutured using 6–0 Prolene. Suturing of the upper eyelid must include several aponeurotic fibers in order to reconstruct the superior palpebral crease.

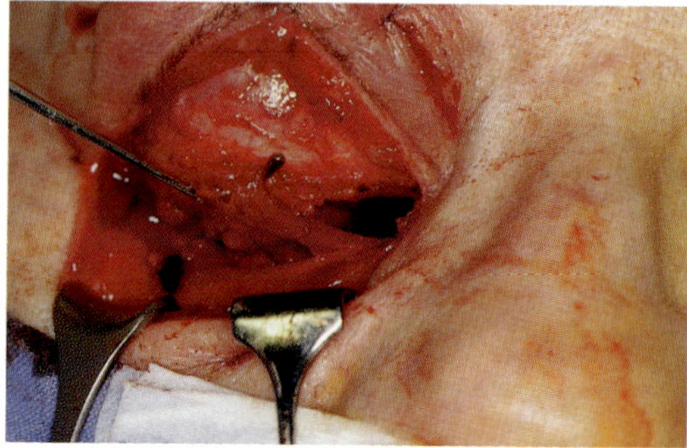

Fig. 10.8. Inferior oblique muscle after fat removal in the inferomedial and inferomedian fat pad areas

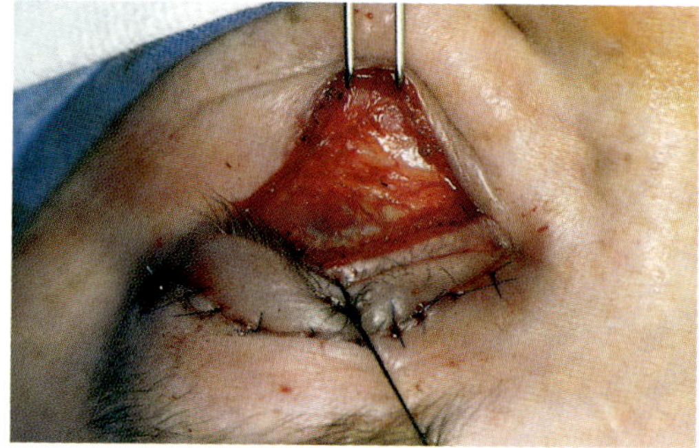

Fig. 10.9. Incision line below the eyelashes in the inferior eyelid

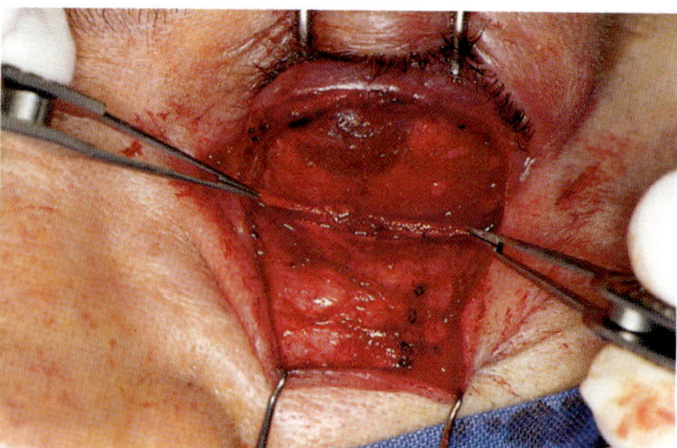

Fig. 10.10. Lower eyelid retractors grasped between two forceps

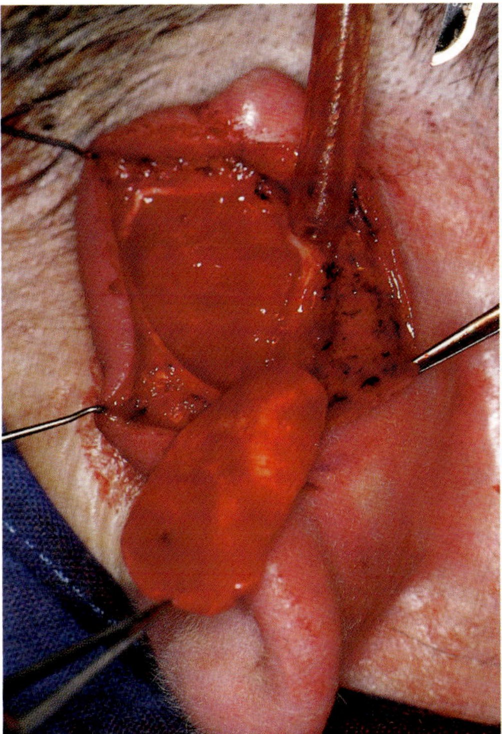

Fig. 10.11. Cartilage harvesting with an incision line behind the ear

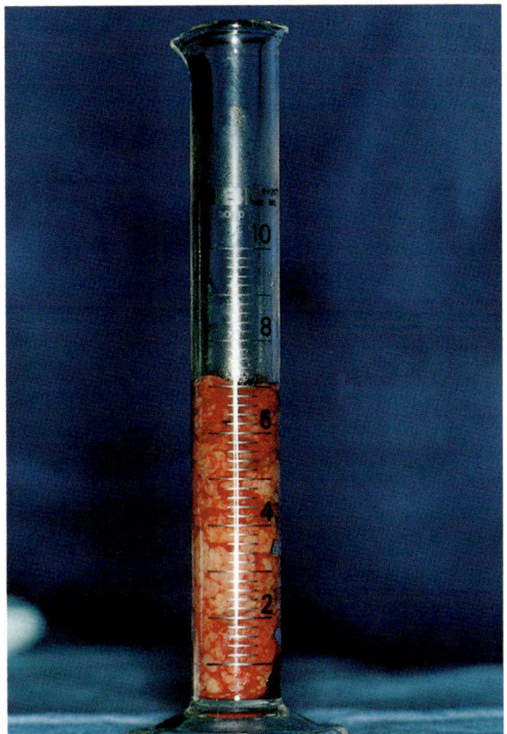

Fig. 10.13. Measure in a tube of the volume of fat excised

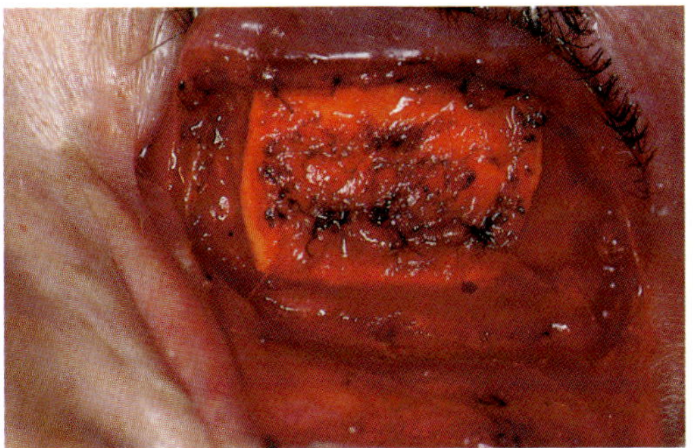

Fig. 10.12. Cartilage graft for treatment of the inferior eyelid retraction

10.2.3 The Volume of Resection

The inferolateral fat pad contains the most adipose tissue and the superomedial fat pad, the least. To satisfactorily reduce the exophthalmos, the total resected volume must be approximately 6–7 cc and is measured in a tube (Fig. 10.13). Frequently 9 cc is removed. In our experience for an average of 6 cc of fat that is removed, exophthalmos is reduced by 4.7 mm [10].

10.2.4 Treatment Program

The surgical approaches of this procedure make it possible to perform other maneuver that are sometimes necessary, such as resection of skin and the orbicularis oculi muscle, eyelid lengthening using a retroauricular cartilage graft, and resection of the inferior rectus muscle or the lower lid retractors. Surgery is performed on only one eye at a time. The second eye can be operated on several days later, after verifying there are no visual complications on the first eye.

Summary for the Clinician

- FROD is performed with the patient under general anesthesia through a blepharoplasty approach
- Extraconical and intraconical fat is removed from the five fat pads, two through the upper eyelid, three from the lower eyelid
- The amount of resected fat is measured retrospectively
- One eye is operated on at a time

10.3 Our Experience

We report here the results of fat removal orbital decompression in a series of patients operated on in our department between 1992 and 2002 and for which binocular vision was studied before and after FROD [10].

10.3.1 Patients

This study involved 64 eyes of 39 Graves' patients, 13 males and 36 females of mean age 52.5 years (27–80 years). Every patient signed an informed consent form and the principles outlined in the Declaration of Helsinki were followed. The indication for surgery was proptosis, eyelid disorders or oculomotor disorders. Patients with optic neuropathy were excluded from the study.

Every patient was operated on after thyroid hormonal equilibrium was stable for at least 6 months. Surgery was proposed after previous treatments of Graves' orbitopathy had failed: 1 month general steroid therapy for every patient and 20 Gy orbital irradiation for eight patients.

10.3.2 Surgical Procedure

Orbital decompression was performed as described by Olivari, under general anesthesia with two aids and modified by using an operating microscope (300-mm terminal lens).

10.3.3 Clinical Data

Clinical data were collected preoperatively, and at 1 week and 6 months postoperatively. Proptosis was measured using Hertel's exophthalmometer. Visual acuity was evaluated using the ETDRS chart. Patients underwent automated static threshold perimetry using Humphrey's Sita standard software (Field Analyzer 750, Carl Zeiss Inc., Le Pecq, France). Every patient was skilled in visual field evaluation from at least three previous tests. Intraocular pressure was measured using Goldmann's applanation tonometer in the primary position of gaze.

10.3.4 Statistics

Clinical data were compared using Pearson's chi-square test, Student's *t*-test, and linear regression analysis.

10.4 Results

10.4.1 Proptosis (Figs. 10.14–10.16)

The mean proptosis was 24.3 ± 2.5 mm preoperatively, and reduced to 19.9 ± 3 mm at 1 week and 19.9 ± 3.1 mm at 6 months. The decrease in proptosis measurements was clinically significant from preoperatively to 1 week, and from preoperatively to 6 months (paired *t*-test, $p<0.001$). However, we found no association between proptosis reduction and the volume of resected fat. Neither was proptosis found as a predictive value for

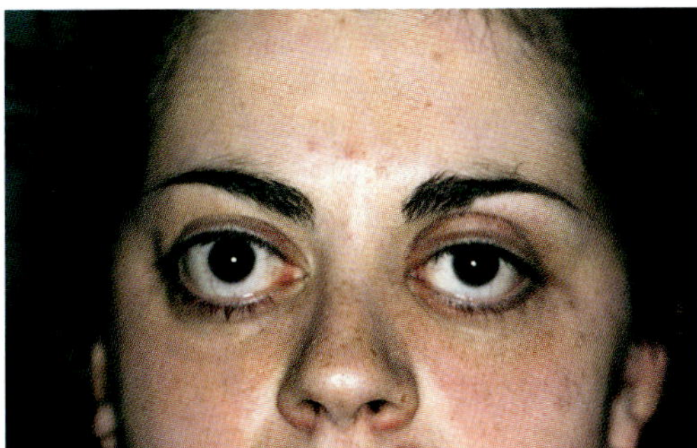

Fig. 10.14. Patient with proptosis and eyelid retraction before fat removal orbital decompression

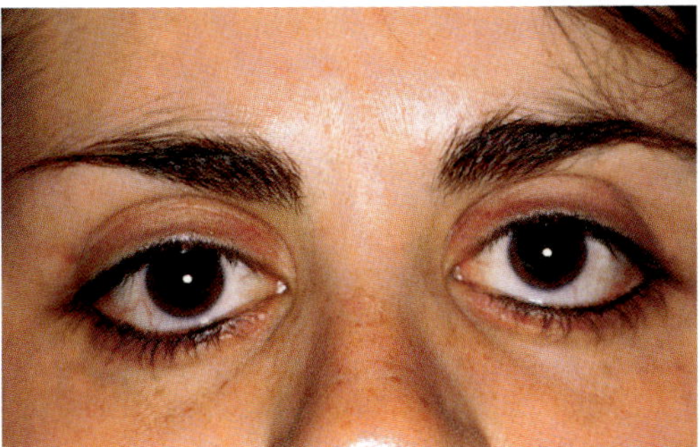

Fig. 10.15. Patient after fat removal orbital decompression

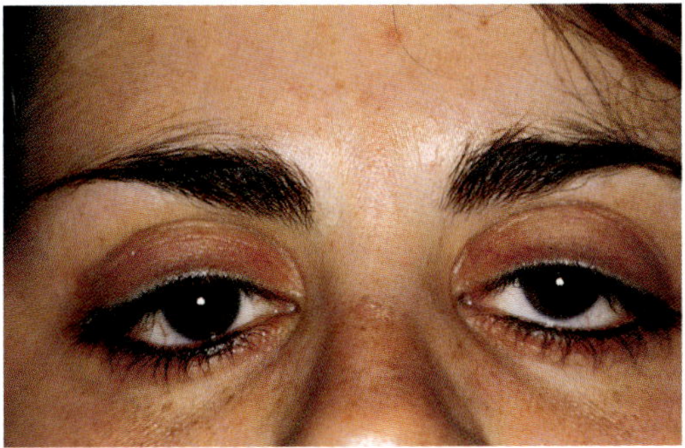

Fig. 10.16. Final aspect of the patient after lower eyelid retraction treatment

proptosis reduction after FROD. It appears that some orbits are fairly well decompressed with a small amount of fat resected, and others poorly decompressed despite a large amount of fat resected. This finding highlights the non-linear pressure-volume relationship of the orbit.

10.4.2 Visual Field

The average mean defect (MD) was -3.3 ± 5.15 dB preoperatively, -3.3 ± 3.7 dB at 1 week and -1.46 ± 3.25 at 6 months. The improvement was statistically significant between preoperative and 6 months (paired *t*-test, $p<0.001$). No significant change of CPSD was shown.

Thirteen eyes were found to have an MD under −3 dB preoperatively. Of these patients, five had complete recovery, four partial recovery, and four no change postoperatively. Every patient with preoperative intraocular pressure (IOP) above 21 mmHg had complete VF recovery.

The defects persisting after FROD featured glaucoma-like scotomas, whereas defects that disappeared after FROD were rather diffuse or altitudinal.

The visual field MD, measured with Humphrey's automated perimetry, was statistically improved in the whole group of patients. On the contrary, no improvement of individual deviation (CPSD) was evidenced. In addition, diffuse or altitudinal defects were significantly lowered in the study, whereas every defect featuring glaucoma-like scotoma persisted after FROD.

Recent studies have highlighted the role of retrobulbar vascular changes in the progression of glaucomatous visual field defects. To explain these two different behaviors, we suggest that compressive optic neuropathy may imply two separate mechanisms: on the one hand, mechanical compression of the optic nerve in the posterior orbit. In this first mechanism, intraorbital pressure and IOP would be high, and compression would induce diffuse or altitudinal scotomas. This kind of optic neuropathy would reduce after FROD. On the other hand, insufficiency of blood supply to the optic nerve during orbital inflammation is implied. This second mechanism would not necessarily be associated with increased intraorbital pressure and IOP, and would rather induce glaucoma-like scotomas. This second kind of lesion is more likely to be definitive and to respond poorly to surgical orbital decompression.

10.4.3 Intraocular Pressure

Mean preoperative IOP was 19.3±4.4 mmHg (12–29 mmHg), and reduced to 17.0±2.9 (10–25) at 1 week and 15.9±3.7 (10–26) at 6 months. The reduction of IOP was significant from preoperatively to 1 week, and from preoperatively to 6 months (paired *t*-test, $p<0.001$).

10.4.4 Volume of Excised Fat

The volume of excised fat was not found to influence any postoperative change, especially proptosis reduction, IOP reduction or MD improvement, even when separately studying patients with and without preoperative elevated IOP. Also, the reduction of IOP was not statistically related to the reduction of proptosis.

10.4.5 Diplopia

Seven patients had preoperative diplopia. Two of them underwent unilateral decompression, and five bilateral decompression with a 6.3-ml resected volume of fat. Every patient maintained a diplopia after surgery, which was successfully corrected by secondary oculomotor surgery.

In the group of 28 patients without preoperative diplopia, 9 presented postoperative diplopia. Two of them had unilateral FROD, and seven bilateral FROD with a 7.4-ml volume of resected fat. In this group, four patients were treated successfully by prisms only, four were operated on, seven patients had no diplopia, one patient persistent diplopia and one was lost to follow-up. Finally 19 patients had no diplopia after surgery, including 8 with unilateral FROD and 11 bilateral FROD with an average of 7.5 ml of resected fat.

These data show no correlation between surgical volume, uni- or bilateral FROD, and the occurrence of postoperative diplopia.

Summary for the Clinician

- **In 64 eyes operated on in 39 patients, FROD allowed significant proptosis reduction, visual field improvement, and IOP decrease**
- **Proptosis reduction was not correlated with the volume of resected fat, showing that the pressure/volume relationship is not linear in the orbit**

10.5 Discussion

10.5.1 Types of Bone Removal Orbital Decompression (BROD) Performed

Various types of surgical bone removal orbital decompression have been performed over the years, but the most commonly used types of modern decompression are:

1. Lateral orbital decompression [12]
2. The two-wall decompression [13] and ethmoidal or antral ethmoidal decompression by various routes:
   - The anterior translid approach
   - The outer canthus and fornix approach
   - The transantral approach [14]
   - The endonasal approach is another possibility for removal of the medial orbital wall and varying amounts of the floor. This approach is best performed by ENT surgeons.

In MacCord's [15] survey of orbital decompression, the two-wall decompression, antral-ethmoidal route was the most frequently performed procedure. Of the antral-ethmoidal decompressions, the transantral route was more effective than the translid route in the management of optic neuropathy because of its ability to decompress the posterior ethmoid.

In terms of dealing with optic neuropathy the equivalence of a transantral and a transfrontal decompression (also a two-wall decompression) was shown by Gorman et al. [16]. Under experimental conditions these two same procedures were compared in terms of their ability to lower intraorbital pressure and were found to be equally effective. Interestingly, bone removal was associated with pressure reduction, whereas incision of the periorbita was associated with proptosis reduction [17].

In three-wall decompression, lateral wall decompression is added to antral-ethmoidal decompression. This procedure is widely used in Europe in two different ways:

1. Using a small horizontal skin incision in the lateral canthus and a larger incision along the whole length of the inferior fornix, allowing the removal of the lateral wall, the floor medially to the infraorbital nerve, and the ethmoidal cells under the origin of the two ethmoidal arteries.
2. Using the coronal approach with a long skin incision from one tragus to the other behind the first rows of hair follicules. This approach allows a good view of the lateral and medial wall but sometimes needs an inferior fornix incision for the floor.

Described by Kennerdell [18], in the "four-wall decompression" the lateral wall portion of the three-wall decompression technique is extended. In the Kennerdell decompression, a large portion of the sphenoid bone in the apex of the orbit and the lateral half of the orbital roof are removed, a process which invariably exposes dura.

The three- and four-wall decompressions have their greatest utility in the management of excessive proptosis.

10.5.2 FROD or BROD?

10.5.2.1 Proptosis Reduction

The average reduction in proptosis is similar in our study and in Olivari's study [2], demonstrating that FROD alone is efficacious in correcting proptosis. We did not find any correlation between proptosis reduction and the volume of excised fat. In the three FROD series [2, 3, 11], the effect on proptosis was quite variable, despite a similar mean volume of excised fat; further studies are necessary to determine other predictive factors.

More interesting will be the study of the influence on proptosis reduction of the volumes of the orbital bony compartment, the volume of the increased muscles, the volume of orbital fat and its relative proportion with the two previous volumes.

10.5.2.2 Optic Neuropathy

Until recently, BROD was considered to be the only available surgical technique with which to address proptosis and optic neuropathy. In 1993, Garrity [18] reported results of 491 BROD in 428 patients. His study comprised 50 % of patients with optic neuropathy. Our study addressed the efficacy of FROD in reducing proptosis and improving the eyelid position. The size of the series is too small to draw any conclusions regarding improvement of the visual function.

The visual field is impaired differently during optic neuropathy depending on the size of the muscles.

If the muscles are stretched and fat volume increased (Fig. 10.17), the visual field is impaired in its superior portion. If the muscles are enlarged at the apex (Fig. 10.18) with compressive neuropathy in this area, the visual field is impaired centrally.

For patients with optic neuropathy, Rootman [19] and ourselves recommend steroids and retrobulbar irradiation before performing orbital surgery when possible.

FROD reduces the IOP in patients with preoperative IOP above 21 mmHg, even after unsuccessful prior treatment with β-blockers. As a hypothetical explanation of this finding, we postulate that FROD might reduce the downstream venous pressure of the eye, which in turn might reduce the IOP.

Considering that FROD effectively reduces IOP in patients with a preoperative IOP above 21 mmHg, it might be indicated in Graves' patients with an elevated IOP threatening the optic nerve if the orbital volume is large and fat pad compartments enlarged.

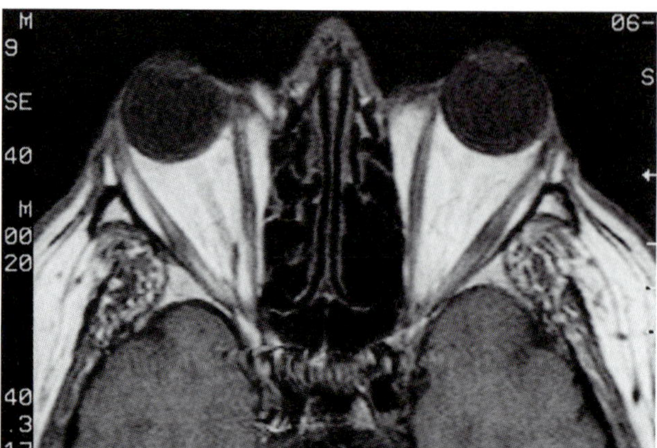

Fig. 10.17. MRI aspect of proptosis with stretched muscles and large fat volume compartment

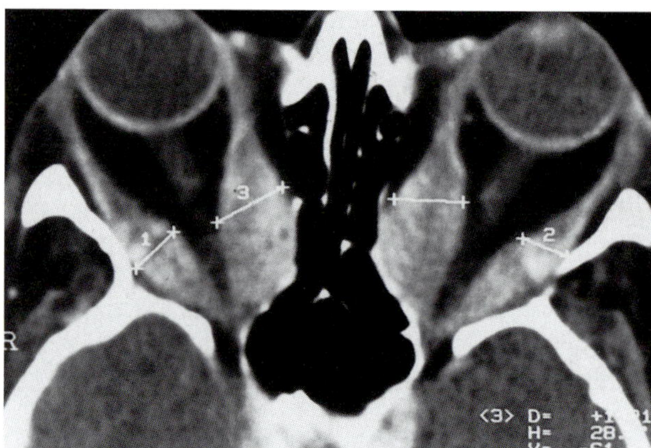

Fig. 10.18. CT scan aspect of proptosis with small bony orbit enlarged muscles at the apex and small fat volume compartments

10.5.2.3 Palpebral Retraction

The results of FROD alone on palpebral retraction are poor. Successful palpebral lengthening may be obtained with combined levator aponeurosis weakening of the upper eyelid, and a cartilage graft on the lower eyelid.

10.5.2.4 Oculomotor Disorders

Oculomotor disorders subsequent to FROD were as follows: Three out of 23 patients (13%) experienced a new diplopia, for which two (9%) required orthoptic therapy. In Garrity's study [20], 74 patients (17%) had new diplopia and 300 (70%) ultimately had surgery for strabismus after BROD. As opposed to BROD, in which it is mostly the inferior and internal walls that are removed, FROD achieves fat removal all around the eye, in a circumferential fashion. This might explain why FROD induces fewer ocular motility disturbances than BROD.

Summary for the Clinician

- **Among BROD techniques, the three-wall and four-wall techniques are probably the most useful in the management of excessive proptosis**
- **FROD is probably best indicated in patients with large orbital volume and fat enlargement**
- **BROD is probably best indicated in patients with small orbital volume and muscle enlargement**

- **Oculomotor and eyelid disorders can be treated together with FROD in a single procedure**

10.6 Conclusion

FROD is efficacious in reducing proptosis in Graves' ophthalmopathy. Although FROD alone fails to reduce palpebral retraction, significant palpebral lengthening can be achieved with combined section of the levator aponeurosis horns in the upper eyelid and/or a cartilage graft in the lower eyelid. FROD leaves the possibility of concomitant palpebral and/or oculomotor surgery.

Further studies are necessary to determine which procedure, FROD or BROD, or combined surgery, should be performed initially, depending on the clinical presentation, radiologic findings, and previous treatments.

However, our impression is that FROD is better indicated in patients:

- With large bony orbital content, large orbital fat volumes and stretched muscles.
- With cosmetic "grotesque" disability

On the contrary BROD is better indicated in patients:

- With small bony orbital volume, small orbital fat volumes and enlarged muscles
- With compressive optic neuropathy

Finally combined FROD and BROD techniques can address nearly all the indications of orbital decompression as a first choice.

References

1. Olivari N (1988) Transpalpebrale Decompression-Operation bei endokriner Orbitopathie (exopthalmus). Wien Med Wochenschr 18:138–142
2. Olivari N (1987) Transpalpebral decompression of endocrine ophthalmopathy (Graves' disease) by removal of intraorbital fat: experience with 147 operations over 5 years. Plast Reconstr Surg 87: 627–641
3. Trokel S, Kazim M, Moore S (1993) Orbital fat removal, decompression for Graves' ophthalmopathy. Ophthalmology 100:674–682
4. Hecht S, Guibor P, Wolfey D, Wiggs E (1984) Orbital dissection defatting technique for Graves' disease. Am J Ophthalmol 4:314–318
5. Roncevic R, Jackson IT (1989) Surgical treatment of thyrotoxic exophthalmos. Plast Reconstr Surg 89:754–760
6. Roncevic R, Roncevic D (1995) Surgical treatment of severe dysthyroid ophthalmopathy – long term results. J Craniomaxillofac Surg 23:355–362
7. Liu GT, Heher KL, Katowitz JA, Kazim M, Maozami G, Moshang T, Teener JW, Sladky J, Volpe NJ, Galetta SL (1996) Prominent proptosis in childhood thyroid eye disease. Ophthalmology 103: 779–784
8. Morax S, Bok C, Chahbi M, Hurbli T (1997) Décompression orbitaire au cours de l'exophtalmie dysthyroïdienne. Ann Chir Plast Esthet 42: 207–215
9. Moreiras JPV, Prada CM (2004) Thyroid orbitopathy. In: Orbit. Examination, microsurgery and pathology, vol 2. Highlights of ophthalmology, pp 947–1036
10. Adenis JP, Robert PY, Lasudry JGH, Dalloul Z (1998) Treatment of proptosis with fat removal orbital decompression in Graves' ophthalmopathy. Eur J Ophthalmol 8:246–252
11. Adenis JP, Camezind P, Robert PY (2003) La diplopie est elle un facteur déterminant du choix de la technique de décompression orbitaire au cours de l'orbitopathie dysthyroïdienne. Bull Acad Natl Med 187:1649–1660
12. Anderson RL, Linberg JV (1981) Transorbital approach to decompression in Graves' disease. Arch Ophthalmol 99:120–124
13. MacCord CDJR (1981) Orbital decompression for Graves' disease; exposure through lateral canthal and inferior fornix incision. Ophthalmology 88: 533–541
14. Ogura JH, Lucente FE (1974) Surgical results of orbital decompression for malignant exophthalmos. Laryngoscope 84:637–644
15. McCord CD (1985) Current trends in orbital decompression. Ophthalmology 92:21–23
16. Gorman CA, de Santo LW, MacCarty CS, Riley FC (1974) Optic neuropathy of Grave's disease. N Engl J Med 290:70–75
17. Stanley RJ, McCaffrey TV, Offord KP, DeSanto LW (1989) Superior and transantral orbital decompression procedures. Arch Otolaryngol Head Neck Surg 115:369–373
18. Kennerdell JS, Maroon JC (1982) An orbital decompression for severe dysthyroid exophthalmos. Ophthalmology 89:467–472

19. Rootman J, Stewart B, Nugnet R, Robertson W (1988) Anatomy of the orbit. In: Rootman J (ed) Diseases of the orbit. JB Lippincott, Philadelphia, pp 241–280
20. Garrity JA, Fatourechi V, Bergstralh EJ, Bartley GB, Beatty CW, DeSanto LW, Gorman CA (1992) Results of transantral orbital decompression in 428 patients with severe Graves' ophthalmopathy. Am J Ophthalmol 116:533–547

Esthetic and Lid Surgery

Update on Upper Lid Blepharoplasty

Markus J. Pfeiffer

Core Messages

- A great variety of anatomical factors must be considered to predict the lid crease level, the most important landmark in blepharoplasty
- The superficial aspect of the eyelid and the skin fold depend more on the deeper layers of orbital anatomy than on the skin itself
- The main key to the patient's satisfaction is the ability to predict the possible result of surgery
- Symmetry and regularity are the primary aims of blepharoplasty
- Simple and complicated cases should be differentiated preoperatively
- The approach to the orbit is safer using a layer by layer technique and separating the different sheaths by hydrodissection
- Most complications are iatrogenic and can be avoided by careful preoperative planning of the blepharoplasty
- If there is doubt about the ideal correction, undercorrection rather than overcorrection should be the approach
- The majority of asymmetry complications are predictable and can be managed by supplementary unilateral interventions
- Associated pathology should be be corrected in all cases of blepharoplasty

11.1 Introduction

Upper lid blepharoplasty can be considered to be one of the most frequent operations carried out by a variety of surgical specialists, ophthalmologists and non-ophthalmologists. The eye's function and expression should play a primary role in the concept of blepharoplasty. Surgery is recommended to be planned in a centrifugal manner, from the eye to the lids. Concern for the eye's function and the eye's protection should be given priority in any eyelid surgery. This chapter is written from an ophthalmologist's point of view. The details of anatomy are described in order to reveal their geometric role in the eyelid appearance and functional dynamics. Instead of proposing a standard technique [5, 6, 18, 22, 28], I will try to analyze the multiple anatomical factors in order to show how the results of upper lid surgery can be made more predictable. The predictability of the result is the main key to the patient's satisfaction because it is the only way to find a realistic balance between the patient's expectations and what is possible for the surgeon [15].

11.2 Surgical Anatomy of the Upper Lid and Upper Orbit

Blepharoplasty requires a profound knowledge of palpebral and orbital anatomy. A basic knowledge can be obtained by "dry" anatomical studies of anatomical textbooks, drawings and anatomical specimens [32, 41]. As the tissues look very different during surgery, it has been necessary to give names to some "wet" surgical observations that are not listed in anatomical textbooks. Bloodless surgery with the carbon dioxide laser provides a far better differentiation of the structures [14, 21, 39]. Use of the laser is combined with hydrodissection by injecting an anesthetic solution under each layer and thus making visible the structures below. The following anatomical observations have been selected according to their surgical relevance in upper lid blepharoplasty.

11.2.1 Relationship of Aperture Plane, Lid Crease and Skin Fold

Blepharoplasty cannot be planned without checking the size and position of eye and orbit. The relationship of orbit and eye can be compared with the relationship of container and content or the relationship of the visual organ and its socket. As the lids form the exterior connection between orbit and eye, they depend on the position of both. Any variation of size and position affects the eyelid appearance. Pronounced proptosis or increased diameter of the globe, enophthalmus or microphthalmus are easily recognized, but discrete alterations may be overlooked and result in postoperative unexpected lid crease positions or asymmetry. The aperture plane is determined by three measurements: (1) the position of the center of the globe, (2) the radius of the globe, and (3) the position of the orbital rim (Fig. 11.1). The lid crease formation depends on the position of the aperture plane. The skin fold covers the lid crease superficially.

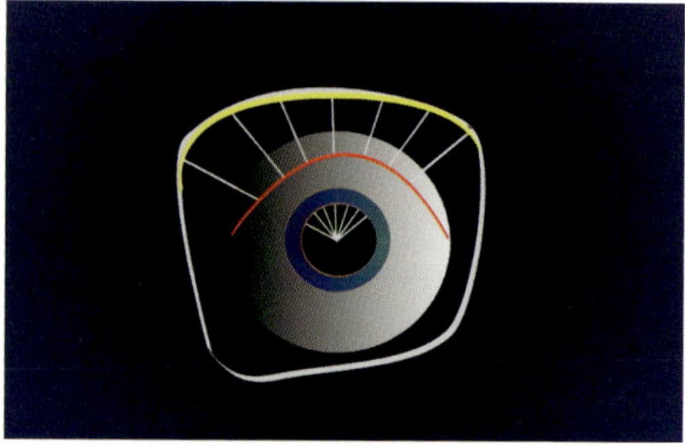

Fig. 11.1. The aperture plane coincides with the shortest distance between the globe surface and the upper orbital rim. The position of the plane can be defined by tracing multiple lines from the center of the globe to the orbital rim

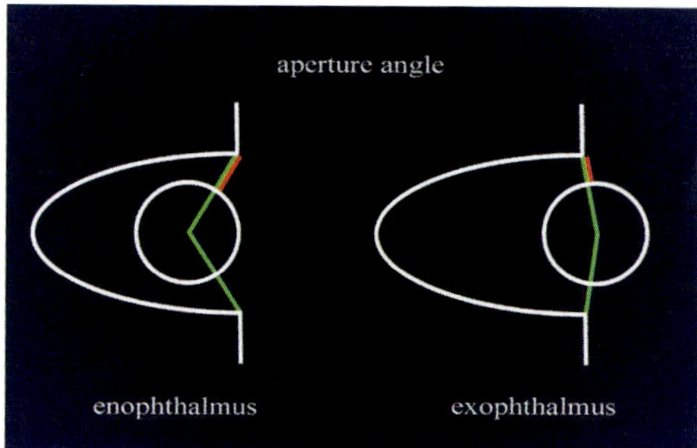

Fig. 11.2. In most normal cases, the aperture plane is inclined in a posterior angle. In enophthalmus, there is a more pronounced posterior inclination. In exophthalmus we can even find an anterior inclination. The globe-rim distance (*red line*) within the aperture plane is the most important distance for the lid crease formation

11.2.2 The Aperture Plane

The aperture plane of the upper orbit defines the relationship of eye and orbit. If we draw multiple straight lines from the center of the globe to the upper orbital rim, they will perforate the surface of the eye in an arcuate line (Fig. 11.1). This line separates two surfaces: (1) the aspherical aperture plane between the upper orbital rim and the meridian on the eyeball and (2) the spherical surface between the meridian and the optical axis. In most normal cases, the aperture plane is inclined in a posterior angle. In enophthalmus, there is a more pronounced posterior inclination. In exophthalmus we can even find an anterior inclination. The globe-rim distance within the aperture plane forms the most important area for the lid crease formation. Before blepharoplasty we have to check the size and the inclination of the aperture plane to be able to plan where the lid crease will be formed (Fig. 11.2).

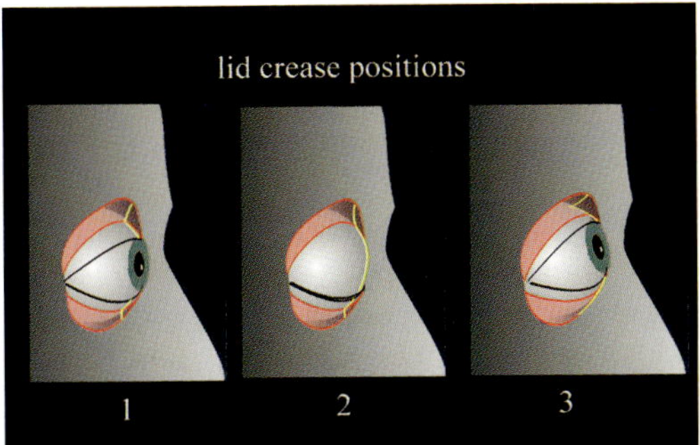

Fig. 11.3. In the primary position of gaze the lid crease covers the basic aperture angle formed by the aperture plane and the ocular surface (*1*). During lid closure the crease is unfolded anteriorly in front of the aperture plane (*2*). In the up gaze position, the lid crease is retracted behind the aperture plane (*3*)

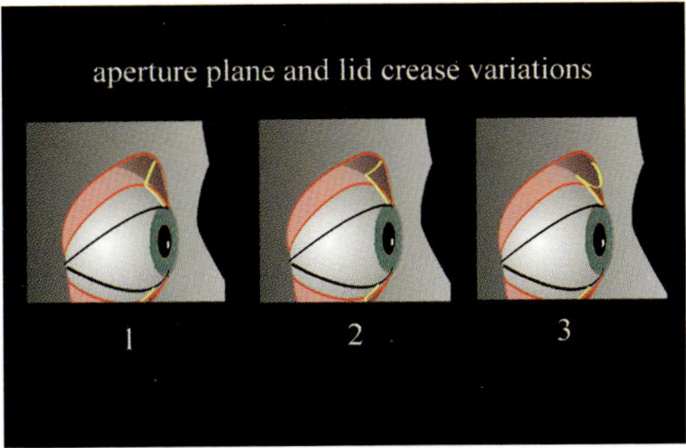

Fig. 11.4. The lid crease normally tends to form in the level of the aperture plane (*1*). If there is little tissue volume within the aperture plane, the skin crease will form at a higher level (*2*). Excessive tissue volume like orbital fat in the aperture plane will lower the lid crease (*3*)

11.2.3 The Upper Lid Crease

The upper lid crease cannot be seen directly, because it is located behind the normal skin fold. After having created a surgical access through the skin, the lid crease can be viewed directly. The lid crease is formed in a dynamic angle in the junction between the preseptal and the pretarsal surface. The angle becomes smaller when the patient looks upward and wider in downward gaze (Fig. 11.3). The individual angle is more dependent on the alterations of the septal surface than the tarsal surface. During surgery we can easily observe the preseptal surface in various gaze positions. The upper lid crease formation is the most important aspect in blepharoplasty, because the position of the skin crease and its symmetry is evaluated more critically by the patient than the brow position or the upper lid level [25]. The position of the lid crease depends on many factors: (1) the position of the aperture plane, (2) the preseptal orbicularis muscle, (3) the anatomy of the orbital septum, (4) the brow position, (5) the sub-brow fatpad (SOOF), (6) the preaponeurotic fat and (7) the levator and its function (Fig. 11.4).

11.2.4 The Skin Fold

For the information of the patient and the planning of blepharoplasty it is important to understand the mechanism of the skin fold formation in the upper lid. We find it useful to describe the vertical section of the fold in the center of the lid like an "N" that is composed of an inward fold and an outward fold. For lid closure the fold has to be able to unfold freely to a straight layer without traction. The inward fold is cosmetically more desirable, because it allows the skin to be stored away posteriorly while the lid is opened. The aim of blepharoplasty can either be the reduction of the outward fold or the enhancement of the inward fold. In most cases both folds have to be corrected, the outward fold by excision of redundant skin and the inward fold by deepening the lid crease. The deepening of the inward fold is achieved by the removal of the lid crease inhibiting tissues like excessive preseptal orbicularis muscle, prolapsed preaponeurotic fat or ptotic SOOF (Fig. 11.5).

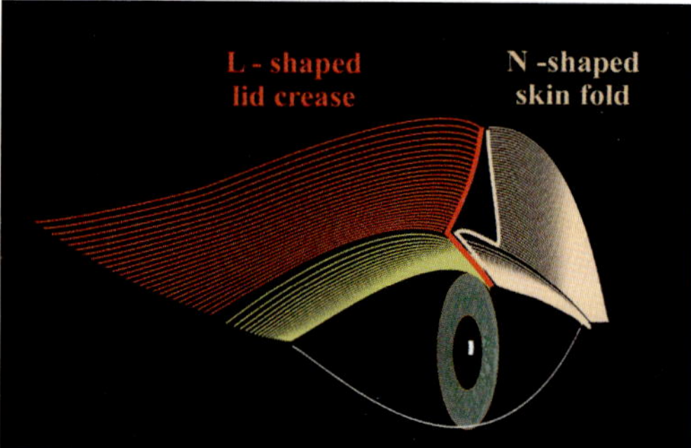

Fig. 11.5. The lid crease is formed by the angle between the ocular surface and the aperture plane whereas the lid crease itself is covered anteriorly by the N-shaped skin fold

11.2.5 The Eyelid Skin

The eyelid skin is the thinnest skin of the body. The subcutaneous fat layers are absent in the area between the eyebrow and the lid margin. However, we can find subcutaneous fat below the eyebrow, medially from the medial canthus and laterally from the lateral canthus. The thin skin allows the formation of a thin skin fold. The skin fold is necessary to permit the eyelid movement. The surgical treatment of the upper lid skin is different in the central, medial and lateral area. In all areas there must be left sufficient skin to permit unrestricted eyelid closure. The aging process of the skin is characterized by a loss of elastic fibers and an increase of laxity. The increased laxity is obvious in dermatochalasia, where excessive skin forms a redundant skin fold. The redundancy of the skin fold can be excised. For normal closure and blinking the central skin needs sufficient extension to cover the distance from the brow to the lid margin without any tension. The medial skin needs enough surface to cover the medial cavity above the medial canthal tendon. If we measure the distance between the lacrimal punctum and the medial brow, the amount of the minimal vertical skin extension has to be at least 1 1/2 of this distance in order to cover the semicircle of this cavity. The edema during surgery and after surgery causes the medial skin to turn out into a prominent bag. We need to be careful not to misinterpret this phenomenon as a medial skin redundancy that must be resected. This error would create an epicanthal fold, which is very difficult to correct. The lateral eyelid skin covers the area between the lateral canthus and the lateral brow. The convex surface and reduced deepness of the lateral lid crease allows more skin resection than medially. Nevertheless any excessive lateral resection would pull the lateral brow downwards or inhibit lateral lid mobility.

11.2.6 Relationship of the Anterior and the Posterior Lid Lamella

The anterior lamella is composed of the skin and the orbicularis muscle. The posterior lamella includes the tarsus, the conjunctiva and the levator.

In the tarsal area the posterior lamella is fused with the anterior lamella (skin and orbicularis muscle). In the septal area the lamellas are separated: the posterior lamella with the levator structures continues backward into the orbit and the anterior lamella continues to the orbital rim below the eyebrow. Between the lamellas we find the preaponeurotic fat. The lid crease forms at the junction between the fused and the separated lamellas.

11.2.7 The Pretarsal Orbicularis Muscle

The pretarsal orbicularis muscle is closely connected to the tarsal surface. The contraction of its rapid fibers results in a quick eyelid closure and enables the eyelid blinking. Blinking has a functional and esthetic importance and should not be inhibited after blepharoplasty. For this reason the pretarsal orbicularis muscle should not be weakened. Only in cases of upper lid entropion, where a detachment and lowering of the pretarsal orbicularis muscle from the tarsal plate is observed, do we try to create a refixation of the muscle on the tarsus. Above the pretarsal area, where the lamellas begin to separate, a redundant muscle bulge can be resected without harming the function. Extensive surgery of the septum and the preseptal muscle can provoke a denervation of the pretarsal muscle in very rare cases. The proper function of the pretarsal orbicularis muscle is only guaranteed if the muscle fibers are running parallel to the curvature of the eye's surface. If the canthal insertions of the muscle are weakened, the muscle can dislocate and provoke an upper lid ectropion or a floppy eyelid. If too much eyelid skin is resected, the downward movement of the lid margin is restricted. The preseptal orbicularis muscle tends to pull the posterior lamella downwards and create an upper lid ectropion.

11.2.8 The Preseptal Orbicularis Muscle

The preseptal orbicularis muscle covers the septum and permits forced eyelid closure. The preseptal muscle can glide downwards to overlap the pretarsal muscle and create an effective protection of the eye. The preseptal muscle tends to undergo more involutional changes and thus disturb the formation of the lid crease. A partial resection is usually necessary in upper lid blepharoplasty to create a better lid crease and an improved skin fold. The resection of these muscle fibers usually weakens the muscle without creating significant functional problems. The medial extension of the preseptal muscle where it originates from the medial canthal area tends to be affected by a fatty degeneration of the muscle fibers or an infiltration of fatty tissue. As the medial area is concave and the fatty tissue tends to swell significantly after the surgery, there will be a postoperative outward bulging of the area, which is often misinterpreted as an insufficient skin resection. Therefore we prefer to eliminate the medial fatty degeneration or the fatty infiltration in this area of the preseptal orbicularis muscle. The lateral extension of the preseptal muscle covers the area over the lacrimal gland and continues into the orbital part of the orbicularis muscle [13].

11.2.9 The Orbital Part of the Orbicularis Muscle

The orbital part of the orbicularis muscle covers the orbital rim. The fibers run semicircular from the medial to the lateral canthus. At the lateral canthus the fibers are directed nearly vertically and act as depressors of the eyebrow. During blepharoplasty we can resect parts of these vertically acting orbital orbicularis fibers in order to elevate the lateral brow. The resection of these fibers has the disadvantage that the covering tissue of the orbital rim is thinned and that the lateral rim can be exposed to form a vertical edge. This vertical edge of the orbital rim appears like a lateral downwards directed prolongation of the skin crease. The ideal skin crease, however, fades laterally in a horizontal direction.

11.2.10 The Suborbicularis Oculi Fat (SOOF)

The SOOF (or sub-brow fat pad) is located under the orbital part of the orbicularis muscle and covers the orbital rim. The function of the SOOF is to allow the brow elevation and depression by an upwards and downwards gliding deformation of the fat pad. The thickness of this fat pad is extremely variable. There are patients where this fat pad is minimal and the orbital rim appears like the bony rim covered by skin. In other cases the SOOF has so much volume that it appears like a fatty lump that overlaps the lid crease. The SOOF usually only disturbs the skin crease in the lateral two-thirds of the upper lid. The SOOF is covered by a bag of fibrous tissue formed by extensions of the periosteum and the orbital septum. The anterior layers of the SOOF are filled with solid fat lobules that can be resected without problems. The posterior layers are situated close to the periosteum and contain a venous network and the neurovascular bundle of the lacrimal nerve and artery. Therefore it is not advisable to perform a deep resection of the lateral SOOF. The medial SOOF should never be approached through a blepharoplasty incision because it is crossed by the supraorbital nerve.

The best approach to the medial SOOF is subperiosteal through a frontal or temporal incision behind the hairline. From an esthetic point of view the SOOF has the benefit of smoothening the contour of the orbital skull. Any procedure on the SOOF should be planned carefully to avoid a sulcus formation in the superolateral orbital area. Any brow elevation technique will also lift the sub-brow fat pad.

11.2.11 The Orbital Septum

The orbital septum is formed by a membrane that separates the anterior eyelid lamella from the orbital space. The septum can also be considered as the entrance into the orbit [26]. A blepharoplasty can be performed with or without opening the septum. It can be opened through a buttonhole incision, or through a wide approach. It plays an important role in the lid crease formation. The upper insertions of the septum are parallel to the orbital rim, where they merge with the fascia of the SOOF and the periosteum. The upper insertion of the septum also depends on the volume and the motility of the sub-brow fat pad. The lower part of the septum fuses with the posterior lid lamella. Therefore the septum can also be defined as a bridge between the container (orbit) and the content (globe). The lower insertion of the septum on the posterior lid lamella is extremely variable. We can find very high insertions into the high aponeurosis where the septum correlates with the aperture plane. Those patients will show a maximal high lid crease. Asian eyelids show a very low insertion of the septum with a very low or non-existent lid crease. The septum can contain various layers of a fibroelastic tissue. It can be tight and straight or dilated and bulged. In most cases the septum is formed like a bag where the anterior layer continues into the posterior layer on the aponeurosis. The fundus of the bag is not always filled with orbital fat. The identification of variations of the septal layers is very important for the safe access to the orbit. On downgaze the septum is stretched and forms a more or less straightened layer. The medial and lateral insertions of the septum follow the direction of the medial and lateral canthal tendon. The unrestricted motility of the septum has to be preserved. It seems unnecessary or even counterproductive for the motility to try to repair a transected septum [38]. In reoperations we observe that the membrane tends to reform in a natural way. It is also not recommended to try to deepen the skin crease by picking up deep tissue since this can result in a shortening of the septum and eyelid retraction.

11.2.12 The Orbital Fat

The orbital fat fills the spaces between the globe, the extraocular muscles, the neurovascular pathways and the orbital wall. The septum forms the anterior limitation of the orbital fat. We can differentiate central, medial and lateral compartments of orbital fat. The fatpads are deformable and change their shape in different gaze positions. There is an age related tendency to protrusion of fat lobules caused by laxity of the septum. Also an age related increase of the fat volume has been observed.

The orbital fat of the upper lid is composed of two different fat pads: the preaponeurotic fat and the medial orbital fat (Fig. 11.6).

11.2.12.1 The Preaponeurotic Orbital Fat

The preaponeurotic fat can often be seen through the septum. If it is not visible, an injection of clear solution under the septum will make it shine through. Sometimes the preaponeurotic fat can be hardly detected and only forms a thin layer above the levator muscle. In other cases it presents as an unsightly bulge. After the septum is dissected and retracted, the fat will prolapse in a semiliquid manner. The preaponeurotic fat is the most flexible and liquid fat of the orbit. A resected lump of preaponeurotic fat will form like a drop of oil on a plane surface due to its homogeneous monolobular structure. The preaponeurotic fat is covered by a few thin transparent membranes. If these membranes are opened, the fat transforms to a flat layer. The lateral part of the

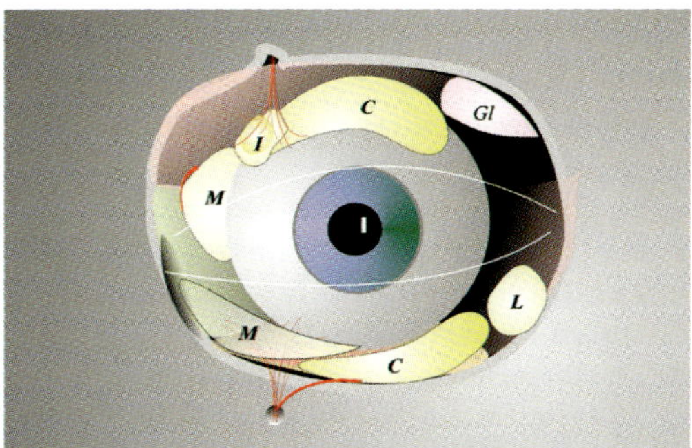

Fig. 11.6. The central preaponeurotic fat (*C*) extends medially to the intermedial orbital fat (*I*) and laterally to the lacrimal gland (*Gl*). The medial orbital fat (*M*) is found in a separate medial orbital compartment

preaponeurotic orbital fat neighbors the lacrimal gland [34]. As it often surrounds the firm gland lobules, care must be taken not to injure the gland during fat resection. The medial part of the preaponeurotic fat is completely different, because it contains much smaller fat lobuli. Branches of the supraorbital neurovascular bundle run through the medial part of the preaponeurotic fat. As the medial part of the preaponeurotic fat has to be recognized and differentiated from the central preaponeurotic fat, we have called it the "intermedial fat pad". The resection of this fat pad can produce two serious complications in blepharoplasty: (1) injury of the neurovascular bundle and (2) formation of an undesired deep excavation of the intermedial lid crease. There is no need to extend the preaponeurotic fat resection backwards into the orbit. In blepharoplasty only the fat that inhibits the lid crease formation has to be reduced. Even if orbital decompression is necessary as in cases of thyroid orbitopathy, resection of the deep portions of the preaponeurotic fat has no significant decompressive effect.

11.2.12.2 The Medial Orbital Fat

The medial orbital fat of the upper lid is found behind the medial extensions of the septum and the aponeurosis, where they continue to the medial canthal tendon. To expose the medial orbital fat, first the septum has to be retracted to expose the medial extension of the aponeurosis. The medial fat pad is located behind these medial fibrous extensions of the aponeurosis. There is only a small area where the fat pad can be approached safely. That is the lateral margin of the fat pad halfway between the medial canthal tendon and the trochlea in order to avoid the vessels running vertically to the medial limit of the fat pad. In cases with a pronounced laxity of the fibrous tissue, the medial fat tends to protrude anteriorly and can be identified easily before opening any fibrous membranes. The medial fat pad has a more stable shape and a brighter whitish colour than the preaponeurotic fat. Any excessive resection from the medial fat pad should be avoided, but it does not cause the complications that we expect by resecting the intermedial fat. Special care should be taken not to confuse intermedial and medial orbital fat.

11.2.13 The Eyebrow

In males the eyebrow tends to follow the horizontal shape of the superior orbital rim. Occasionally the lateral brow is turned downwards parallel to the lateral orbital rim. In females the brow covers the orbital rim medially and rises upwards laterally to cross above the lateral orbital rim. For this reason the contour of the superolateral orbital rim can usually be seen below the brow in females. The shape of the orbital rim is smoothened by the presence of the SOOF. Some females like to enhance this surface by epilating the inferior brow margin.

11.2.14 The Frontalis Muscle and Its Antagonists

The shape of the upper eyelid crease depends considerably on the frontalis activity.

The frontalis muscle can produce an elevation of the brow and the SOOF of more than 20 mm. Every individual has a different pattern of frontalis activity. Only few cases have an independent unilateral innervation of the frontalis muscle. In the majority of cases the frontal branch of the facial nerve shows bilateral simul-

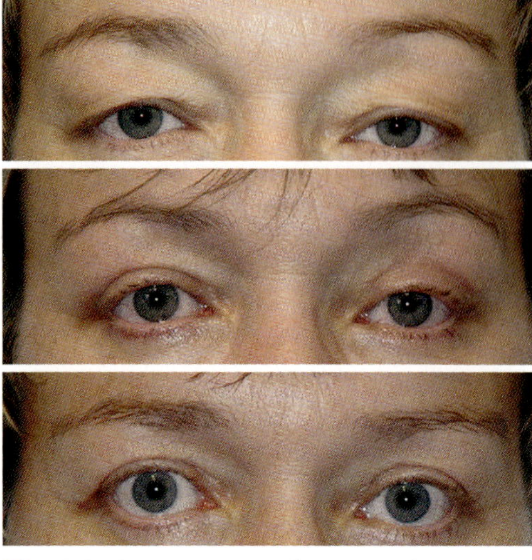

Fig. 11.7. Symmetry: *1* nearly symmetric preoperative appearance; the small ptosis on the left is not treated; *2* postoperatively: lid crease asymmetry is revealed due to left ptosis and brow overactivity; *3* improved symmetry after injection of botulinum toxin into the left frontalis muscle

taneous activity. The antagonists (orbicularis muscle and procerus muscle) can be activated unilaterally. This explains why we often find a marked brow asymmetry in cases with symmetric frontalis innervation. As any brow asymmetry will disturb our intentions to achieve a symmetric blepharoplasty result, we need to find out whether we can eliminate the cause before we have to intervene on the brow. Often we observe a unilateral compensatory brow elevation due to unilateral ptosis or pseudoptosis. The correction of ptosis would secondarily reduce the brow elevation [12] (Fig. 11.7).

11.2.15 The Posterior Lid Lamella

The tarsoconjunctiva is the essential structure that enables the lid to function as a protective "lid" on the cornea. The inner surface of the tarsal plate corresponds to the corneal surface. Any eyelid surgery should primarily respect and never disturb this relationship of the lid and the ocular surface.

Summary for the Clinician

- **The skin fold is N-shaped with an anterior and posterior plication and covers the lid crease anteriorly**
- **The lid crease forms at the junction of the tarsal and the septal surface of the lid**
- **The lid crease forms at the junction of the anterior and posterior lamella**
- **The tarsal surface of the lid is convex; the septal surface of the lid is medially concave and laterally convex**
- **Surgical dissection should respect anatomical layers. Surgical exposure "layer by layer" or "open sky" are safer than "button hole" approaches**

11.3 Preoperative Evaluation and Surgical Planning

11.3.1 The Patient's Expectation

We all know the kind of patient who wishes to have the same operation that has been performed successfully on another patient. The patient's expectation is based on the presumed similarity of any orbital region, any aging process and any recommended eyelid surgery. If an esthetic improvement of the eyelid region is noticed, it is often difficult to explain what exactly has changed. Most patients are therefore unable to describe in detail what they wish to have corrected. Even if we show all our photographs of pre- and postoperative examples, there will be no case that can be used as a reliable reference for an individual situation. A normal patient will usually not be able to recognize the relevant details that are responsible for the improvement of his or her lids. On the other hand the patient is able to differentiate thousands of individual faces. This paradox explains the main difficulty in blepharoplasty: (1) the patient expects an improvement without being conscious of the changed anatomical details and (2) the patient and their social environment will be very critical about any change in individual facial expression. The preoperative evaluation has to consider this paradox when the operation is planned. The convergence of the patient's "what do I want?" and the surgeon's "what can I do?" can never be aimed at an ideal. The ideal can, however, be reduced to some basic guidelines that are commonly accepted in the occidental population: (1) the upper lid surface is divided into two surfaces, the pretarsal and preseptal surface, (2) both surfaces should be visible in the primary position and separated by the skin crease, (3) the visible size of the two surfaces in the primary position is dependent on individual anatomical factors, and (4) both surfaces should be regular and uninterrupted [10].

11.3.2 Evaluation of the Lid Crease Symmetry

Symmetry is one of the main demands in upper lid blepharoplasty. Symmetry and regularity are the fundamental esthetic principles. Asymmetry after upper lid blepharoplasty is much less readily tolerated in comparison to other esthetic procedures. As the orbital area is the main target for individual facial recognition, asymmetry is easily recognized. Physiologic studies have analyzed the eye movements while another person's face is observed. The observer's point of fixation oscillates from one eye to the other, creating a permanent comparison of both orbital regions. The most critical structure where symmetry is expected is the lid crease and the overlying skin fold position. Differences in the lid crease position seem to disturb patients more than differences of the MRD (margin reflex distance) or the brow level. On the other hand, the lid crease position depends primarily on the MRD and the brow level. The lid crease cannot be seen preoperatively. The postoperative lid crease position can be calculated approximately by using the preoperative data of lid level (MRD) and brow level. The three landmarks (1) lid level (MRD), (2) brow level and (3) lid crease level form a triangle in sagittal section. To calculate the approximate skin crease position we have to evaluate the position of each point in relation to the other two points: (1) the lid level (MRD) affects the skin crease level and the brow level in an inverse manner. A drop of lid level makes the skin crease rise. A drop of the lid level also makes the brow rise by compensatory innervation of the frontalis muscle. (2) The brow level only affects the lid crease level and has no effect on the lid level. (3) The lid crease level has no effect on the other two landmarks. As the lid crease is hidden before and revealed after surgery, any preexistent asymmetry will be hidden before and revealed after surgery. I have the experience that patients usually tolerate a 1-mm asymmetry, but are quite concerned about a 2-mm asymmetry. Patients seem to be much more concerned about lid crease asymmetry than asymmetry of the lid level or the brow level (Fig. 11.7).

11.3.3 Preoperative Examination

The preoperative evaluation should include a complete ophthalmologic examination. It is very important to measure the refraction, visual acuity and visual field. The refraction is needed to exclude any anisometropia with asymmetry of the axial length affecting the aperture plane. The exclusion of amblyopia is also necessary to understand the existence or absence of any unilateral compensatory activity of the frontal muscle. A strabismologic examination is needed primarily to exclude a vertical deviation that could result in an important lid crease difference. The position of the lid margin (MRD), the skin crease and the eyebrow is measured in millimeters distance from the corneal reflex in the primary position. These three measurements determine the most important landmarks for planning blepharoplasty. They are compared and confirmed by the measurements from the digital photography. If ptosis is present, we also measure the function of the levator and the orbicularis muscle and Bell's phenomenon [1] (Fig. 11.8).

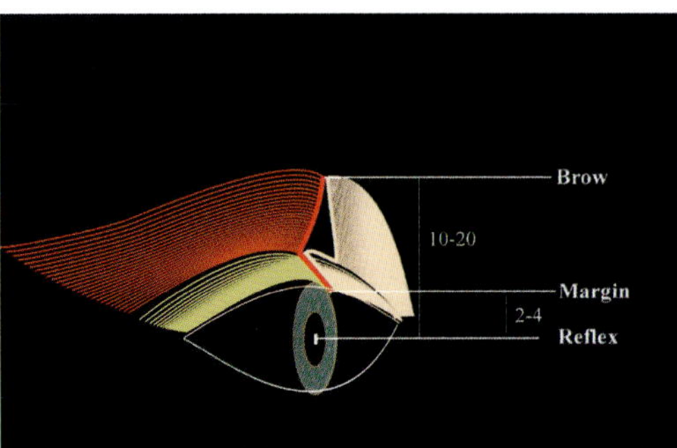

Fig. 11.8. The most important preoperative measurements are the distance between the corneal reflex and the upper lid margin (*MRD*) and the distance between the corneal reflex and the brow

11.3.4 Differentiation of Simple and Complicated Cases

Simple and complicated cases can appear similar unless they are examined more precisely. It is extremely important to differentiate simple and complicated cases, because this is the only way to avoid undesired results. In the simple group of blepharoplasty patients we find almost symmetric measurements without great deviations of the MRD and brow level. The simple blepharoplasty patient shows an MRD of 3–4 mm, an MRD asymmetry of a maximal 0.5 mm, a brow level of 12–20 mm and a brow asymmetry of a maximal 1 mm. In the simple group we can proceed to a standard blepharoplasty procedure without having to concern ourselves about asymmetric results, or under- or overcorrection. The standard blepharoplasty procedure can also be defined as the most frequently applied technique.

The complicated group of blepharoplasty patients show an MRD of less than 3 mm or more than 4 mm or an MRD asymmetry of >0.5 mm. Their brow level will be <12 mm or >20 mm or show an asymmetry of >2 mm. Patients with associated pathology such as ptosis, ptosis of the eyelashes, upper lid entropion, thyroid orbitopathy, upper lid retraction, proptosis, floppy eyelid syndrome or blepharochalasia also form part of the complicated group because the associated pathology must be corrected in conjunction with the blepharoplasty [8, 24, 27, 31, 36].

11.3.5 Planning Blepharoplasty According to the Typology of Cases

As I have mentioned above, it is impossible to find a similar case out of 1,000 blepharoplasty cases that could serve as a reliable reference or example for a new patient. There will be always something different that has to be addressed differently in planning surgery. Therefore I have simplified the typology of the examples to describe roughly two pairs of qualities, the "thick/thin" eyelid and the "wide/narrow" eyelid.

11.3.5.1 The Thick Eyelid

The thick eyelid can either be a congenital variation, often observed in young children, or an age related phenomenon. The congenital thick eyelid is due to an increased volume of subcutaneous tissue, orbicularis muscle and sub-brow fat. These cases have a bulky bolster over their orbital rim and septum with a normal intraorbital anatomy. The age related thick eyelid is primarily caused by a laxity of the orbital fibrous tissue that allows the orbital fat to herniate and the sub-brow fat to descend. It is reported, however, that orbital fat can gain volume with age. Thyroid orbitopathy must be ruled out. Orbitopathy patients may present with a swelling of both the subcutaneous and the intraorbital tissue. To plan the surgical procedure we should be able to differentiate the congenital and the age related thick eyelid. Young age photographs of the patient can be very helpful. Congenital cases with a thickened orbicularis muscle and sub-brow fat cannot simply be transformed into thin upper lids. The preseptal area and the lower sub-brow area can be thinned, but the debulking of the higher and deeper sub-brow area can interfere with the frontal and orbicular innervation (Figs. 11.9, 11.10).

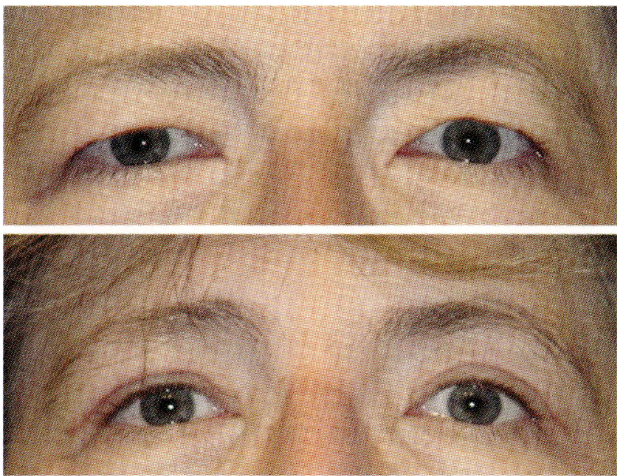

Fig. 11.9. If a brow lift is not planned, narrow and thick eyelids present the greatest difficulty in achieving a sufficient lid crease. The thickness of the eyelids is reduced by resection of orbicularis muscle, sub-brow fat and preaponeurotic fat

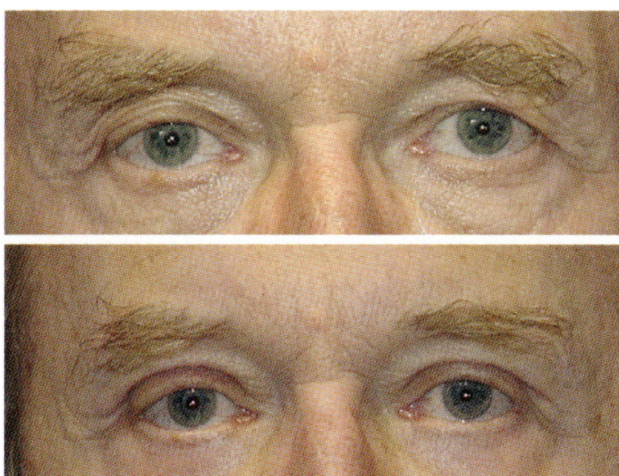

Fig. 11.11. Narrow and thin eyelids are common in males. As the aperture plane is frequently inclined posteriorly, there is enough distance left to elevate the skin crease sufficiently without the need to lift the brow. In this case the 1-mm ptosis on the right was corrected to prevent a lid crease asymmetry

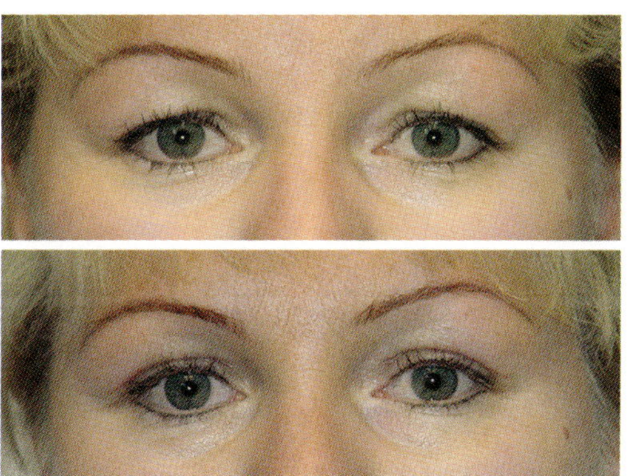

Fig. 11.10. In wide and thick eyelids the lid crease can be formed easily by reduction of sub-brow fat, orbicularis muscle and preaponeurotic fat. Excessive resection must be avoided

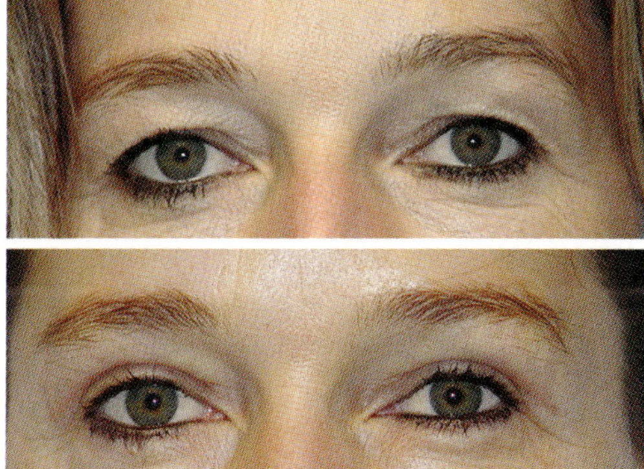

Fig. 11.12. Blepharoplasty in wide and thin eyelids tends to result in an undesired high lid crease and a demarcation of the orbital rim. To avoid this problem resection has to be limited

11.3.5.2 The Thin Eyelid

The thin eyelid shows a thin layer of orbicularis muscle and sub-brow fat [4, 7]. The orbital fibrous tissues are also thinner than normal and there is an increased tendency of aponeurotic ptosis. The volume of the orbital fat is usually not increased in these cases. There is usually no central preaponeurotic fat herniation, but the medial fat pad tends to protrude anteriorly because it is not retained by the lax fibrous tissue. The plan of the procedure would include a resection of the excessive skin without orbicularis muscle and resection of the herniated medial fat. As these patients usually show a high lid crease, the preaponeurotic fat pad may not have to be touched. Also the intermedial fat should not be resected in order to avoid a deep intermedial sulcus (Figs. 11.11, 11.12).

11.3.5.3
The Narrow Eyelid

The narrow eyelid is characterized by a reduced vertical distance of <10 mm between the lid margin and the brow. If a marked brow ptosis interferes with the visual field, we will have to plan a brow lift combined with a blepharoplasty. There are cases where the benefit of the brow lift is questionable, because there is a limited maximal aperture due to the relationship of the orbital rim and globe (aperture, see above). If the eyebrow does not interfere with this preexistent aperture, it must not be lifted. To predict whether a blepharoplasty will be successful without brow lift we have to look at the lateral aspect of the orbit in a primary position of gaze and estimate the shortest distance between the superior orbital rim and the globe. If the aperture plane angle is inclined posteriorly, there is often enough space to perform a blepharoplasty and create a lid crease. This option is suitable for males, where a low eyebrow is not usually considered an esthetic problem. In females, however, a brow lift [12, 19, 23, 29] is much more frequently indicated to create a lateral widening of the upper lid with parallelity or divergence of lash line and brow line (Figs. 11.9, 11.11).

11.3.5.4
The Wide Eyelid

The lateral widening of the eyelid with parallelity or even divergence of lash line and brow line is desirable on the one hand but demands some caution on the other hand when we plan the surgery. As the superolateral rim of the orbit will not be covered by the brow, its contour can show through and create an undesired downward projection or lateral rounding of lid crease. In these cases we would rather resect sub-brow fat in order to keep the superolateral rim smooth and allow the skin crease to fade laterally in a horizontal direction (Figs. 11.10, 11.12).

Summary for the Clinician

- **The most important measurements in the preoperative examination are the lid level (MRD), the brow level and the lid crease position**
- **The width of the inclined aperture plane (the shortest distance between the orbital rim and the surface of the globe) shows the available space for blepharoplasty**
- **Narrow and thin eyelids with low brows can often be treated with simple blepharoplasty without a brow lift**
- **Narrow and thick eyelids tend to have a very low lid crease, if a brow lift or debulking of the SOOF is not performed**
- **Wide and thin eyelids tend to have a excessively high lid crease level**
- **Wide and thick eyelids tend to have a normal lid crease level**

11.4
Surgical Technique of the Most Frequent Types of Upper Lid Blepharoplasty

11.4.1
Marking the Outlines of Incisions

Before the tissue is deformed by the injection of local anesthetic, we mark the outlines of the skin incisions with a pen. There is no need to do this with the patient in an upright position, as the amount of excision has been planned preoperatively and the situation can be compared with the photographs of the patient. The lower skin incision is marked first in the center of the eyelid at a distance of 7–11 mm from the lid margin. Sometimes this point coincides with the inward plication of the skin fold. In our cases the average distance is 8.5 mm depending on the size of the eye and the orbit. From this point a line is drawn medially and laterally in the direction towards the insertions of the medial and lateral canthal tendon. Then the skin is grasped without tension with a blunt forceps to measure the amount of excessive skin. We have to determine in every individual case a definite incision line in order to place it in the junction between the tarsal and the septal surface, where the lid crease will form postoperatively and thus hide a possible scar (Fig. 11.13).

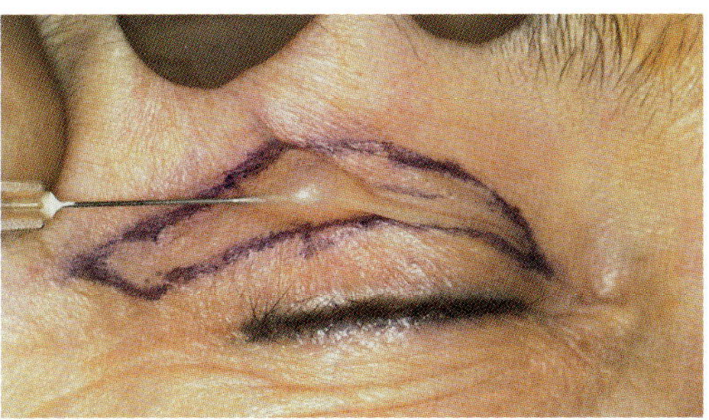

Fig. 11.13. After having outlined the borders of the excision, the skin is subcutaneously hydrodissected with a local anesthetic to separate the skin from the orbicularis muscle

11.4.2
Local Anaesthesia

With appropriate sedation the intervention is much more comfortable for patients and the pain of the local anesthetic injection is reduced significantly. The second purpose of the local injection is to separate tissues by hydrodissection. Every layer can be separated from the underlying layer by this method (Fig. 11.13).

11.4.3
Skin Incision

The skin can be excised with a blade, a radiofrequency needle or a CO_2 laser. The medial angle of the incision should be small and not extended medially to the lacrimal punctum. We must be aware that the medial upper lid skin rarely needs to be shortened, because it will be needed to fill the medial cavity. The lateral angle of the incision commonly ends above the lateral canthus. Sometimes the incision is carried out further laterally to approach the lateral subcutaneous tissues [8, 22, 24].

11.4.4
Skin Excision

The skin is excised with scissors, a laser or a radiofrequency needle, leaving the underlying orbicularis muscle intact. The previous hydrodissection facilitates the separation of the tissues. Only if we have planned to excise the entire exposed surface of the underlying muscle can we excise both layers simultaneously.

11.4.5
Orbicularis Separation

The orbicularis muscle has to be separated to expose the septum. In cases with thin orbicularis muscle or compromised orbicularis function, the muscle is only separated by a horizontal incision without any excision of muscle fibers. The selected level of the orbicularis separation can affect the position of the lid crease to some degree. If we do not know at this step whether an orbicularis excision will be necessary, we can start with the orbicularis separation, proceed through the septum and orbital fat, check the level of lid crease formation and decide about the orbicularis excision afterwards.

11.4.6
Orbicularis Excision

For the majority of cases, a controlled excision of orbicularis fibers will improve the lid crease formation. After having removed the skin and exposed the preseptal orbicularis muscle, the patient is asked to open the lids. At this stage it is possible to view the lid crease and decide if we want to eliminate the orbicularis fibers. The level and the width of the excision are important for the location of the crease.

11.4.7
Identification of the Septum

For all further surgery it is necessary to identify the orbital septum to create an approach into the orbit. In most cases the septum can easily be identified as the underlying membrane with orbital fat shining through it after the orbicularis muscle has been separated or partially resected. As the septum is multilayered and shaped like a bag overlying the aponeurosis, it can sometimes

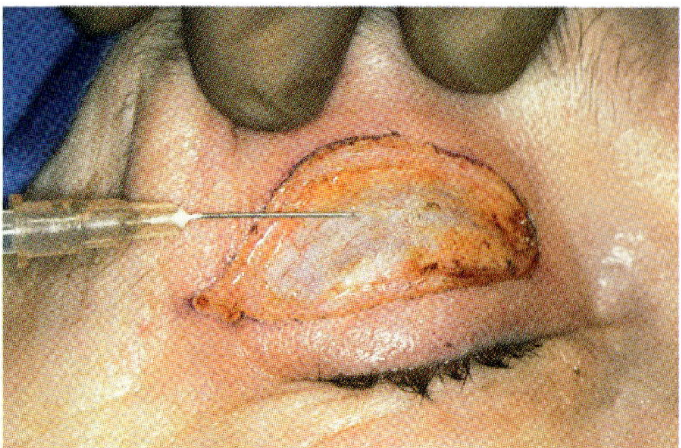

Fig. 11.14. After having resected a portion of the orbicularis muscle, the septum is exposed and an anesthetic solution is injected below to visualize the underlying orbital anatomy

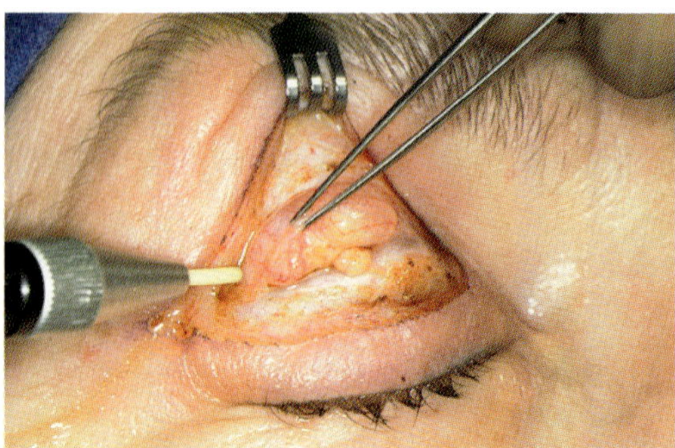

Fig. 11.15. After a wide "open sky" section of the orbital septum, the preaponeurotic fat can be visualized and reduced laterally, centrally or intermedially

be more difficult to identify. In these cases we recommend choosing a higher level of septum penetration and first injecting liquid under the membrane to improve the visibility below (Fig. 11.14).

11.4.8 Dissection of the Septum

The section of the septum is performed for two reasons. First we can create an approach into the orbit to expose the orbital fat. I prefer the wide "open sky" section of the septum to visualize the different fat compartments. The second advantage of the "open sky" section is its benefit on the lid crease formation. We can observe during surgery that the wide section of the septum creates a much better definition of the lid crease. We never intend to suture the opened septum. The orbital fat can alternatively be approached and resected through buttonhole incisions [26, 38].

11.4.9 Management of the Preaponeurotic Fat

The preaponeurotic fat pad is the most easily approached compartment in the orbit. As it is semiliquid it can dislocate medially or laterally. The best area to begin the resection is the central part of the fat pat, where vessels are rare. Care must be taken in the neighborhood of the intermedial area, where we get very close to the supraorbital neurovascular bundle, and in the lateral area, where we need to preserve the lacrimal gland [34]. The fat lobuli can be lifted gently with a forceps and cut with scissors, a radiofrequency needle or laser [27, 31, 36]. To avoid any traction, we prefer not to clamp the fat with a forceps (Fig. 11.15).

11.4.10 Management of the Intermedial Orbital Fat

The intermedial orbital fat is identical to the medial extension of preaponeurotic fat. We prefer to differentiate this area well, because the fat looks different with smaller, irregular lobuli. Its resection can cause two serious complications. The first risk is the injury of the supraorbital neurovascular structures. The second risk is related to the tendency that the lid crease in this area can become excavated into a deep sulcus after surgery (Fig. 11.16).

11.4.11 Exposure of the Medial Orbital Fat

The medial orbital fat is covered by two fibrous membranes, the medial extensions of the septum and the medial extensions of the aponeurosis. The two layers can be encountered separate-

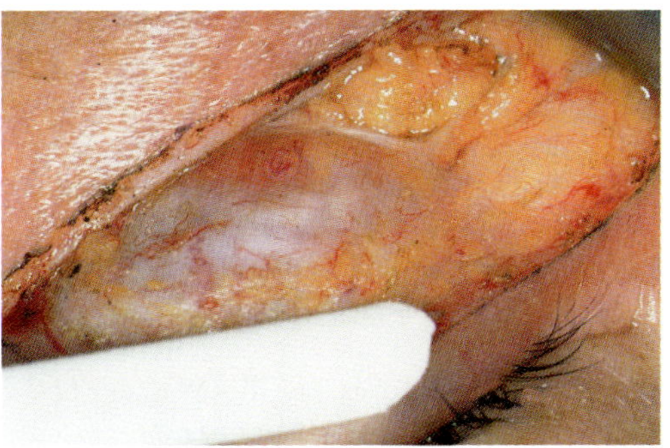

Fig. 11.16. The intermedial part of the preaponeurotic fat is exposed, while the medial orbital fat is still covered by a fibrous membrane

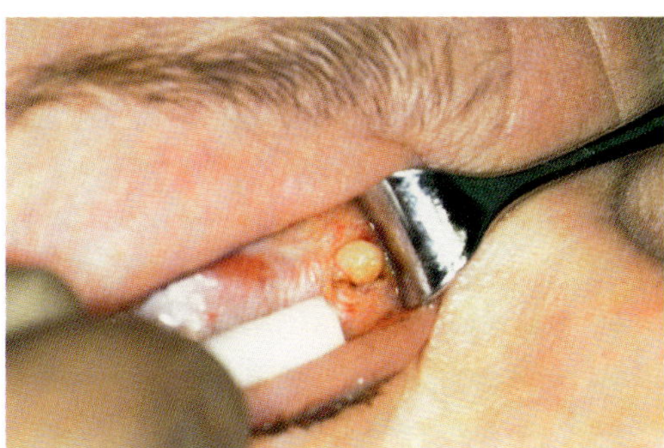

Fig. 11.17. Medial orbital fat protrudes after the careful section of the anterior fibrous membranes

ly or found to be fused into one layer. The approach is much easier in cases with thin eyelids, where the medial fat pad tends to herniate. The dilated and thinned anterior fibrous membranes are transparent and let the fat shine through. After the incision of the membranes the fat protrudes and can be resected. When the fibrous membranes show a greater density, the approach to the medial fat can be achieved by retracting the septum medially upwards and medially downwards with two small Desmarres retractors. Thus the small anterior membrane of the medial fat pad can be exposed. With the injection of an anesthetic solution beyond the fibrous membrane, the medial fat compartment is visualized before the membrane is incised in a semicircular manner. The apex of the semicircular incision is placed laterally in order to preserve the medial wall of the compartment, where vessels are running from the supraorbital vascular supply downwards to the medial canthal tendon to connect with the tarsal arcade.

11.4.12 Resection of the Medial Orbital Fat

After exposure of the medial orbital fat, it will not prolapse, because it is covered by another proper transparent membrane. After the incision of this membrane the fat lobules protrude and can be excised without having to perform any traction. The medial fat lobules are more solid and more pale than the preaponeurotic fat modules. They form a sausage-like structure that continues backwards into the orbit. They can also be resected more extensively with the intention of decompressing the orbit (Fig. 11.17).

11.4.13 Resection of the Medial Subcutaneous Fat

Medially above the lacrimal punctum we frequently find a fatty infiltration in the layer of the medial preseptal orbicularis muscle, which is responsible for a postoperative prolonged swelling and protrusion of the tissue. The medial subcutaneous fat can be resected while the overlying skin has to be preserved carefully. This is achieved by stretching the skin like a tent to carry out the subcutaneous debulking. Any skin resection in this area should be avoided (Fig. 11.18).

11.4.14 SOOF Resection

The sub-brow fat or suborbicularis oculi fat (SOOF) can easily be approached laterally after having separated the preseptal orbicularis muscle. The SOOF is covered by its proper fibrous membrane, which has to be opened to expose the fat lobules. The resection should only include the anterior and inferior redundant lobules, as the profound dissection down to the orbital rim can cause a laceration of the deep vascular network and the lacrimal nerve.

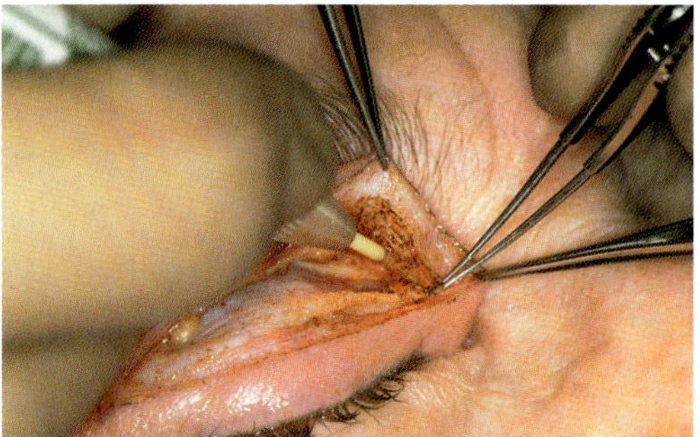

Fig. 11.18. A subcutaneous fatty degeneration in the level of the medial orbicularis muscle is resected

11.4.15 Sutures

We do not recommend deep translamellar or invaginating sutures from the skin to the posterior lamella as they create a permanent fixed crease that will be incompatible with the natural dynamic lid crease. We only suture the skin to close the wound. The preferred suture material is 6–0 or 7–0 monofilament nylon or 7–0 braided nylon. Running or single sutures can be used taking care that the skin margins are just aligned but not compressed. The material is removed after 5 days or in the case of laser surgery after 7 days. For intracutaneous sutures we can use a 5–0 or 6–0 monofilament nylon.

11.4.16 Laser Blepharoplasty

The carbon dioxide laser can be used as a cutting or a skin resurfacing instrument [14, 21, 39]. Usually we do not apply the resurfacing mode on the upper lid, because the redundant skin is removed in any case. The resurfacing mode, however, finds its best applications on the lower lid skin. To use the carbon dioxide as a cutting instrument has some advantages and some disadvantages. If both are compared after having performed about the same amount of surgery with and without a laser, I find that it is more reasonable to use a laser in upper lid blepharoplasty. There are two main advantages of the laser application related to bleeding. The first is that we save the time that would be lost by cautery. The second is more important because the identification of the orbital anatomical structures is made much safer. In upper lid blepharoplasty, the location to enter into the medial orbit must be identified exactly. Without the use of a laser we sometimes risk blood staining under the medial septum and aponeurosis, which obscures the safe approach to the underlying orbital structures. The disadvantage of the laser application is related to prolonged wound healing and postoperative late onset edema (see Sect. 11.4.11).

Summary for the Clinician

- **The skin incision is placed at the level where the lid crease is expected to form**
- **After the skin excision enough skin must be left to form the posterior plication of the lid crease and the medial cavity of the upper lid**
- **The wide "open sky" incision of the septum allows a more pronounced lid crease formation and a better exposure of the orbital fat**
- **The treatment of the different components of orbital fatty tissue has to be planned individually**

11.5 Complications in Upper Lid Blepharoplasty: Prevention and Management

The majority of upper lid blepharoplasty complications are caused by the surgery concept and can be avoided by careful planning. For this reason I have included extensive sections about relevant anatomical evaluation and surgical planning. There are some other complications, however, that cannot be predicted by the analysis of the patient or prevented by the surgeon [9, 11, 16, 17, 30, 37, 40].

11.5.1 Undercorrection

Even if the patient will be unhappy and might need another intervention, undercorrection must not be considered as a severe complication. If the patient has been informed preoperatively that the most common cause of a severe overcorrection was the attempt to prevent any undercorrection, he or she will be grateful not to belong to the overcorrected group. While overcorrection can create unrepairable defects, undercorrection can always be relieved. The most frequent form of undercorrection results when thick eyelids are treated with simple skin excision.

11.5.2 Overcorrection

As the major surgical process in upper lid blepharoplasty is the resection of tissue, the surgeon is likely to be seduced into associating a larger resection with a better result. The second cause of overcorrection is the fear of producing an undercorrected result and therefore performing an excessive resection.

11.5.3 Excessive Skin Resection

11.5.3.1 Excessive Resection of Central Skin

As the central eyelid skin is the main area to permit the formation of the skin crease, a small surplus of skin is needed for an unlimited plication of the fold. We have to be aware that we initially want to create a skin crease and we need enough skin to fill the crease. Excessive resection also creates the functional problems of lid lag, defective closure and restricted blinking. Skin has to be replaced by skin grafting. The best cosmetic results of grafting are achieved if autologous eyelid skin can be harvested elsewhere and transplanted over a healthy orbicularis muscle. If eyelid skin is not available, we can obtain retroauricular skin as a second choice. Any graft of eyelid or retroauricular skin must be separated cautiously from all subcutaneous tissue before it is inserted. As the grafted area will be less flexible than the natural eyelid skin, the graft should not be placed in front of the lid crease. It should be inserted above or below the crease.

11.5.3.2 Excessive Resection of Medial Skin

An excessive medial resection will inhibit the skin lining of the medial cavity. The skin will not be sufficient to cover the orbicularis muscle surface and will be lifted off in the form of a traction fold. The fold forms in the direction of the traction. If the central blepharoplasty incision has been extended too far medially and has created a medial skin deficiency, the incision line will be perpendicular to the lack of skin. Any traction on a wound can cause a scar formation and an increased traction. The condition is not easy to resolve, because a preexistent scar may disturb the healing of a skin graft or skin flaps. A free skin graft should be the first choice for the problem, because a Z-plasty might produce a new traction in a perpendicular direction.

11.5.3.3 Excessive Resection of Lateral Skin

The excessive resection of lateral eyelid skin causes less severe complications than the central and medial resection, because we have a shallow lateral lid crease and a convex lateral eyelid surface. The resection can therefore be extended so far that the elevation of the lateral brow and the closure of the lid are not inhibited. Especially the desired lateral eyebrow level has to be considered before resecting skin. Lateral skin can also best be replaced by a free graft.

11.5.4 Excessive Orbicularis Muscle Resection

If the pretarsal muscle is not preserved, severe functional problems with defective eyelid closure and insufficient blinking can result. An extremely broad resection of the preseptal muscle can produce a denervation of the pretarsal muscle. The consequences are severe, because an insufficient orbicularis muscle function cannot be repaired. Another problem after the extensive resection of the preseptal and orbital muscle is the excavated "round eye" appearance by the exposure of the lateral and superior orbital rim.

The excavation can be camouflaged to some extent by the transposition of a flap of SOOF into the sulcus. Another option is the transplantation of small fat lobules of orbital or periumbilical fat.

11.5.5 Excessive SOOF Resection

Excessive resection of sub-brow fat will also cause a local depression or exposure of the orbital rim. To refill the lost volume we can try to transplant fat lobules or inject a filling material under the periosteal fibrous sheath. Hyaluronic acid can be injected as a probatory filler material. Another consequence of excessive SOOF resection can be the lesion of the supraorbital or lacrimal neurovascular structures.

11.5.6 Excessive Resection of Preaponeurotic Fat

The hyperresection of the central part of the preaponeurotic fat creates fewer problems than the resection of the lateral and intermedial fat. The lateral lobules of the preaponeurotic fat surround the lacrimal gland and the lacrimal neurovascular structures. If the lacrimal gland is not identified, it can be resected with the fat, causing a serious problem of xerophthalmia. The intermedial orbital fat surrounds the supraorbital neurovascular structures. Its resection can cause severe hemorrhage and injury to the supraorbital nerve. The resection also tends to create an undesired deep excavation of the intermedial area.

11.5.7 Excessive Resection of Medial Orbital Fat

Excessive medial fat resection has a decompressive effect on the orbit and can be used for this purpose. We have rarely found any excavation problems of the medial area, presumably because the anterior membranes of the septum and the extensions of the aponeurosis reform sufficiently to build a firm barrier.

11.5.8 Asymmetry

The resection of redundant skin uncovers the lid crease. After the intervention we do not always find the creases at the same level. We have mentioned above that a lid crease asymmetry of 1 mm may be tolerable, whereas a difference of 2 mm should be corrected. If a 2-mm asymmetry has occurred, we have to decide whether we want to lower the higher crease or elevate the lower crease. Usually the patient's complaint will be addressed to only one side. The patient will probably interpret the lower crease as an undercorrection and the higher crease as a persistent swelling. To solve the problem we need to analyze the balance of the frontal muscle activity on the brows and the levator innervation. Due to Hering's law the levator innervation is bilaterally equalized. The brow elevation can, however, show a unilateral overactivity.

11.5.8.1 Unilateral High Lid Crease

The problem is often caused by a unilateral ptosis. If a small ptosis of 0.5 mm or 1 mm has been not detected and not corrected during blepharoplasty, we often produce an asymmetric lid crease elevation of 2 mm or more enhanced by the brow elevation. The most adequate way to manage the problem would be a ptosis correction [2, 3, 20, 35]. If a reoperation is not considered, we can use botulinum toxin to relax the frontal muscle and lower the brow and the lid crease. The botulinum toxin can even create a long term effect after the patient has learned to relax the frontal muscle.

11.5.8.2 Unilateral Low Lid Crease

A low lid crease can be caused by upper lid retraction or by brow ptosis. If the problem has not been detected and corrected during blepharoplasty, the patients will need a second procedure to lift the brow or to lower the lid. The direct brow lift by a supra-brow excision is often impossible because the scar cannot be hidden close to the hairline of the brow. The brow elevation can also be achieved by indirect transpalpebral or transfrontal procedures. In some cases the lid crease can be elevated by resecting prolapsed SOOF or by weakening the lateral fibers of the orbicularis muscle, as they act as an antagonist to the frontalis muscle.

11.5.9 Double Skin Fold

A undesired double skin fold can be produced when the skin is invaginated by sutures that pick up deep tissue of the posterior lamella. The first normal fold will develop anteriorly to the natural lid crease. The second fold will be formed by the invagination technique with skin crease deepening sutures [11, 30, 33]. The natural fold will unfold completely in downgaze or lid closure whereas the invaginated fold stays visible.

11.5.10 Posterior Lamella Lacerations

As the layers of the conjoined fascia, the orbital septum and the aponeurosis are confluent and superimposed in the lid crease area, confusion of the anatomy is possible with the consequence of a posterior lamella lesion. The accidental section of the aponeurosis in a limited area does not affect the lid level. A deeper laceration of the posterior lamella can, however, cause a hematoma of Müller's muscle, ptosis or upper lid retraction.

11.5.11 Failure to Correct Associated Pathology

The oculoplastic surgeon should always look for associated pathology such as ptosis, brow ptosis, thyroid eye disease, retraction, upper lid entropion, blepharitis, lash ptosis, floppy eyelid syndrome, facial palsy, and blepharospasm. If associated pathology is missed and not corrected, we can face serious complications or deceptive results. The most common fault is not to correct associated ptosis, which will create an unexpected high skin crease.

11.5.12 Hemorrhage, Edema and Scar Formation

Severe postoperative hemorrhage is very rare in upper lid surgery, although we found some increase in patients after CO_2 laser surgery. CO_2 laser surgery may also be responsible for a postoperative late onset edema in 0.3% of patients after 4–5 days, a complication we never observed after surgery without laser. Scars are extremely rare after conventional upper lid blepharoplasty and seem to be even less probable if a CO_2 laser is used. After the laser incision, the wound takes 2 days longer to heal but suture nodule formation is less common.

Summary for the Clinician

- **Excessive resection is the most frequent iatrogenic error and can produce unrepairable defects**
- **A >1-mm asymmetry of the lid crease level is not accepted in most cases and can be corrected by subsequent surgery**
- **Laser surgery with a layer by layer approach facilitates the correct anatomical identification and reduces the risk of inadvertent lacerations**
- **Ptosis, pseudoptosis, lash ptosis, entropion and proptosis should be corrected in conjunction with the blepharoplasty**

References

1. American Academy of Ophthalmology (1991) Functional indications for upper and lower eyelid blepharoplasty. Ophthalmology 98:1461–1463
2. Anderson RL, Beard C (1971) The levator aponeurosis. Arch Ophthalmol 95:1437–1441
3. Anderson RL, Dixon RS (1979) Aponeurotic ptosis surgery. Arch Ophthalmol 97:1123–1128
4. Bergin DJ, McCord CD, Berger T, Friedberg H, Waterhouse W (1988) Blepharochalasis. Br J Ophthalmol 72:863–867
5. Bosniak SL (1990) Cosmetic blepharoplasty. Raven Press, New York
6. Callahan MA (1979) Ophthalmic plastic and orbital surgery. Aesculapius Publishing Co., Birmingham, AL
7. Collin JR (1991) Blepharochalasis. A review of 30 cases. Ophthal Plast Reconstr Surg 7:153–157

8. Colton JJ, Beekhuis GJ (1986) Blepharoplasty. In: Cummings CW, Krause CJ (eds) Otolaryngology – head and neck surgery, vol 1. Mosby, St. Louis, pp 487–510
9. Demere M, Wood T, Austin W (1974) Eye complications with blepharoplasty or other eyelid surgery. Plast Reconstr Surg 53:634–637
10. Flowers RS (1987) The art of eyelid and orbital aesthetics: multiracial surgical considerations. Clin Plast Surg 14:703–721
11. Flowers RS (1993) Upper blepharoplasty by eyelid invagination. Anchor blepharoplasty. Clin Plast Surg 20:193–207
12. Flowers RS, Caputy GG, Flowers SS (1993) The biomechanics of brow and frontalis function and its effect on blepharoplasty. Clin Plast Surg 20: 255–268
13. Fumas DW (1981) The orbicularis oculi muscle – management in blepharoplasty. Clin Plast Surg 8:687–715
14. Kang DH, Koo SH, Choi JH, Park SH (2001) Laser blepharoplasty for making double eyelids in Asians. Plast Reconstr Surg 107:1884–1889
15. Katzen LB (1986) The history of cosmetic blepharoplasty. Adv Ophthalmic Plast Reconstr Surg 5:89–96
16. Levine MR, Boynton J, Tenzel RR, Miller GR (1975) Complications of blepharoplasty. Ophthalmic Surg 6:53–57
17. Lisman RD, Hyde K, Smith B (1988) Complications of blepharoplasty. Clin Plast Surg 115:309–335
18. McCord CD (1995) Eyelid surgery, principles and techniques. Lippincott-Raven, New York
19. McCord CD, Doxanas MT (1990) Browplasty and browpexy: an adjunct to blepharoplasty. Plast Reconstr Surg 86:248–254
20. Millay DJ, Larrabee WF Jr (1989) Ptosis and blepharoplasty surgery. Arch Otolaryngol Head Neck Surg 115:198–201
21. Morrow DM, Morrow LB (1992) CO_2 laser blepharoplasty. A comparison with cold-steel surgery. J Dermatol Surg Oncol 18:307–313
22. Owsley JQ (1994) Aesthetic facial surgery. WB Saunders, Philadelphia
23. Paul MD (2001) The evolution of the brow lift in aesthetic plastic surgery. Plast Reconstr Surg 108:1409–1424
24. Pfeiffer MJ (2003) Blepharoplastik der Oberlider. Ophthalmo-Chirurgie 15:317–323
25. Putterman AM, Urist MJ (1974) Reconstruction of the upper eyelid crease and fold. Arch Ophthalmol 94:1941–1954
26. Putterman AM, Urist MJ (1974) Surgical anatomy of the orbital septum. Ann Ophthalmol 8:290–294
27. Rathburn JE (1989) Eyelid surgery. Little, Brown and Co., Toronto
28. Rees TD (1980) Aesthetic plastic surgery, vol 2. WB Saunders, Philadelphia
29. Rees TD, Aston SJ, Thorne CHM (1990) Blepharoplasty and facial plasty including forehead-browlift. In: McCarthy JG (ed) Plastic surgery, vol 3. WB Saunders, Philadelphia, pp 2320–2358
30. Sheen JH (1977) A change in the technique of supratarsal fixation in upper blepharoplasty. Plast Reconstr Surg 59:831–835
31. Siegel RJ (1984) Advanced blepharoplasty. In: Regnault P, Daniel RK (eds) Aesthetic plastic surgery. Little, Brown and Co., Boston, p 354
32. Siegel RJ (1993) Essential anatomy for contemporary upper lid blepharoplasty. Clin Plast Surg 20:209–212
33. Small RG (1979) Supratarsal fixation in ophthalmic plastic surgery. Ophthalmic Surg 9:73–85
34. Smith B, Lisman RD (1983) Dacryoadenopexy as a recognized factor in upper lid blepharoplasty. Plast Reconstr Surg 71:629–632
35. Stasior OG, Ballitch HA (1993) 2d: Ptosis repair in aesthetic blepharoplasty. Clin Plast Surg 20:269–273
36. Tebbetts JB (1992) Blepharoplasty. A refined technique emphasizing accuracy and control. Clin Plast Surg 19:329–349
37. Tenzel RR (1969) Surgical techniques and problems in cosmetic blepharoplasty. Trans Am Acad Ophthalmol Otolaryngol 73:1154–1161
38. Tipton JB (1972) Should incisions in the orbital septum be sutured in blepharoplasty? Plast Reconstr Surg 49:613–615
39. Trelles MA, Velez M, Sanchez J, Sala P, Bell G (1991) Carbon dioxide laser blepharoplasty – advantages and disadvantages. Ann Plast Surg 27:180–181
40. Wilkins RB, Byrd WA (1985) Complications of blepharoplasty. Ophthal Plast Reconstr Surg 1: 195–198
41. Zide BM, Jelks GW (1985) Surgical anatomy of the orbit. Raven Press, New York

Update on Lasers in Oculoplastic Surgery

Julie A. Woodward, Aerlyn G. Dawn

Core Messages

- The use of laser technology for incisional surgery, skin resurfacing and other applications is a rapidly advancing area within oculoplastic surgery
- The carbon dioxide (CO_2) laser is frequently used for upper and lower eyelid blepharoplasty. Advantages of the CO_2 laser for incisional surgery include reduced total intraoperative time, excellent hemostasis, and enhanced visualization of relevant anatomy
- In many instances, laser skin resurfacing with the CO_2 laser or the erbium:yttrium aluminum garnet (Er:YAG) laser is the treatment of choice over chemical peels and dermabrasion for photoaged skin
- Non-ablative laser technologies are being used as alternative methods of improving photoaged skin with minimal healing time. These include the 580–590-nm fast-pulsed dye laser, the 595-nm pulsed dye laser, the 1,320-nm neodymium:YAG laser, and the 1,450-nm diode laser
- Various non-laser technologies that also use electromagnetic radiation to heat tissue are being used for skin rejuvenation including broad spectrum light and radiofrequency
- Vascular lesions can now be safely and effectively treated using a variety of lasers in the 488–638 nm range, or using broad spectrum light
- Q-switched lasers, including the 532-nm fd Nd:YAG, the 755-nm alexandrite laser, and the 1,064-nm Nd:YAG laser are effective in removing tattoo pigments
- In lacrimal surgery, the potassium titanyl phosphate (KTP) laser and holmium laser can be used to perform endonasal laser dacryocystorhinostomy and laser canaliculoplasty
- Laser hair removal with the 694-nm ruby laser, the 755-nm alexandrite laser, the 810-nm diode laser, the long pulsed 1,064-nm Nd:YAG, or broad spectrum light can be successful in the reduction of pigmented hair follicles
- The development of lasers with longer pulse widths and improved cooling devices allows treatment of darker skin types

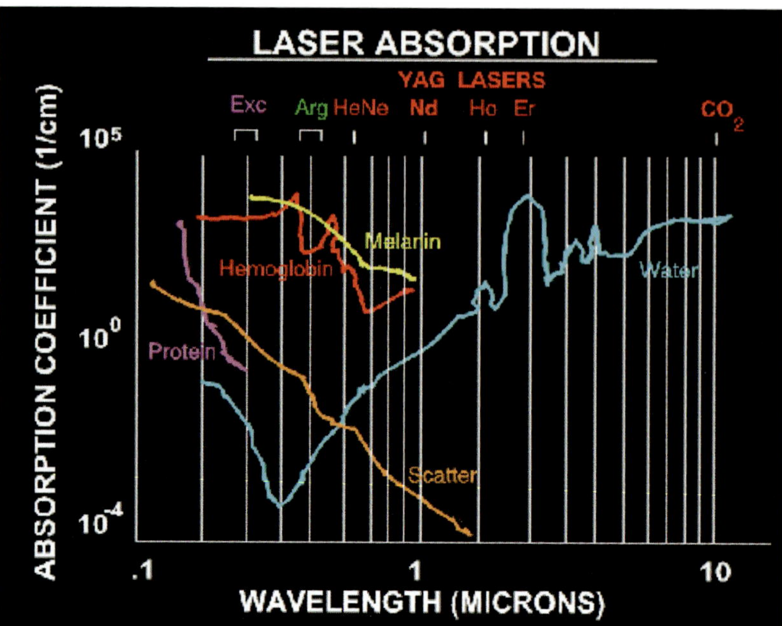

Fig. 12.1. The laser absorption curve

12.1 Introduction

Lasers have been used extensively in ophthalmology for both anterior and posterior segment surgery. In recent years, lasers have greatly enhanced the field of oculoplastic surgery.

The theory of selective photothermolysis describes the basic interaction between lasers and human tissue [1]. Individual molecules in human tissue, termed chromophores, absorb each wavelength of electromagnetic radiation with a different affinity. The three commonly presented chromophores in human tissue that are noted to specifically absorb laser energy are water, hemoglobin, and melanin. The conceptualization of the laser absorption curve is important to understanding the basic principles of how lasers can be used in the surgical treatment of patients as seen in Fig. 12.1. Because of these principles, lasers can be used to heat water in cells, hemoglobin in vessels, or melanin in hair follicles with minimal damage to the surrounding tissues.

The first ever laser treatment in humans was performed with ruby and neodymium lasers in 1962 to create thermal necrosis of a malignant melanoma prior to excision [2]. Treatment of non-pigmented tissue became possible after the development of the invisible 10,600-nm continuous wave CO_2 laser by Patel in 1964 [3]. The use of the CO_2 laser for incisional blepharoplasty surgery was developed in 1980 by Baker [4]. Laser skin resurfacing with the CO_2 laser was developed in the late 1980s. The erbium:YAG laser was not FDA approved for laser resurfacing until 1996; yet there have been more than 20 different manufacturers of these lasers. Many applications of laser technology have developed in recent years, and they are likely to play an increasingly important role in oculoplastic surgery and other related specialties in the coming decades. This chapter outlines the current major applications of lasers in oculoplastic surgery, including incisional laser surgery, laser skin resurfacing, laser treatment of vascular lesions, laser tattoo removal, laser hair removal, and laser assisted dacryocystorhinostomy.

12.2 Incisional Laser Surgery

Incisional devices used in periorbital surgery include the traditional steel blade, radiofrequency, needlepoint monopolar cautery, and the CO_2 laser. The goals for the ideal incisional instrument are patient safety, minimal local tissue trauma, excellent hemostasis, rapid surgical time, rapid wound healing, wounds with excellent tensile strength, superior final appearance of healed wounds, and, ultimately, high patient satisfaction. The lack of tactile feedback from the laser is an important difference between performing incisional surgery with a laser versus a traditional scalpel blade. Traditional surgical techniques provide non-visual stimuli that help the surgeon to determine wound depth. Laser surgery, in contrast, requires visual recognition of tissue planes without tactile stimuli [4].

The CO_2 laser produces three zones of thermal injury: (1) central, (2) surrounding, and (3) peripheral. The central zone corresponds to the actual incision where the tissue is precisely vaporized. The surrounding zone is irreversible thermal damage consisting of coagulation necrosis and denatured, melted, and contracted collagen. The peripheral zone is reversible thermal damage.

There are several advantages of lasers for incisional surgery. Total intraoperative time is reduced because the laser handpiece acts as a cutting tool, a cautery, and a blunt dissection instrument. A shorter surgical time makes the procedure much more tolerable to patients. Hemorrhage can rapidly obscure the anatomic detail of eyelid structures; thus, the excellent hemostasis achieved with laser incisions greatly enhances the visualization of important anatomy and increases the efficiency and precision of surgery [5]. This may also reduce the incidence of postoperative blindness, which is most commonly associated with orbital hemorrhage. These unique qualities of incisional laser surgery make it a desirable instrument for many surgeons to use not only for blepharoplasty, but also for ptosis repair, ectropion and entropion repair, thyroid decompression, and other orbital surgeries.

There are some disadvantages to incisional laser surgery. First, a laser costs significantly more than a scalpel; however, many surgery centers already have CO_2 lasers that are perfectly suitable. Special sandblasted metal instruments must be purchased to protect the patient and operating room staff. In addition, the surgeon must undertake the significant learning curve required not only to learn how to perform the surgery, but also how to train operating room staff. Usually, training the nursing staff demands much greater effort than learning how to perform the surgery, but once these hurdles are overcome the surgeon will enjoy the benefits of using the laser.

12.2.1 CO_2 Laser

The first use of the 10,600-nm CO_2 laser for cutaneous incisional surgery was in the 1960s and 1970s. By the late 1970s, CO_2 lasers were being used by gynecologists, otorhinolaryngologists, neurosurgeons, plastic surgeons, and dermatologists. Histologic studies revealed that the CO_2 laser was able to seal lymphatic vessels and small nerve endings and coagulate vessels up to 0.5 mm in diameter [1]. This is important in oculoplastic surgery because most blood vessels in the periorbital region are less than 0.5 mm in diameter. However, one of the major problems with such continuous wave CO_2 lasers was that the 1.0-mm spot size caused a broad zone of thermal injury at the wound edges (200–500 µm) [6]. Baker performed the first laser-assisted blepharoplasty in 1980 [4]. However, many oculoplastic surgeons at that time felt that CO_2 lasers produced too much thermal damage to be useful in cutaneous surgery.

Smaller diameter (0.2 mm) high frequency pulsed beam (superpulsed) CO_2 lasers were developed in the 1980s. These produced a smaller zone of thermal injury (115 µm) than previous CO_2 lasers. This expanded the use of CO_2 lasers for cutaneous incisional surgery [5]. Carbon dioxide lasers are used in continuous wave mode, or the newer high-frequency superpulsed beam that has a frequency of 3,000 pulses/s. Such lasers include the UltraPulse Encore

(Lumenis, Santa Clara, CA) and Unipulse 1040 (Nidek Inc., Fremont, CA). The zone of thermal injury with these lasers has been reduced to only about 110–115 μm. This makes them ideal tools for periorbital surgery. The ultimate clinical appearance of healed wounds after cutaneous surgery with a superpulsed CO_2 laser is generally impossible to differentiate from wounds following traditional cold steel surgery [5].

12.2.1.1 Current Uses of the CO_2 Laser

The CO_2 laser has two modes – incisional and resurfacing. The laser has a focused delivery system for incisional purposes where the diameter of the beam is controlled by the distance that the laser is held from the target tissue. There is usually a handpiece with a focal length of $f = 125$ mm at which the beam diameter is 0.2 mm. When the laser is defocused a few centimeters from the target tissue, the spot size increases, so the fluence (J/cm^2) decreases, which creates more thermocoagulation instead of vaporization, which provides hemostasis. The high absorption of the CO_2 laser by water allows the oculoplastic surgeon to perform precise incisional procedures.

The CO_2 laser can also be used in a resurfacing mode. This is often the treatment of choice for wrinkles and sundamaged skin. It can also be used to tighten lower lid festoons. Resurfacing lasers may be either focused or collimated. They are delivered via a computer pattern generator in either a series of pulses, or in a continuous wave beam that is swept across the tissue very quickly. The focused delivery systems must be held a set distance from the skin. The collimated systems are easier to work with because they will produce the same spot size no matter what distance they are held from the skin. This will be further discussed in Sect. 12.3.

12.2.1.2 CO_2 Laser – Technique and Complications

Before the laser is turned on, a laser safe environment is a requirement. This includes providing protective eyewear for everyone in the operating room, turning off any supplemental oxygen on the field, providing a laser-safe drape of wet towels or sterile aluminum foil, and placing a "caution laser in use" sign on the entry door to the operating room. "Laser safe" instruments are required that are anodized or sandblasted to provide a rough surface that reduces specular reflection of laser beams.

When using the CO_2 laser for incisional purposes, it is important to understand that the speed that the laser is moved over the skin and the distance that the laser is held from the tissue are the key factors in determining what reaction will be produced in the target tissue. The surgeon's use of the laser is based on visual feedback, instead of tactile feedback. A laser moved over skin rapidly will make a much more shallow incision than one moved slowly.

The laser's spot size is smallest and therefore most precise when the laser handpiece tip is held 1 mm from the skin. This is desirable for making incisions. When the laser is held in a slightly defocused mode, 1–2 cm from the tissue, the spot size is larger, but more hemostasis is notable. This is best for removing a skin/muscle flap. Bleeding vessels may be coagulated by using the laser in the defocused mode, at about 5–8 cm from the target tissue.

Not only is hand-eye coordination important for laser blepharoplasty, but also foot-eye coordination since the laser is delivered when the foot pedal is depressed. The surgeon will create stray marks on the skin if the laser is pulled away from the target tissue before the foot pedal is released.

Any carbon dioxide laser that delivers at least 6 W of power and has a 0.2-mm focused delivery handpiece may be used. The laser should be ergonomically positioned so that the surgeon is comfortable and does not feel any tension on the hand piece. The balance should be set so that if the hand piece were to be released, it would either stay in place or very slowly rise. Most surgeons use the laser at 6 W to perform laser blepharoplasty. One of the commonly used lasers, the Lumenis UltraPulse, actually produces a high frequency pulsed beam when set in continuous wave mode. This creates similar tissue effects as when the laser is set in pulsed mode to make an incision. Incisional laser surgery can also be performed with a laser set in a high fre-

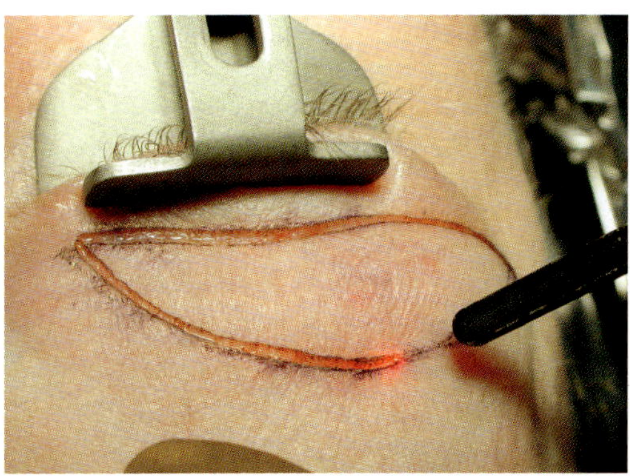

Fig. 12.2. In this example of a laser upper lid blepharoplasty, the globe is protected with a David-Baker lid clamp. Notice the bloodless incision

quency pulsed mode. As one would anticipate, this will produce less lateral thermal damage than a continuous wave beam but may yield less hemostasis.

For upper blepharoplasty, the David-Baker lid clamp (Oculo-plastik, Vancouver, BC) is used to protect the globe. It is placed with a gentle stretch placed on the lid, and the laser is used to make an incision along the inferior portion of the previously marked ellipse (see Fig. 12.2). Care is taken not to extend the incision too deeply laterally so as not to divide one of the terminal branches of lacrimal artery which passes between the skin and orbicularis muscle at the level of the lateral orbital rim. The superior incision is made in a similar fashion. Next, toothed forceps are used to elevate the temporal end of the ellipse so that a skin flap may be dissected with the laser. This is easily accomplished if the surgeon remembers to move the hand holding the skin flap more than the hand holding the laser. The flap should be kept on a taught tension and constantly moved from superior to inferior as the laser is cutting. Wet gauze should be placed behind the flap to absorb stray laser rays. Some surgeons prefer to elevate a skin flap only until the orbital rim has been crossed, at which point the flap is deepened to include orbicularis muscle. The dissection should always stay above the level of the orbital septum.

After the skin flap is removed, the surgeon may choose to open the orbital septum to remove a portion of the pre-aponeurotic fat pad. The septum will be a clearly visible shiny white structure. It can be divided by elevating a portion of it over a wet cotton tipped applicator with small forceps. The laser can then be used to buttonhole the septum centrally, allowing the fat to be exposed. The applicator is then inserted into the potential space beneath the septum so that the laser can be used to open the septum over its full extent laterally and then medially. The fat is then teased out and then draped over the wet applicator and divided with the laser. Care should be taken to remove only fat that easily prolapses. Over-resection of fat may result in a hollow sulcus, which is very difficult to treat. If the patient has a prominent nasal fat pad, the laser may be used to approach this area. The nasal fat pad is easily recognized as being separate from the pre-aponeurotic fat pad due to its more white color. Great care should be taken if approaching this area because damage to trochlear vessels can result in bleeding that may be difficult to control.

Hemostasis must be maintained in a meticulous fashion throughout the entire procedure to avoid orbital hemorrhage and the possibility of secondary blindness. In most cases, this may be achieved by simply defocusing the laser by pulling the hand piece away from the bleeding vessel. If the vessel is greater than 1 mm, a bipolar cautery may be required. Although often not required, a bipolar should be available during every case. Wound closure is usually done with a 6–0 non-absorbable monofilament suture and left in place for 7 days.

A transconjunctival lower lid blepharoplasty may be performed while protecting the globe with a laser safe Jaeger plate as the assistant everts the lower lid. The laser is then used at 6 W in continuous wave mode. In a focused mode and curvilinear fashion, an incision is made from the lateral fornix to about 3 mm away from the caruncle. The incision is carried through the conjunctiva and lower lid retractors. The incision is made 1–2 mm superior to the vascular arcade that is visible in the conjunctiva of the inferior fornix, which is about 3–4 mm inferior to the inferior border of the tarsal plate. Next the

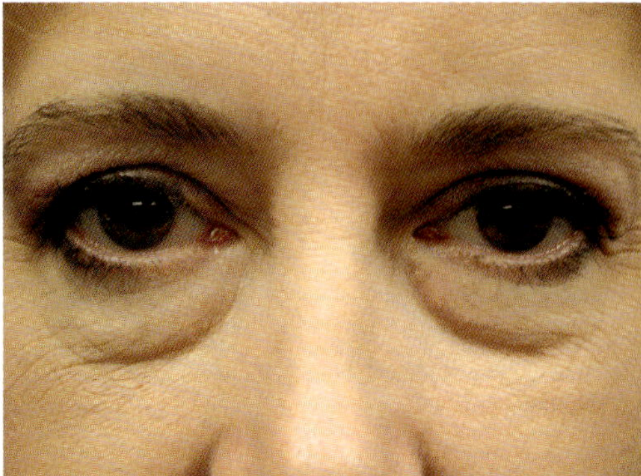
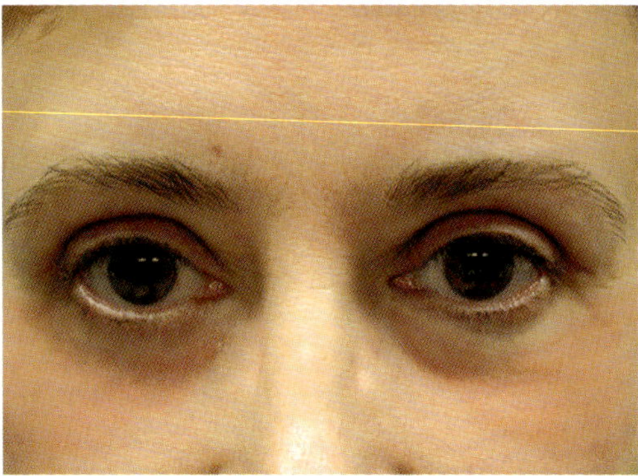

Fig. 12.3. Preoperative and 1 month postoperative photos following bilateral upper lid blepharoplasty, bilateral lower lid blepharoplasty, bilateral lower lid laser resurfacing, and endoscopic brow lift

assistant takes hold of the Jaeger plate and retracts the lower lid with a laser safe Desmarres lid retractor. The surgeon is then able to use the laser finger and forceps to access each of the three fat pads in the lower lid. Each fat pad is encased in a thin sheath that contains vessels. When the sheath is opened with the laser, the fat should then prolapse with a gentle pull with the forceps where it can then be removed with the laser in a slightly defocused mode in front of the Desmarres retractor. The inferior oblique muscle may be visualized between the nasal and central fat pads. When the fat pads are resected the surgeon will observe the remaining stump retract into the orbit. Care must be taken never to allow a bleeding fat pad to retract into the orbit since retrieving the pad to achieve hemostasis may be difficult. Bleeding vessels must be either coagulated with the laser in a defocused mode or with the bipolar before the fat retracts into the orbit. Periocular laser resurfacing may be provided at the same time as the blepharoplasty as seen in Fig. 12.3.

12.2.1.3 Diamond Laser Scalpel

The recently introduced diamond scalpel laser (Diamond Laser Knife, Clinicon Co., Carlsbad, CA) combines the superior cutting performance of a traditional scalpel blade with the hemostatic properties of a CO_2 laser. Some surgeons desire subtle tactile feedback from the surgical wound; however, no tactile feedback is produced when using the CO_2 laser. The diamond scalpel laser system preserves the tactile feedback offered by a traditional surgical blade. Compared to a needle point cautery or non-tactile continuous wave CO_2 laser incision, the diamond laser scalpel reduces collateral thermal damage by 40–60%. The laser energy is delivered through a wave-guide to a diamond blade and is conducted through the blade's facets to produce hemostasis. The diamond laser scalpel permits the option of cutting with or without hemostasis [7].

12.2.2 Erbium:YAG Laser

The 2,940-nm erbium:YAG (Er:YAG) laser was developed to provide laser skin resurfacing with a smaller zone of thermal injury. Because it proved to be a successful resurfacing tool, as will be described in Sect. 12.3.2, surgeons sought out incisional applications as well. The challenge was that the Er:YAG laser did not provide enough hemostasis to offer any advantages during surgery. Sciton (Palo Alto, CA) was the first to create an incisional Er:YAG laser in the late 1990s. This was accomplished by placing two laser heads in one unit that alternately fire, the first at an ablative threshold with short pulse duration (<1 ms) for cutting, and the other at a subablative threshold with long pulse duration (8 ms) to provide hemostasis. The spot size is 0.25 mm. The zone of thermal injury is about 70 µm, which is less than that of the CO_2 laser at 115 µm.

Although the tool will work for incisional surgery, it does have some disadvantages. First, the erbium laser cuts tissue much more slowly because it operates at lower frequency. The incision is also more "choppy" and not as smooth as that of the CO_2 laser. Some surgeons still feel that it does not provide adequate hemostasis. Also, the addition of the incisional handpiece to the laser unit is very expensive [8].

12.2.3 Neodymium: YAG Laser

Lasers may be used as a free beam, such as CO_2 and erbium:YAG lasers, or in contact mode with sapphire tip technology such as 1,064-nm neodymium:YAG (Nd:YAG) lasers. The Nd:YAG laser can be transmitted through an optical fiber delivery system to a synthetic sapphire surgical probe, which can then be used as a surgical scalpel. The sapphire tip concentrates the Nd:YAG laser energy onto a small area at the end of the scalpel and enables precise incisions with excellent hemostasis. However, contact laser tips create larger zones of thermal injury than CO_2 lasers or cold steel. According to the manufacturers, contact laser tips (cutting tips) create at least 300–500 µm of tissue necrosis, which is too large to be useful for skin incisions but may have applications for subcutaneous dissection [9].

12.3 Laser Skin Resurfacing

Over the past decade, public interest in facial rejuvenation has increased dramatically. In recent years, laser technologies have replaced chemical peels and dermabrasion as the treatment of choice for photoaged skin. Laser resurfacing has well documented benefits for photoaging. The CO_2 and Er:YAG lasers effectively ablate damaged tissue and promote contraction of underlying collagen and formation of new collagen, which lead to tissue tightening and reduction in wrinkles [10, 11]. One of the challenges for patients undergoing laser resurfacing is the long time required to heal – usually 10 days off from work for the CO_2 laser and 8 days for the erbium laser. More recently, non-ablative laser applications for treatment of photoaged skin have been developed in an effort to reduce healing time. These will be discussed in Sect. 12.3.4.

Laser skin resurfacing of the periorbital region can be performed as an isolated procedure, as part full-face laser resurfacing, or in conjunction with transconjunctival blepharoplasty. The laser procedure itself is not a particularly challenging technique for cosmetic surgeons. The skill mainly lies in proper preoperative assessment and consultation as well as postoperative care to avoid complications. Preoperative evaluation for both CO_2 and Er:YAG lasers is very similar.

Candidates for laser skin resurfacing include patients with cosmetically unattractive rhytids, patients with moderate to severe photoaging including those with actinic keratoses and dyschromia, or patients with rhinophyma. Patients should understand that the laser is best for static rhytids that are present when the face is still, as opposed to dynamic rhytids that are best treated with botulinum toxin [12]. Patients with acne scars may expect only a 20–25% improvement of their scars. Laser resurfacing will not shrink the size of pores, minimize telangiectasia, or reduce unwanted facial hair.

Various factors should be considered relative contraindications in selecting patients for laser resurfacing. The Fitzpatrick skin type (Table 12.1) is important because patients with skin types I and II are the best candidates for laser resurfacing. Patients with skin types III and IV may undergo resurfacing but may have a greater risk of hyperpigmentation, which should be addressed with the patient in preoperative discussions [13]. Those at risk for hyperpigmentation may be better candidates for the erbium laser, which causes less thermal damage and thus triggers less hyperpigmentation. Hyperpigmentation also may be reduced with topical hydroquinone 4% daily. True melasma may temporarily improve after resurfacing, but will frequently return and may not be responsive to hydroquinone. Patients with a history of herpes simplex 1 dermatitis on the face should be observed closely for reactivation during the postoperative period.

Table 12.1. Fitzpatrick classification for sun-reactive skin types [48]

Skin type	Reaction to sun	Colour/examples
Type I	Always burns, never tans	Very white or freckled Caucasian
Type II	Burns easily, tans minimally	Fair skinned, fair haired Caucasian
Type III	Sometimes burns, slowly tans to light brown	White to olive skin, darker Caucasian, light Asian
Type IV	Rarely burns, always tans to moderate brown	Moderate brown, Mediterranean-type Caucasian, Asian, Hispanic
Type V	Very rarely burns, tans easily	Dark brown, Middle Eastern, Latin, light-skinned Black, Indian
Type VI	Never burns, always tans	Black, dark-skinned Black

All patients undergoing laser resurfacing should be placed on valacyclovir 1,000 mg PO daily beginning on the morning of surgery through postoperative day 10. Preoperative antibiotics are not required. If patients develop any signs of HSV dermatitis, the dose should be doubled to 1,000 mg PO twice per day. Laser resurfacing may be contraindicated in patients with histories of radiation or deep phenol peels because they may not have a sufficient reserve of epithelial cells in their skin appendages (hair follicles and pores) to be able to re-epithelialize their skin after surgery. The surgeon can examine the skin appendages in the slit lamp to determine if they appear adequate to heal the epithelial surface. Patients who have lifestyles that include significant sun exposure need to be aware that they must drastically decrease their time in the sun after laser resurfacing. Suspicious lesions should be biopsied prior to laser resurfacing.

There are absolute contraindications to laser resurfacing. Patients with scleroderma, vitiligo, and use of oral accutane within the past year are at risk of scarring. Non-facial skin such as that on the neck and hands is also not a candidate for resurfacing because it too has a high risk of scarring. Patients with unrealistic expectations or an active infection are also not candidates.

After surgery, patients may wear an occlusive dressing such as Flexzan (Delasco, Council Bluffs, IA), Silon-TSR (Bio Med Sciences, Inc., Allentown, PA), or resurfacing recovery system (RRS, Neutrogena, Los Angeles, CA) following a specific regimen for 2–3 days. When this is removed, soaks are performed using a mixture of one cup of water to one teaspoon distilled white vinegar every 2–4 h while awake followed by application of Aquaphor ointment (Beiersdorf, Charlotte, NC). This is continued until postoperative day 10. The skin produces a serous transudate in the first 24 h. Patients may expect their skin to look the worst on postoperative day 3 or 4 with scattered areas of crusting, edema and erythema. By postoperative day 10, the skin should be epithelialized, although edema and erythema will persist.

Complications of laser resurfacing include scarring, hyperpigmentation, hypopigmentation, prolonged erythema, petechiae, acne, milia, enlarged pores, itching, ectropion, and demarcation lines. Scarring can result from laser treatment that penetrates too deep into the reticular dermis, an infection, or possibly from a severe contact dermatitis to topical ointments. Patients typically do not complain of pain after resurfacing. Complaints of pain should, therefore, be taken very seriously. Such patients should be seen immediately and appropriate cultures should be obtained. Topical ointments should be changed to petroleum jelly, and oral or intravenous antibiotics should be started. Hypopigmentation is permanent and is difficult to treat. Erythema is usually gone by 4–6 months, but can persist up to 1 year. Petechiae are common in the first month after the procedure and will usually resolve in 4–5 days. Patients should be reminded not to touch their face. Acne may require antibiotics. Milia are common and may be removed with a needle and forceps. Itching may be treated with topical steroids, but steroids should not be started until after postoperative day 10.

12.3.1 CO_2 Laser Skin Resurfacing

The development of CO_2 lasers with short-pulsed high-peak power for use in laser skin resurfacing has considerably enhanced physicians' ability to treat photodamaged skin in a precise and reproducible manner. Laser resurfacing permits laser reduction of inferior lid festoons or malar bags without creating lower eyelid scars, as can be seen with conventional scalpel surgery [14].

Water is the main chromophore in human tissue that is absorbed by the CO_2 laser thereby producing heat. When intracellular and extracellular water is rapidly heated to a vaporizing temperature, the laser precisely vaporizes the superficial layers of tissue so quickly that there is not enough time for the heat produced to create a burn in the deeper tissue layers. Thermal energy is dissipated in part by conduction to adjacent tissue along the edges of the wound to produce a zone of thermally devitalized tissue, known as the *berm*. The vaporization of water in the target layer of the skin generates the resurfacing applications of the CO_2 laser. This requires a fluence of 4.5–5.0 J/cm^2. The amount of thermal energy conducted to adjacent tissue is determined by how rapidly vaporization is achieved. The thermal relaxation time of skin is about 800 μm. If vaporization occurs in less than 800 μm, most of the resulting thermal energy will not be conducted to adjacent tissue, thereby limiting the amount of thermally damaged tissue. This is an important goal of laser resurfacing because a burn with a scar can result if too much heat is conducted into surrounding tissues [14].

Carbon dioxide lasers achieve limited thermal damage adjacent to the site of application by using two types of computer pattern generators (CPGs) – sweep or pulsed. Using "sweep" technology, the duration of laser energy applied to an area of skin is determined by mechanically sweeping a focused laser beam at a speed sufficiently fast to limit exposure of any specific area of target skin to less than the thermal relaxation time. Pulsed technology rapidly delivers a high energy beam as a pulse. Pulsed applications vary by the pulse duration, the diameter of the beam, and the relative overlap of adjacent pulses [14].

Skin resurfacing lasers are also designed with either focused or collimated delivery systems. Focused systems must be held a set distance from the skin to ensure the desired fluence. Collimated systems may be held any distance from the skin without changing the spot size.

The surgeon should thoroughly understand the laser being used and how to select appropriate settings. Suggested settings are beyond the scope of this chapter because there are too many lasers from which to choose. When performing laser resurfacing, the surgeon should place each square immediately adjacent to the next but should avoid any overlap. Pattern overlap may lead to deeper burns that require more time to heal and are cosmetically unattractive during postoperative healing [15]. The surgeon should cool and hydrate as well as remove the desiccated tissue with moist saline gauze. After removal of the epidermis, the skin should appear reddish-pink in colour. Usually, between two and four passes are delivered.

When performing laser resurfacing on the eyelids, it is particularly important to evaluate the integrity of the lower eyelid and its supporting structures. CO_2 laser resurfacing may cause the eyelid skin to shrink by as much as 20–30 %. This can lead to scalloping or ectropion [15]. The tightness of the eyelid skin should be evaluated by a "snap" or pull-down retraction test. In some cases, tarsal tightening surgery may be necessary prior to laser resurfacing to prevent lower eyelid deformity.

The advantages of CO_2 laser resurfacing over erbium laser resurfacing include more uniform cosmetic improvement, less bleeding, and fewer passes required [16]. The major disadvantages of CO_2 laser skin resurfacing include operative pain, prolonged erythema, slow re-epithelialization, scarring, and risk of hypopigmentation, particularly in darker skinned patients (Fitzpatrick skin types III–VI). Almost all patients experience erythema following CO_2 laser resurfacing. Healing time typically lasts approximately 3 months but erythema may persist up to 12 months following some procedures. Despite these disadvantages, however, the CO_2 laser may be safer than the erbium laser for the novice surgeon because maximally organized fibroplasia and wound contraction is produced with a minimum depth of initial injury [17]. Because of the limited ablation at typical resurfacing fluences, the uniform zone of thermal damage produces more predictable wound healing [16].

There is still a strong desire for patients to achieve improvement in rhytids without the prolonged healing time typical for CO_2 laser resurfacing. For this reason, Lumenis, Inc. has developed the Ultrapulse Encore with CO_2 Lite that provides skin rejuvenation with a single subablative pass, in which the epithelium is not removed. This provides a superficial resurfacing [18].

12.3.2 Erbium:YAG Laser Skin Resurfacing

The short pulsed erbium:YAG 2,920-nm laser minimizes some of the disadvantages associated with CO_2 laser skin resurfacing. Skin resurfaced with erbium laser epithelializes faster, has less erythema, and less risk of hyperpigmentation or hypopigmentation; however, the erbium laser tends not to improve facial rhytids as much as the CO_2 laser [19]. Because there is so much interest in non-ablative resurfacing, and because the CO_2 laser has proven to be the gold standard for ablative resurfacing, some of the major laser companies have stopped producing the erbium laser.

Intraoperative documentation for the CO_2 laser includes the laser settings for each pass with a description of the cooling and hydration between passes. In contrast, documentation for the erbium laser includes the cumulative fluence used in each facial area. If the laser unit does not display the fluence to the surgeon, the fluence should be calculated in J/cm^2.

In clinical practice, the erbium laser works primarily as an ablating tool. The amount of energy absorbed by tissue water is approximately 12 times greater for the erbium laser than the CO_2 laser. The explosive yet very precise ablation induced by the erbium laser typically causes the ejection of skin debris at supersonic velocities, which is associated with a loud pop during surgery and coating of the erbium laser handpiece with debris. Unlike the CO_2 laser, the erbium laser does not require hydration and cooling in between passes. It comes in either focused or collimated delivery systems, with and without CPGs, so the surgeon must be familiar with the specific machine being used [11].

Unlike the CO_2 laser, most of the energy of the erbium laser is used to produce ablation rather than tissue heating. The zone of adjacent thermal damage is small (20–50 µm). At the typical fluences used for laser skin resurfacing, the CO_2 laser essentially produces a controlled col-

Table 12.2. Average thickness of facial epidermis and dermis at various locations [48]

Location	Epidermis (µm)	Dermis (µm)	Total
Neck	115	138	253
Eyelids	130	215	345
Root of nose	144	324	468
Cheek	141	909	1,050
Lobule of nose	111	918	1,029
Forehead	202	969	1,171
Lower lip	113	973	1,086
Upper lip	156	1,061	1,217
Mental region	149	1,375	1,524

lagen melt, whereas the erbium laser produces a dermal tissue effect similar to mechanical tissue wounds. However, the role of thermal damage in wound healing is not completely understood. Unlike the CO_2 laser, there is little tissue shrinkage during ablation with the erbium laser. Re-epithelialization is almost complete by about 5–8 days following erbium ablation.

In the periocular area, the dermis is relatively thin (300 μm), and atrophic scarring secondary to transdermal injury is more common than hypertrophic scarring (see Table 12.2). Consequently, the surgeon should apply no more than three passes with the erbium laser in the infraorbital and medial canthal areas [11].

The Contour laser (Sciton Inc., Palo Alto, CA) contains both a short pulsed and a long pulsed erbium laser in one unit in an attempt to create zones of thermocoagulation that are somewhere between that of the CO_2 and erbium lasers [20, 21]. This type of laser is termed a variable pulsed erbium. When using this laser, the surgeon can set the ablative short pulsed laser independently from the long pulsed subablative laser. It is an all erbium laser that has a variable pulse width so the cosmetic effect can be made more similar to a CO_2 than a short pulsed erbium, but with a side effect profile closer to the short pulsed erbium.

12.3.3 Combined CO_2 and Erbium Laser Resurfacing

Carbon dioxide and erbium lasers can be used to complement each other in treating the same patient in the same setting. In this way, the surgeon can combine the heating properties of the CO_2 laser with the ablative properties of the erbium laser. For example, in patients with severe acne scarring, the CO_2 laser can be used to remove the epidermis with a single pass, the erbium laser can be used to sculpt the acne scars, and the CO_2 laser can be used on the exposed dermis to tighten the tissue. In patients with photodamage, the CO_2 laser can be used to resurface areas of maximal photodamage, such as the periocular skin, and the erbium laser can be used to resurface areas with milder photodamage.

The DermaK laser (ESC, Lumenis, Santa Clara, CA) is a unit that contains both a CO_2 laser and an Er:YAG laser that can fire simultaneously. It contains an incisional handpiece for the CO_2 component as well [21].

12.3.4 Non-ablative Resurfacing

Traditional skin rejuvenation for photoaged skin can include invasive methods such as dermabrasion, chemical peels, and ablative laser skin resurfacing with the CO_2 and erbium:YAG lasers. These methods remove epidermis and superficial papillary dermis and are thought to improve rhytids by stimulating long term wound healing with dermal collagen synthesis [22, 23]. Such approaches produce improvement in rhytids; however, they generate open wounds and require extended recovery time of at least 10 days off from work. There are also uncommon but significant risks associated with these methods such as prolonged erythema, hyperpigmentation, hypopigmentation, and scarring [19, 24]. There is growing interest in non-invasive methods for skin rejuvenation of photodamaged skin. Non-ablative skin resurfacing is a topic of much discussion since recent studies have reported improvement in rhytids with minimal healing time and minimal risk of complications. Although many non-ablative technologies are accomplished with lasers, much of the current technology involves other forms of electromagnetic radiation. Due to their similar goals they are all included in the same discussion.

The goal of non-ablative photorejuvenation is to produce useful and controlled minimally aggressive thermal damage in the superficial and reticular dermis while sparing the epidermis. Recent evidence suggests that non-ablative applications of electromagnetic radiation can also produce a dermal wound healing response effective for the treatment of facial rhytids. There is ample evidence that adverse effects are less common with non-ablative techniques; however, cosmetic improvement is often subtle, and patients may require repeated treatments over a 6- to 12-month period to achieve the desired benefits. Nevertheless, such non-invasive methods of facial rejuvenation are likely to play an increasingly important role because of patient demand for treatments with shorter healing times.

Non-ablative technologies include broad spectrum light, lasers, and radiofrequency. These frequently offer cooling devices such as cryogen spray or sapphire crystal chill tips to keep the epidermis cool. Non-ablative devices can be used to treat not only rhytids, but also other signs of photoaging such as dyschromias, telangiectasia, generalized flushing, and large pore size. A common observation of many of the non-ablative technologies is that they frequently show an obvious improvement in collagen production in tissue histology; however, this does not always correlate with clinical improvement of rhytids [25].

12.3.4.1 Broad Spectrum or Intense Pulsed Light

The development of broad spectrum light, also known as intense pulsed light (IPL), provides an alternative method of producing thermal damage without epidermal injury. Non-ablative photorejuvenation with broad spectrum light, first described by Bitter, has demonstrated varying efficacy as an alternative to laser skin resurfacing but has few adverse side effects [26]. The FotoFacial RF is a registered trademark by Patrick Bitter, MD, that describes his technique for non-ablative skin rejuvenation.

Intense pulsed light consists of a powerful pulse of broad-spectrum white light from a flashlamp, which produces simultaneous wavelengths in a large range of 500–1,200 nm delivered along a fiberoptic arm. The use of appropriate filters permits the irradiation of dermal tissue through the epidermis. The use of such filters cuts off shorter wavelengths while allowing the passage of non-specific longer infrared wavelengths to treat wrinkles associated with photoaging. In addition, the filters permit passage of longer wavelengths to treat vascular, pigmentary, and dyschromic conditions. IPL has demonstrated more success in the treatment of vascular and pigmented lesions than in appearance of rhytids [27]. Because of its increased popularity, Lumenis, Inc., now produce five versions of intense pulsed light machines. They are popular because they can be used not only for non-ablative resurfacing, but also for removal of unwanted hair, vascular lesions, and pigmented lesions. Syneron Medical, Ltd., makes three machines that employ broad spectrum light.

Because the results of IPL vary from patient to patient and they do not always correlate with histological improvement, patients must be properly counseled about realistic expectations. Goldberg et al. demonstrated substantial improvement in wrinkle severity 6 months after final treatment with IPL in 9 of 30 patients and apparent clinical improvement in 16 of 30 patients [27]. A comparative study of IPL and the Q-switched Nd:YAG laser demonstrated no statistically significant difference in the subjective degree of improvement between the treatment groups [28]. However, treatment with intense pulsed light has been associated with the lowest rate of adverse effects. The main side effects reported with use of IPL for photorejuvenation have been blistering and transient erythema [26]. Recent reports on the use of IPL for non-ablative photorejuvenation have used a wide range of filter, fluence, and pulse parameters. Variations in such parameters most likely contribute to differences in the reported efficacy of intense pulsed light.

12.3.4.2 Non-ablative Lasers

The Q-switched 1,064/532-nm Nd:YAG laser was the first laser used as a non-ablative device for skin rejuvenation. The most common side effects associated with the Q-switched Nd:YAG laser are pinpoint bleeding, transient erythema, and postinflammatory hyperpigmentation. Treatment with the non-ablative Nd:YAG laser is thought to promote collagen synthesis through selective papillary dermal injury and long-term wound healing without removing the epidermis. In contrast to ablative lasers, the Nd:YAG laser produces thermal damage to the papillary dermis and superficial reticular dermis, while dynamic cooling protects the epidermis. Several studies demonstrated the efficacy of the Q-switched Nd:YAG laser for improving

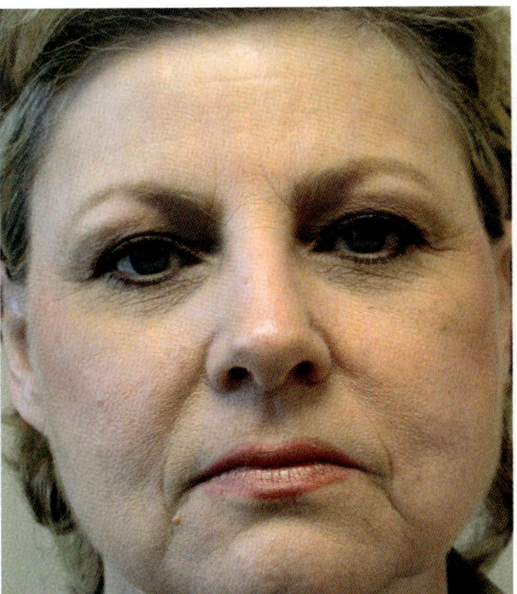

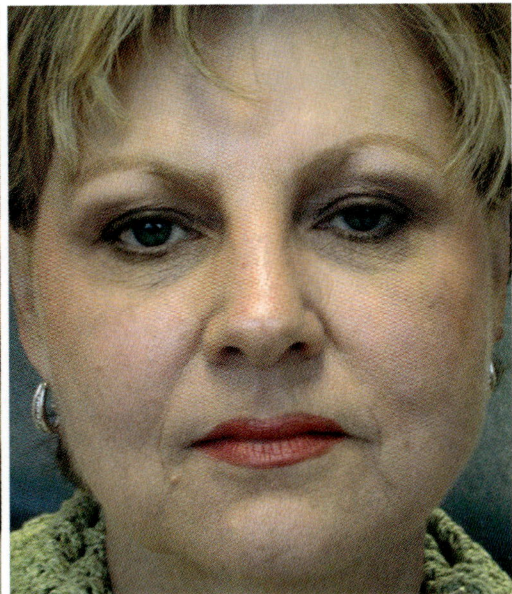

Fig. 12.4. Preoperative and postoperative photos following non-ablative resurfacing treatment with radiofrequency thermage of lower face and neck

wrinkles, skin texture, and skin elasticity; however, the Q-switched Nd:YAG laser is less effective than the CO_2 laser for most patients [29, 30].

The majority of studies have involved the 1,320-nm Nd:YAG CoolTouch laser with a dynamic cooling device (CoolTouch Laser, Roseville, CA). The 1,320-nm Nd:YAG laser was the first commercially available system designed exclusively for non-ablative facial rejuvenation. In dynamic cooling, the epidermis is protected from extensive damage by a spurt of cryogen delivered onto the skin for tens of milliseconds immediately prior to laser activation. However, the efficacy of the 1,320-nm Nd:YAG laser for facial rejuvenation appears to be limited. Menaker et al. demonstrated that four of ten patients experienced improvement in wrinkles of 1 point on a 5-point scale at 3 months post-treatment. However, complications included hyperpigmentation and scarring. Levy et al. treated 13 patients with the 1,320-nm Nd:YAG laser in the periocular region. Histologic findings were promising; however, very few patients demonstrated a subjective improvement in wrinkles [31–33].

The 580–590 nm N-lite laser (USA Photonics, Inc.) is a fast-pulsed dye laser that was FDA approved for non-ablative skin rejuvenation. It emits a yellow light that heats small vessels that stimulate new collage formation and kills *P. acnes* bacteria to treat acne. The 1,450-nm Smoothbeam and the 595-nm pulsed dye V-beam (Candella Co., Wayland, MA) are also non-ablative lasers that can be used to treat rhytids. The Smoothbeam is also used to treat acne whereas the V-beam is used to treat vascular lesions.

12.3.4.3 Radiofrequency

Recently, radiofrequency tissue tightening has been introduced as another alternative to laser therapy. In radiofrequency technology, the electrical resistance of the tissue converts electric current into thermal energy deep within the dermis. It appears that radiofrequency technology can produce dermal heating as shallow as the papillary dermis or as deep as subcutaneous fat [34]. This thermal injury denatures collagen within the deep tissues leading to immediate tissue contraction. Later, new collagen formation leads to further tissue tightening and reduction in wrinkles (see Fig. 12.4). A recent multicenter study examined the application of non-ablative radiofrequency technology for treatment of periorbital wrinkles. Based on independent scoring of blinded photographs, 83% of treated areas demonstrated improvement in periorbital wrinkles at 6 months following a single treatment session. The overall incidence of second degree burns was less than 1 in 200 radiofrequency applications [16].

A new non-ablative monopolar radiofrequency device, ThermalCool TC System (Thermage, Inc., Hayward, CA), has been developed to tighten deeper dermal structures without epidermal damage [34]. This technology uses controlled cryogen cooling to protect the epidermis while uniformly dispersing higher energy fluences to a greater volume of dermal tissue than do non-ablative lasers. One study showed that 50% or patients were satisfied, and 61% noticed at least 0.5 mm elevation of their brow [16]. Although these authors report minimal side effects, critics argue that this technology may penetrate too deeply and do too much damage to the subcutaneous fat that can result in areas of displeasing atrophy.

The Galaxy (Syneron Medical Ltd., Yokneam Illit, Israel) with elos (electro-optical) technology combines broad spectrum light with bipolar radiofrequency technology. The bipolar technology has the advantage of limiting the penetration of the radiofrequency from travelling deeper than 4 mm into the tissue, which may lead to less damage to subcutaneous fat.

Some physicians use the Thermage and the Syneron systems to complement each other. The first is used to provide a deeper tightening and the second for the FotoFacial RF effect.

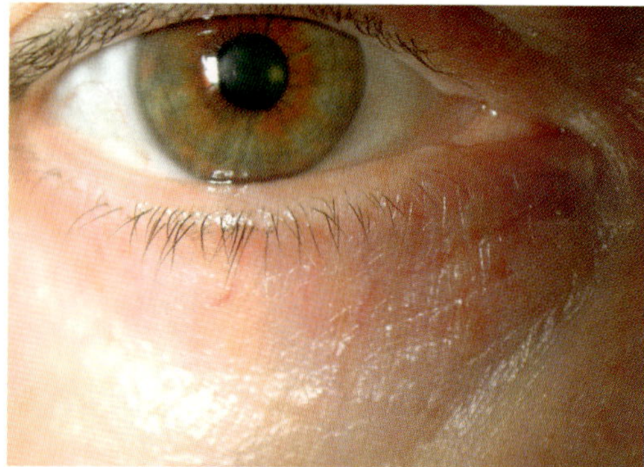

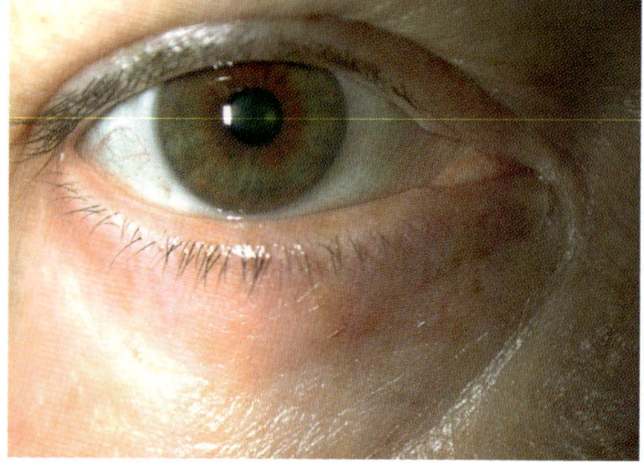

Fig. 12.5. Preoperative and 1 day postoperative photos following treatment of subtle lower lid telangiectasia with the long-pulse 532-nm fd Nd:YAG laser. In this case, telangiectasia arose 3 months after transconjunctival blepharoplasty. The globe is protected with a Jaeger plate as the laser is used to remove telangiectasia

12.4 Laser Treatment of Cutaneous Vascular Lesions

Cutaneous vascular lesions ranging from telangiectasia to port wine stains can now be safely and effectively treated using a variety of lasers in the 488–638 nm range. Hemoglobin in red blood cells best absorbs electromagnetic radiation at approximately 577 nm. This is most successful when done at longer pulse widths that slowly heat the hemoglobin in the vessel. The challenge is to do this without damaging melanocytes in surrounding tissue. Intense pulsed light can also be used to treat such vascular lesions with the use of filters for the above wavelengths.

The 488–514 nm argon laser has been used to treat vascular lesions; however, it is associated with adverse effects including scarring, hypopigmentation, hyperpigmentation and recurrence of veins [35]. This is because melanin in the epidermis and superficial dermis competes for the absorption of these wavelengths.

The 532-nm frequency-doubled Nd:YAG (fd Nd:YAG), otherwise known as potassium titanyl phosphate (KTP), laser is very successful at treating telangiectasia on the face without producing purpura or hypopigmentation as seen in Fig. 12.5. It is more readily absorbed by hemoglobin and less by melanin. It has an ability to modify the pulse duration up to 50 ms, which permits removal of the lesions with less associated purpura than seen with other lasers such as the pulsed dye laser. Typical settings are a 4-mm spot size, 30-ms pulse width, and 15 J/cm^2. Some units deliver the laser along a fiberoptic arm then through a cooled sapphire tip which protects the epidermis from undesired heating of melanin. The KTP laser has been found to cause less swelling, pain, bruising, and redness than the pulsed dye laser [36].

The 585-nm flashlamp-pumped pulsed dye laser (FPPDL) is successful at removing facial telangiectasia but produces a purpuric tissue response with a variable degree of reactive hyperemia.

The argon pumped tunable dye laser is capable of producing continuously tunable wavelengths from 577 nm to 638 nm. It has been found to have a slightly lower incidence of hyper- and hypopigmentation than the pulsed dye laser [37].

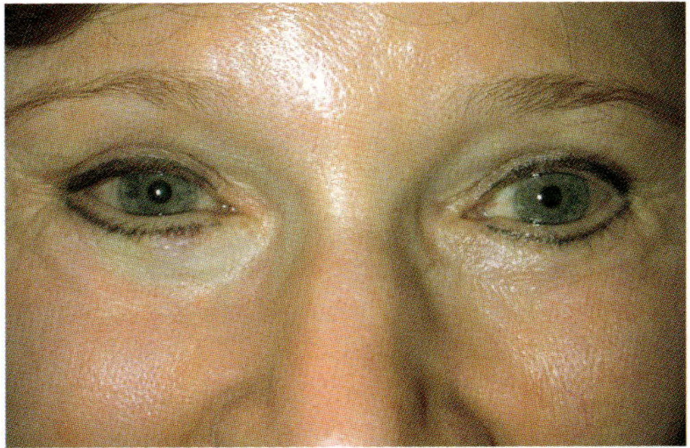

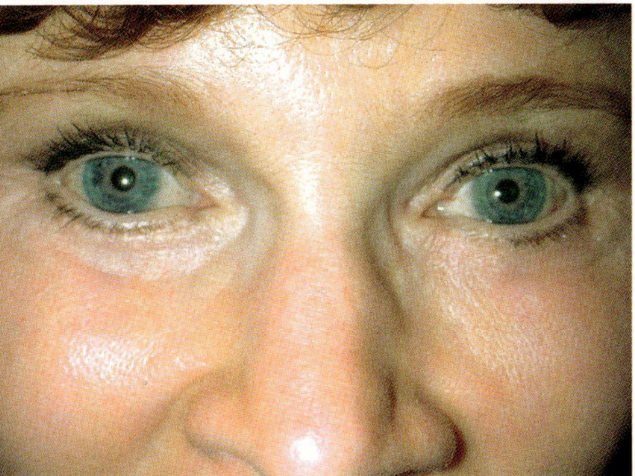

Fig. 12.6. Preoperative and 2-month postoperative photos following two treatments with the 1,064-nm Nd:YAG laser to remove bilateral lower eyelid tattoo pigment

12.5 Laser Treatment of Tattoos

The popularity of tattoos appears to be increasing over time. Currently more than 10 million Americans have at least one tattoo, and about half of these individuals desire tattoo removal. Micropigmentation is the term used for permanent makeup that is ever increasing in popularity. Some patients are not pleased with the results of their permanent makeup. If so, it is possible to remove the pigments with the use of a tattoo removal laser as seen in Fig. 12.6. This is typically performed under local anesthesia with lidocaine 2% and a Jaeger plate to protect the globe [38].

For laser tattoo removal, the principle of selective photothermolysis applies wherein the color of the tattoo ink determines what wavelength of electromagnetic radiation is used. In this case, Q-switched (QS) lasers are used that have pulse widths measured in nanoseconds. They shatter the pigments in pigment containing cells such as fibroblasts, macrophages, and mast cells to rupture and cause a photoacoustic effect. This leads to a neutrophilic response where the shattered pigments are then carried away by macrophages.

Each time a treatment is performed, a small amount of pigment is removed. Treatments are spaced about 1 month apart, and satisfactory removal of the tattoo pigment usually requires 4 to 12 treatments. Most tattoos noted in oculoplastic surgery are blue-black in color, which is the color that has the greatest success in being removed.

Professional tattoos are typically placed more deeply in the dermis with greater pigment density. In addition, multiple color combinations often make it difficult to select the appropriate lasers. Black pigment can be treated with the Q-switched 1,064-nm Nd:YAG, ruby, or QS

755-nm alexandrite lasers. Blue and green pigments can be treated with Q-switched 755-nm alexandrite and QS 694-nm ruby lasers. Red pigment can be treated with the Q-switched fd 532-nm Nd:YAG [39].

Cosmetic tattoos, such as lipliner, eyeliner, and eyebrow tattoos, are becoming increasingly common. Most are off-white, reddish-brown, red, skin-colored, or dull orange. Many of such cosmetic tattoos consist of iron pigments. In some cases, treatment with a Q-switched laser may lead to paradoxical darkening of the tattoo. This results from reduction of red-brown ferric oxide to black ferrous oxide. The resulting gray or black pigment often requires multiple laser treatments to remove; therefore, the laser surgeon should perform a test treatment of all cosmetic tattoos [40].

The most common adverse effects following laser tattoo removal with Q-switched lasers include scarring, pigmentary alteration, textural change, and allergic reactions. Although higher fluences may be more effective in removing tattoo pigment, they are also associated with greater risk of adverse effects.

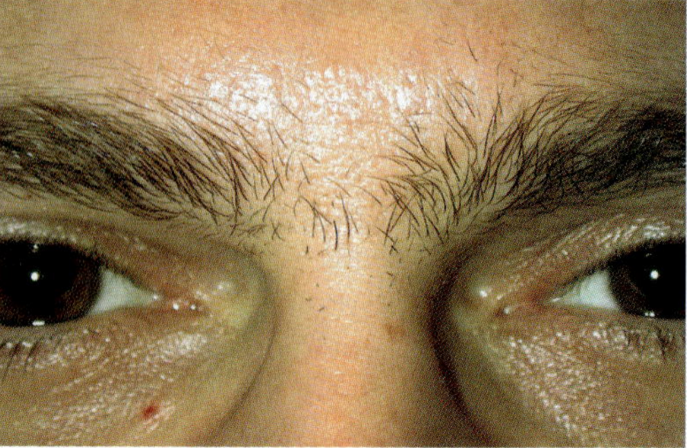

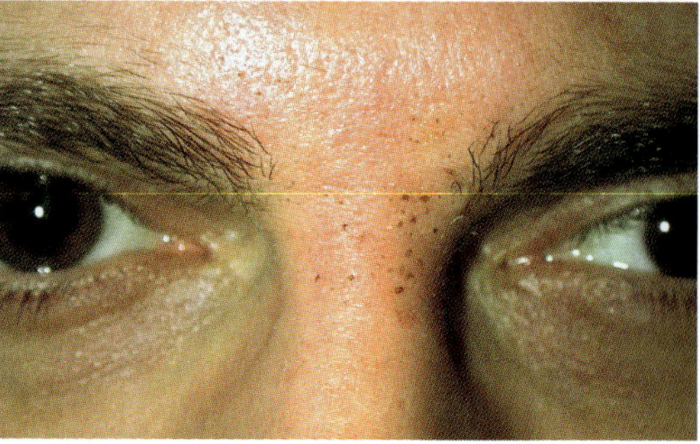

Fig. 12.7. Preoperative and immediately postoperative photos following a second treatment for laser hair removal of the brow. Notice the small amounts of char in the postoperative photo, which are a sign of successful destruction of the hair follicle without damage to surrounding skin

12.6 Laser Hair Removal

Many oculoplastic surgeons have incorporated laser hair removal into their practices. The 694-nm ruby, the 755-nm alexandrite, the 810-nm diode, and the 1,064-nm fd Nd:YAG lasers, as well as intense pulsed light, are used for hair removal. Laser hair removal works by heating the dark melanin pigment in the bulb of the hair follicle to the point of thermocoagulation that damages the follicle. For this reason, white hairs cannot be lasered. Typically three to four treatments are required because the hairs can only be damaged in their anagen (growth) phase and not the catagen or telogen phases. One must wait for the hairs to enter the growth phase.

The obvious challenge for laser hair removal is to selectively heat the melanin in the follicles in the deeper dermis without damaging the melanocytes in the epidermis. This is accomplished with the use of either cryogen spray or a ChillTip to cool the epidermis. A higher fluence may be used with lighter skinned patients while a lower fluence is generally recommended for darker patients. The Lightsheer 800-nm diode (Lumenis, Inc., Santa Clara, CA) provides a very long pulse width that has been successful in removing follicles in Fitzpatrick skin type V patients without causing hypopigmentation [46]. A proper appearance of slightly charred follicles with a small amount of surrounding edema is seen in Fig. 12.7 after hair removal with the Lightsheer.

12.7 Laser Dacryocystorhinostomy

Dacryocystorhinostomy (DCR) is performed to create a connection between the lacrimal sac and the nasal cavity in order to bypass an obstruction of the lacrimal sac or nasolacrimal duct. Traditionally, DCR has been performed via the external approach; however, surgeons may alternatively use an endonasal technique, with or without laser assistance. Endonasal laser dacryocystorhinostomy is now a well-established approach for the treatment of nasolacrimal duct obstruction. Although laser DCR generally has a lower success rate than external DCR, recent studies suggest that the procedure is well tolerated by most patients. Moreover, laser DCR may be particularly appropriate for younger patients, patients who have not undergone previous surgical interventions, patients with a short duration of symptoms, and patients with a higher bleeding tendency [41, 42].

12.7.1 Holmium Laser

The 2,000-nm holmium:YAG laser has been used for laser-assisted dacryocystorhinostomy and laser canaliculoplasty. The primary advantages of the holmium laser are that it is fiber-optic compatible for endoscopic applications and that it produces excellent hemostasis. The holmium laser has been reported to have a success rate as high as 85% for laser-assisted DCR in some studies [42]. However, other studies report symptomatic success of only 60–71%, compared to 95% for external DCR [43, 44]. Endoscopic endonasal laser (EEL) using the holmium:YAG laser may be able to reduce the operating time by up to 50% [44]. A recent study found that 65% of patients declared themselves completely cured following endoscopic endonasal DCR with the holmium:YAG laser, and over 90% achieved anatomical success by the procedure. Over 85% of patients recommended the procedure. Of note, patients with a shorter duration of symptoms, patients who had not previously undergone other surgical interventions, and younger patients all demonstrated a significantly higher complete cure rate [41].

The holmium:YAG laser is thought to be less likely than the Nd:YAG laser to produce thermal injury to soft tissues in the process of removing bone from the lateral nasal wall [42]. The holmium laser has also been used to conduct laser canaliculoplasty as a substitute for the standard Jones-type bypass. Although slightly less effective than a Jones tube, laser canaliculoplasty with the holmium laser avoids the complications and patient dissatisfaction associated with a Jones tube [44].

12.7.2 Potassium Titanyl Phosphate Laser

The potassium titanyl phosphate (KTP) laser provides a cutting fiber device that permits accurate removal of skin, fat, or lesions in the periorbital region with very few side effects. The KTP laser has been used for brow lifting, dacryocystorhinostomy, and transconjunctival blepharoplasty. The KTP laser can be used for both external DCR and endoscopic DCR. It appears that KTP laser-assisted DCR has a lower success rate than standard DCR. A recent study found that endonasal KTP laser-assisted DCR had a success rate of only 64%, compared to 94% for primary external DCR. However, the KTP laser success rate improves to 82% when including revision procedures [45].

Summary for the Clinician

- **Lasers have been used extensively in ophthalmology, and laser applications in oculoplastic surgery have grown dramatically in recent years**
- **Laser applications in oculoplastic surgery include incisional surgery, laser skin resurfacing, treatment of vascular lesions, tattoo removal, hair removal, and dacryocystorhinostomy, among others**
- **Skin resurfacing using the CO_2 laser remains the gold standard for treatment of photoaging; however, improvements in non-ablative technologies such as radiofrequency and broad spectrum pulsed light will likely lead such technologies to play an increasingly important role in the future because of their superior side effect profile**
- **Improvement in technologies that cool the epidermis allows a broader range of skin types to be treated**
- **Laser surgery is a rapidly advancing field and ongoing improvements in laser and related technologies will continue to drive new potential uses in oculoplastic surgery**

References

1. Goldman MP, Fitzpatrick RE (1994) Cutaneous laser surgery: the art and science of selective photothermolysis. Mosby, St. Louis
2. Goldman I (1966) Laser treatment of malignant melanoma. In: Goldman I (ed) Laser cancer research. Springer, New York Berlin Heidelberg
3. Patel CKN (1964) Continuous-wave laser action in vibrational-rotational transitions of carbon dioxide. Phys Rev 136:A1187–1193
4. Baker SS, Muenzler WS, Small RG, Leonard JE (1984) Carbon dioxide laser blepharoplasty. Ophthalmology 91:238–244
5. Biesman BS (2000) Lasers play a useful role in periorbital incisional surgery. Dermatol Surg 26: 883–886
6. Ben-Bassat M, Ben-Bassat J, Kaplan I (1976) An ultrastructural study of the cut edges of skin and mucous membrane specimens excised by carbon dioxide laser. In: Kaplan I (ed) Laser surgery II. Academic Press, Jerusalem
7. Baker SS, Hunnewell JM, Muenzler WS, Hunter GJ (2002) Laser blepharoplasty: diamond laser scalpel compared to the free beam CO_2 laser. Dermatol Surg 28:127
8. Biesman BS, Bernstein E (1999) The Er:YAG laser as a soft tissue incisional device. Lasers Surg Med Suppl 11:64
9. Dickson JB, Flanagan JC, Federman JL (1989) Contact neodymium:YAG laser. Experimental studies and oculoplastic applications. Ophthalmic Plast Reconstr Surg 5:17–26
10. Fitzpatrick RE, Goldman MP, Satur NM, Tope WD (1996) Pulsed carbon dioxide laser resurfacing of photo-aged facial skin. Arch Dermatol 132:395– 402
11. Ross EV, Anderson RR (1999) The erbium laser in skin resurfacing. In: Alster TS, Apfelberg DB (ed) Cosmetic laser surgery. Wiley-Liss, New York
12. Zimbler MS, Holds JB, Kokoska MS, et al. (2001) Effect of botulinum toxin pretreatment on laser resurfacing results: a prospective, randomized, blinded trial. Arch Facial Plast Surg 3:165–169
13. Ho C, Nguyen Q, Lowe NJ, Griffin ME, Lask G (1995) Laser resurfacing in pigmented skin. Dermatol Surg 21:1035–1037
14. Baker SS, Woodward JA (1999) Carbon dioxide laser blepharoplasty, ptosis correction, and treatment of festoons. In: Alster TS, Apfelberg DB (ed) Cosmetic laser surgery. Wiley-Liss, New York
15. Apfelberg DB (1999) Skin resurfacing with high-energy short-pulsed carbon dioxide lasers: preoperative assessment, patient evaluation, sequency of procedure, and adjunctive care. In: Alster TS, Apfelberg DB (eds) Cosmetic laser surgery. Wiley-Liss, New York
16. Fitzpatrick R, Geronemus R, Goldberg D, Kaminer M, Kilmer S, Ruiz-Esparza J (2003) Multicenter study of noninvasive radiofrequency for periorbital tissue tightening. Lasers Surg Med 33:232–242
17. Ross E, Naseef G, Skrobal M, Grevelink J, Anderson R (1996) In vivo dermal collagen shrinkage and remodeling following CO_2 laser resurfacing. Lasers Surg Med 18:38
18. Lumenis, Inc. (2004) UltraPulse Encore. www.aesthetic.lumenis.com/wt/content/ultrapulse
19. Hamilton MM (2004) Carbon dioxide laser resurfacing. Facial Plast Surg Clin North Am 12:289–295
20. Tanzer EL, Alster TS (2003) Side effects and complications of variable-pulsed erbium:yttrium-aluminum-garnet laser skin resurfacing: extended experience with 50 patients. Plast Reconstr Surg 111:1524–1529
21. Weinstein D (2000) Simultaneously combined Er: YAG and carbon dioxide laser (derma K) for skin resurfacing. Clin Plast Surg 27:273–285
22. Nelson BR, Metz RD, Majmudar G, et al. (1996) A comparison of wire brush and diamond fraise superficial dermabrasion for photoaged skin. A clinical, immunohistologic, and biochemical study. J Am Acad Dermatol 34:235–243
23. Cotton J, Hood AF, Gonin R, Beesen WH, Hanke CW (1996) Histologic evaluation of preauricular and postauricular human skin after high-energy, short-pulse carbon dioxide laser. Arch Dermatol 132:425–428
24. Lowe NJ, Lask G, Griffin ME, Maxwell A, Lowe P, Quilada F (1995) Skin resurfacing with the Ultrapulse carbon dioxide laser. Observations on 100 patients. Dermatol Surg 21:1025–1029
25. Levy JL, Trelles M, Lagarde JM, Borrel MT, Mordon S (2001) Treatment of wrinkles with the nonablative 1,320-nm Nd:YAG laser. Ann Plast Surg 47:482–488
26. Bitter PH (2000) Noninvasive rejuvenation of photodamaged skin using serial, full-face intense pulsed light treatments. Dermatol Surg 26:835–842; discussion 843
27. Goldberg DJ, Cutler KB (2000) Nonablative treatment of rhytids with intense pulsed light. Lasers Surg Med 26:196–200
28. Goldberg DJ, Samady JA (2001) Intense pulsed light and Nd:YAG laser non-ablative treatment of facial rhytids. Lasers Surg Med 28:141–144
29. Goldberg D, Metzler C (1999) Skin resurfacing utilizing a low-fluence Nd:YAG laser. J Cutan Laser Ther 1:23–27
30. Goldberg DJ, Silapunt S (2001) Histologic evaluation of a Q-switched Nd:YAG laser in the nonablative treatment of wrinkles. Dermatol Surg 27:744–746

31. Grema H, Greve B, Raulin C (2003) Facial rhytides – subsurfacing or resurfacing? A review. Lasers Surg Med 32:405–412
32. Menaker GM, Wrone DA, Williams RM, Moy RL (1999) Treatment of facial rhytids with a nonablative laser: a clinical and histologic study [see comment]. Dermatol Surg 25:440–444
33. Kelly DM, Nelson JS, Lask GP, Geronemus RG, Bernstein LJ (1999) Cryogen spray cooling in combination with nonablative laser treatment of facial rhytides. Arch Dermatol 135:691–694
34. Hardaway CA, Ross EV (2002) Nonablative laser skin remodeling. Dermatol Clin 20:97–111
35. Dixon JA, Huether S, Rotering R (1984) Hypertrophic scarring in argon laser treatment of port-wine stains. Plast Reconstr Surg 73:771–779
36. Keller GS (1992) Use of the KTP laser in cosmetic surgery. Am J Cosmet Surg 9:177
37. Dover JS, Geronemus R, Stern RS, O'Hare D, Arndt KA (1995) Dye laser treatment of port-wine stains: comparison of the continuous-wave dye laser with a robotized scanning device and the pulsed dye laser. J Am Acad Dermatol 32:237–240
38. Geronemus RG (1996) Surgical pearl: Q-switched Nd:YAG laser removal of eyeliner tattoo. J Am Acad Dermatol 35:101–102
39. Kuperman-Beade M, Levine VJ, Ashinoff R (2001) Laser removal of tattoos. Am J Clin Dermatol 2: 21–25
40. Anderson RR, Geronemus R, Kilmer SL, Farinelli W, Fitzpatrick RE (1993) Cosmetic tattoo ink darkening. A complication of Q-switched and pulsed-laser treatment. Arch Dermatol 129:1010–1014
41. Tripathi A, Lesser TH, O'Donnell NP, White S (2002) Local anaesthetic endonasal endoscopic laser dacryocystorhinostomy: analysis of patients' acceptability and various factors affecting the success of this procedure. Eye 16:146–149
42. Metson R, Woog JJ, Puliafito CA (1994) Endoscopic laser dacryocystorhinostomy. Laryngoscope 104:269–274
43. Moore WM, Bentley CR, Olver JM (2002) Functional and anatomic results after two types of endoscopic endonasal dacryocystorhinostomy: surgical and holmium laser. Ophthalmology 109: 1575–1582
44. Dutton JJ, Holck DE (1996) Holmium laser canaliculoplasty. Ophthalmic Plast Reconstr Surg 12:211–217
45. Mirza S, Al-Barmani A, Douglas SA, Bearn MA, Robson AK (2002) A retrospective comparison of endonasal KTP laser dacryocystorhinostomy versus external dacryocystorhinostomy. Clin Otolaryngol 27:347–351
46. Battle EFJ, Hobbs LM (2004) Laser-assisted hair removal for darker skin types. Dermatol Ther 17:177–183
47. Fitzpatrick TB (1988) The validity and practicality of sun-reactive skin types I through VI. Arch Dermatol 124:869–871
48. Gonzalez-Ulloa M, Castillo A, Stevens E, Alvarez Fuertes G, Leonelli F, Ubaldo F (1954) Preliminary study of the total restoration of the facial skin. Plast Reconstr Surg 13:151–161

Update on the Endoscopic Brow Lift: Pearls and Nuances

Bhupendra C.K. Patel

Core Messages

- The endoscopic brow lift is now the preferred technique for brow lifts
- Scalp incisions can be placed differently in men and women, taking into account the hairline and direction of pull desired
- The endoscope is used to identify the neurovascular bundles and sentinel veins: most of the remaining dissection can be safely performed without the endoscope
- Effective release of the periosteum from the supraorbital rims and nasal bridge is critical to the success of endoscopic brow lifts
- Several different methods of fixation are available: no one method of fixation has been shown to be superior to the others

13.1 Introduction

In 1951, the French philosopher Albert Camus complained of the vanity of ageing adolescents. To these same young persons, now baby boomers, has been ascribed the recent fervor for all things cosmetic. Baby boomers could not be blamed for taking a dim view of George Orwell, who, in rather a fatalistic mood, as the last entry in his notebooks stated, that 'at fifty, everyone has the face he deserves'. Plato, possibly in more enlightened times, chose to observe that the purpose of life was 'to be beautiful, healthy and become rich by honest means'. Whatever one's philosophies, the 'fatal gift of beauty' can be surgically enticed to linger, despite the passage of time. This is most profoundly seen in careful restorative surgery of the forehead, brow and eyelid region. The basic aim is to correct brow ptosis along with reduction of horizontal wrinkles and vertical frown lines around the glabella and to restore the curve of the brow to a more desirable shape.

Since the first description of the endoscopic forehead lift by Vasconez in 1994, endoscopic brow elevation has flourished to become the procedure of choice for the vast majority of patients requiring surgical rejuvenation of the forehead. This supersession of the procedure is largely because of its advantages which include use of small incisions, preservation of sensation, reduction in operative time and blood loss, decreased incidence of pruritus, less ecchymosis and decreased risk of incisional alopecia. However, the coronal brow lift remains the litmus test of brow elevation. It is only by a process of continuous evolution and refinement that one may attain results which approach the superb results that are obtained with the coronal lift.

The technique of endoscopic brow elevation is, by now, familiar to most surgeons. It consists of a variable number of small incisions behind the hairline, a forehead dissection, a temporal dissection, release of the periosteum from the superior and superotemporal orbital rim, ablation or attenuation of the brow depressor muscles and fixation of the brow at an elevated position. Many variations of the planes of dissection have been described. The subperiosteal plane of dissection is a safe and effective one and is our preferred approach. In this chapter it is assumed that the reader is familiar with forehead anatomy and the basic endoscopic brow lift procedure as described by various authors in the early and mid-1990s, and we describe some refinements of this approach.

13.2 Number of Scalp Incisions

Initial endoscopic approaches described as many as eight scalp incisions; five incisions are still most commonly used. We have found that most patients undergoing a full brow-lift or a combined brow and midface lift require four incisions: two paracentral and two temporal (Fig. 13.1 A). After experimentation with incision placements, we found that by choosing the paracentral incisions carefully, the medial and the central brows could be effectively elevated avoiding the central incision. These incisions are placed over the site of the maximal desired brow elevation, which is frequently just lateral to the middle of the brow, but varies from patient to patient. The patient is examined upright and vertical lines drawn from these points mark the incision site. Many authors advocate that the incisions be made about 1.5–2 cm behind the hairline. As the amount of brow lift obtained decreases the further away from the brow the incision is placed, we started to place incisions just behind the hairline. We found that any depression of tissues directly in front of the incision settles quickly following surgery.

13.3 Sites of Scalp Incisions

In balding men, placing the incisions in the scalp can result in scars that are fairly visible, as the scalp in the previously hair-bearing areas is fairly smooth. Even slight indentations in this area can be cosmetically unacceptable. We have been utilizing small horizontal incisions in the superiormost forehead crease, performing the subperiosteal dissection through these incisions (Fig. 13.1 B). Fixation may be achieved with bone tunnels with retraction of the horizontal incisions. In fact, as the point of fixation for elevation of the brow tends to be closer to the

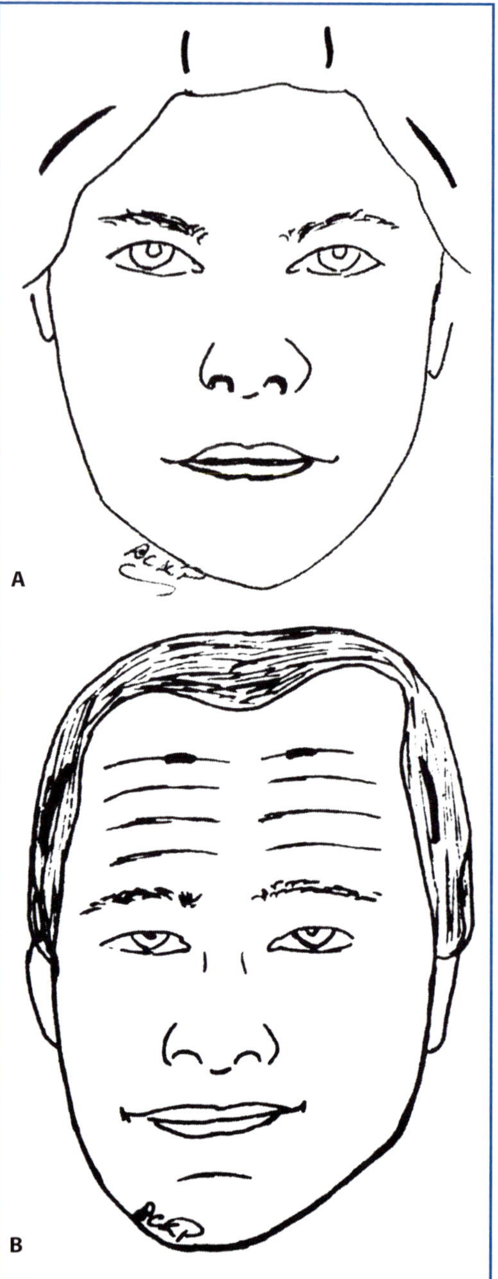

Fig. 13.1. A Typical incisions during endoscopic brow lift. In a female, the temporal incisions are relatively higher than in men. The paracentral incision sites are chosen to reflect the best vector of desired brow elevation. **B** In men with male pattern balding and frontal hair recession, the paracentral incisions are placed within the uppermost rhytid. The temporal incisions are lower than in women

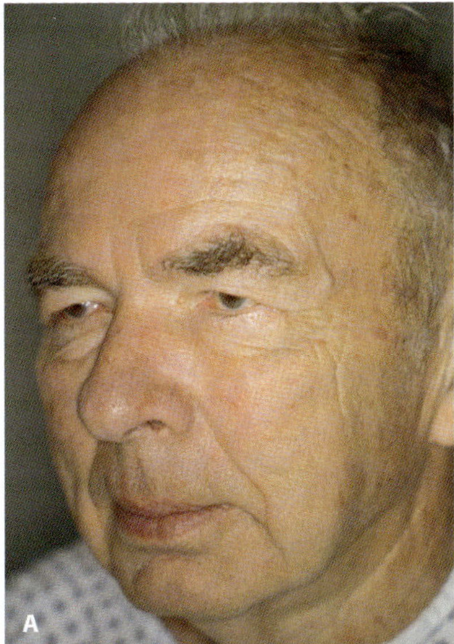

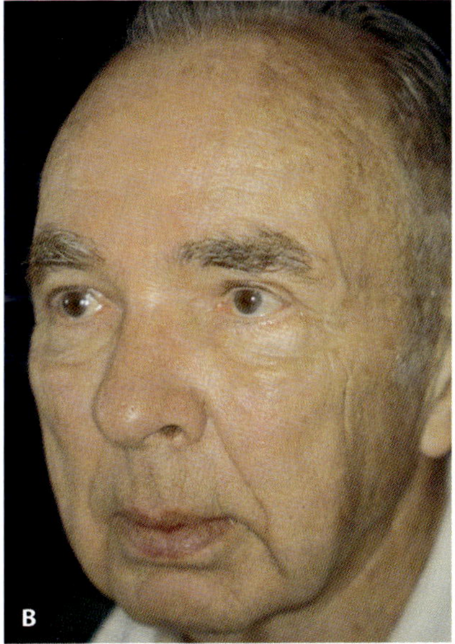

Fig. 13.2. A Sixty-three-year old male with severe asymmetric sickled brow ptosis. There is glabellar muscle overaction, secondary dermatochalasis and upper eyelid ptosis. **B** Four months following male-pattern incision approach endoscopic brow elevation, attenuation of glabellar muscles, ptosis repair and removal of a small strip of upper eyelid skin. These can be challenging because of the heavy sebaceous male forehead skin and Herculean glabellar muscles. Although the asymmetric preoperative brow positions have been reasonably well corrected in this patient, it is generally not quite as successful in most brow asymmetries

brows, the degree of brow elevation is more powerful. This approach may be used even in men with a respectable head of hair to avoid any elevation of the hairline (Fig. 13.2). Successful surgery in many such patients will replace the Brutus brow with a noble brow.

We have also found that instead of placing the temporal incisions at prescribed positions as proposed by various texts, we once again examine the patient sitting up and look for the direction of best lift and support for the tail of the brow. At times, this temporal incision may be fairly low laterally. When combining brow lifts and midface lifts, the angle of the temporal incision may be changed to best achieve the lift, both temporally for the brow as well as vertically for the cheek. This may allow one to achieve a satisfactory pull of the lateral midface and the jowls, which can often be improved to a very reasonable extent. The length of the temporal incisions can vary from 1.5 cm to as long as 3 cm, again depending upon vectors and extent of lift desired. These incisions are usually placed 3–4 cm behind the temporal hairline.

The temporal incisions are kept within the temporal hair. In men, the temporal incisions are kept lower (closer to the ears) than in women, as the brows need to be supported adequately rather than given the elegant effeminate flare which requires a higher lift. In women, the higher temporal incisions allow more manipulation of the temporal one-third of the brow.

13.4 Forehead Dissection

It is well known that the temporal line of fusion should be released only from the temporal dissection to the medial dissection to avoid trauma to the frontal branch of the facial nerve. An attempt at dissecting in the reverse direction runs the risk of dissecting in a more superficial plane, damaging the nerve. Most surgeons approach this dissection from the temporal to central plane rather gingerly and with some trepidation. We have found an easy way to dissect this safely.

A subperiosteal dissection posteriorly about 8 cm and down to about 1.5 cm above the supra-

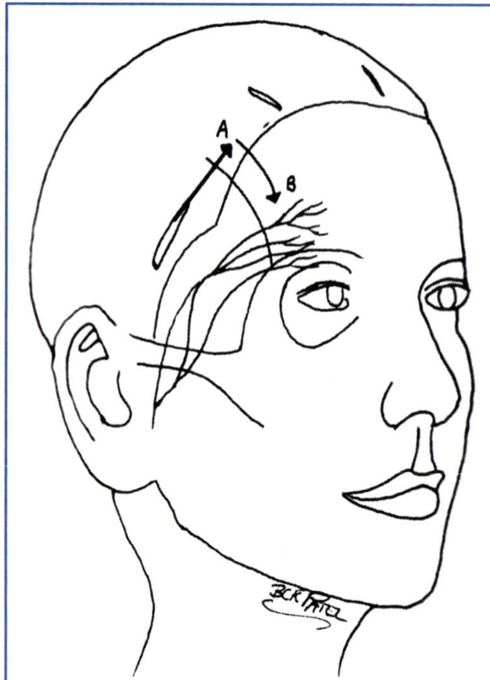

Fig. 13.3. *A* The temporal line of fusion is released high on the forehead, well above the frontal branches of the facial nerve, connecting the temporal and central subperiosteal planes. *B* The elevator is swept downwards, "unzipping" the temporal line safely and effectively

orbital rim is carried out. The temporal incision goes through the temporoparietal fascia down to the glistening superficial layer of the deep temporal fascia. As soon as this plane is seen, we use the forefinger to make the temporal pocket to within a centimeter of the superolateral orbital rim and to the temporal line of fusion. The connection between the temporal fossa and the central subperiosteal plane is made high up along the temporal line of fusion, well above the frontal nerve (Fig. 13.3). In fact this dissection is performed almost level with the superior end of the temporal incision. This release of the temporal line of fusion can be achieved with sharp dissection or, in many cases, with the forefinger. Once this connection is made, the temporal fusion line can be safely "unzipped" with the aid of a freer elevator down to the superolateral orbital rim. We have found that this maneuver reduces time as well as the degree of manipulation of the forehead tissues, reducing the risk of injury to the frontal nerve. The endoscope is used to identify the sentinel vein (sometimes two) just superolateral to the lateral orbital rim. This vein is close to the temporal branch of the facial nerve (which runs superficially within the temporoparietal fascia).

13.5 Release of Periosteum

Much is made of fixation of the released forehead tissues. However, effective release of the periosteum is just as important a component of the endoscopic brow lift. The periosteum needs to be released from one lateral canthal area to the other to create a mobile composite forehead flap. Some surgeons have suggested release of the periosteum within the orbital rim. It is safer and just as effective to release the periosteum at the arcus marginalis or even just above it. Once an opening in the periosteum has been achieved laterally, further release may be obtained by rotating the elevator or using endoscopic scissors. We used to cut the periosteum with angled microscissors that unfortunately dulled quickly secondary to the manly ministrations necessary. We find that a curved periosteal elevator can be successfully used to tear the periosteum while protecting the neurovascular structures. Over the supraorbital and supratrochlear neurovascular bundles, a spreading motion is used to separate the periosteum without injuring the neurovascular structures [1]. We have found that dissecting the periosteum off the nasal bridge, often all the way down the nasal bone, gives a pleasing elevation of the horizontal nasal rhytids and corrects nasal tissue ptosis (Fig. 13.4A–D).

When treating brow ptosis in facial palsy, we connect the periosteal release from the eyelid approach to the endoscopic approach to create a completely mobile forehead, which can then be placed appropriately with fixation. This creates a truly mobile composite forehead flap, which can be elevated and fixed using cable suture techniques. Such aggressive release is usually not required in patients without facial palsy.

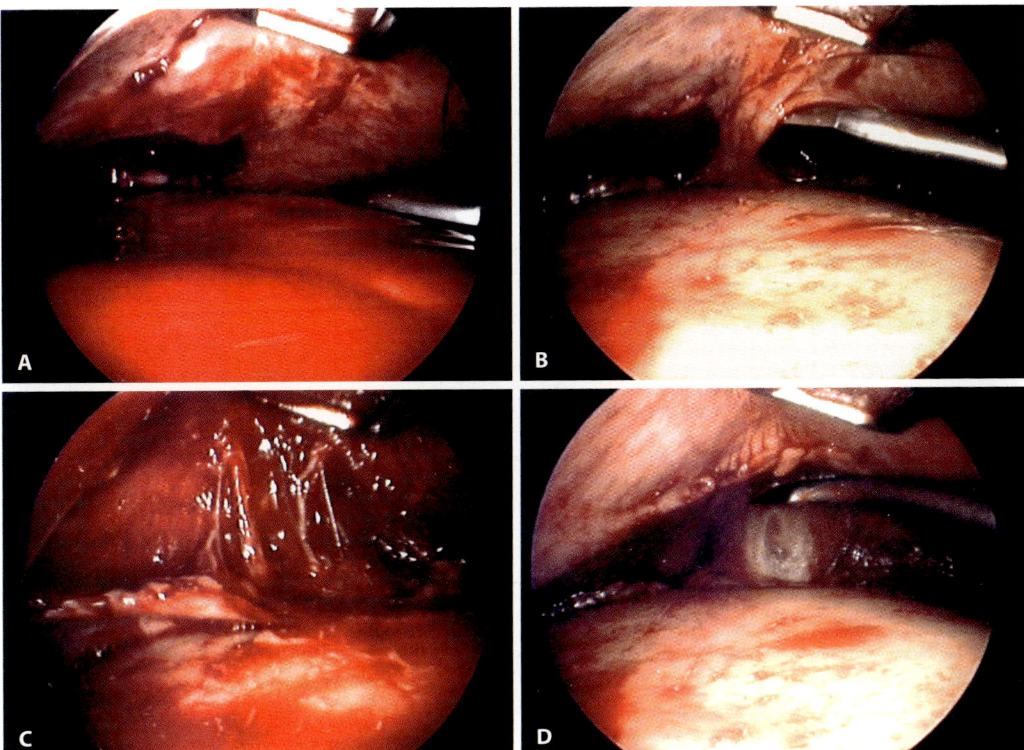

Fig. 13.4. **A** The periosteum can be incised using a sharp elevator with separation of sharp-ended scissors. **B** A rotational motion of the endoscopic elevator will tear the periosteum without injuring the surrounding nerves and vessels. **C** The supraorbital neurovascular bundle can be safely separated from the surrounding corrugator muscle which is then weakened. **D** Dissection of the procerus muscle and skin off the nasal bridge all the way down the nasal bone will allow correction of horizontal rhytids as well as nasal skin ptosis

13.6 Weakening of the Forehead Muscles

There has been considerable debate about the relative actions of the corrugator, procerus, orbital orbicularis and supercili muscles [2,3]. The debate has involved the relative merits of selective weakening of each of these muscles. We feel it is much more productive to think of these muscles as a complex with the muscles acting in harmony resulting in an overall downward shift of the central third of the lower forehead. With this concept in mind, it makes perfect sense to selectively weaken these muscles. Preservation of some action of the muscles allows a more natural appearance while reducing frown lines. It is rarely possible to completely weaken any of these muscles even with tedious and meticulous endoscopic dissection; this has frequently been stated to be a major limitation of the endoscopic approach. However, when complete removal of the depressor muscles is carried out, there is a very real risk of achieving an immobile central third of the forehead and also a depression between the brows. We have also seen patients with irregular bumps (sometimes called diablo horns) when incomplete excision of the corrugator muscles is achieved. If one accepts that weakening rather than annihilation of the muscles is the goal, a perfectly reasonable result may be obtained [4]. Postoperative botulinum toxin may be used as desired for individual patients [5].

The endoscope is used to identify the supraorbital neurovascular bundle while the corrugator muscle is weakened. Once the dissection is medial to the supraorbital neurovascular bundle, the insertion of the corrugator and the procerus muscle may be weakened by using long Mayo scissors in a crosshatch manner. Some of the supratrochlear nerves may be sacrificed in this maneuver. We have not found long-term anesthesia to be a problem using this technique. Not avulsing and removing the muscles in the glabellar region also avoids a depressed glabella. Finally, excessive weakening of the corrugator muscles has been blamed for separation of the medial ends of the brows. We have found that some degree of separation of the medial ends of the brows is desirable to overcome the medially and inferiorly pulled brows; an appropriate degree of such separation may be achieved using the above-described technique of weakening rather than avulsing the muscles.

13.7 Fixation of the Mobilized Forehead: How Long Is Fixation Necessary?

Some surgeons advocated simply weakening the glabellar muscles with no mode of fixation. We tried this technique on our first few patients and quickly realized that the brow and forehead will descend without adequate fixation. Precise control of the brow positioning is also not possible. Subsequently it was thought that 7–14 days was sufficient for the forehead periosteum to reattach to bone. However, it was noted by us and others that the brows and forehead frequently settled and descended to unpredictable levels in some patients after such short fixation. We used the externalized screw fixation technique in more than 30 patients and noted that late slippage of the brows was seen even when the screws were left in place for more than 2 weeks. Indeed, we had occasion to reinsert a permanent suture in a bone tunnel (see below) 3 weeks following surgery and were surprised to find that most of the subperiosteal dissection could be performed with minimal effort. This implies that in the presence of inadequate or short-term fixation, further ptosis is almost inevitable. We subsequently come to the conclusion in the mid-1990s that the best way to achieve a reliable result is to permanently fixate the brow during surgery. Recent studies in pigs have shown that it takes at least 30 days for there to be adequate periosteal refixation to bone after elevation.

13.8 Methods of Fixation

Myriad techniques of fixation have been proposed, and may be divided into temporary and permanent fixation techniques. Temporary fixation techniques that are still used include external bolsters, externalized screws, V-Y plasty of the scalp incisions, and transgaleal suturing techniques. Permanent fixation may be achieved with Mitek anchor screw fixation, bioabsorbable screw fixation, glue, use of buried metallic screws and plates and K-wires for fixation. We have tried most of these fixation techniques. Currently, the most popular technique of fixation among surgeons continues to be positioning of the elevated forehead with staples behind temporary screws. We have encountered significant local alopecia using this approach. Slippage has been discussed above. Patient inconvenience and discomfort are also factors. We therefore believed that permanent fixation was the best approach and used buried metallic screws, around which sutures were tied. Bioabsorbable screws and Mitek anchor screws were also used. All of these work well, but are costly and require permanent placement of hardware in some cases. We currently use three different methods of fixation in our practice, determined by patient needs, instrument availability and convenience.

When harvesting cranial bone for reconstructive surgery, we experimented with drilling tunnels and found that with a 1.5–2.0 mm drill or cutting burr, it was possible to rapidly design appropriate drill holes in the form of a tunnel. At about this time we tried various drills and drill-bits on cadaver skulls and developed a technique which takes us approximately 1 min per side and results in permanent fixation without insertion of any permanent hardware.

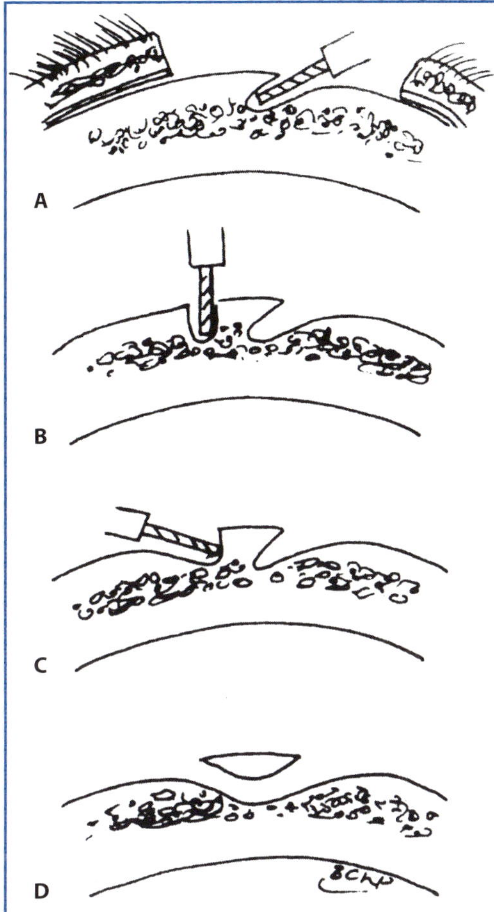

Fig. 13.5. **A** The first hole (distal) is drilled using a 1.5–2 mm burr or drill bit at an angle of 45 degrees to a depth of approximately 4 mm. Note the safety stop at 5 mm. **B** The second hole is drilled 4–5 mm posteriorly to a depth of 2–3 mm with the drill at 90 degrees to the skull. **C** The posterior lip is burred down and the angle of the drill bit is changed to 45 degrees. **D** The bone tunnel is completed and the anterior and posterior lips are beveled to allow easy passage of the needle

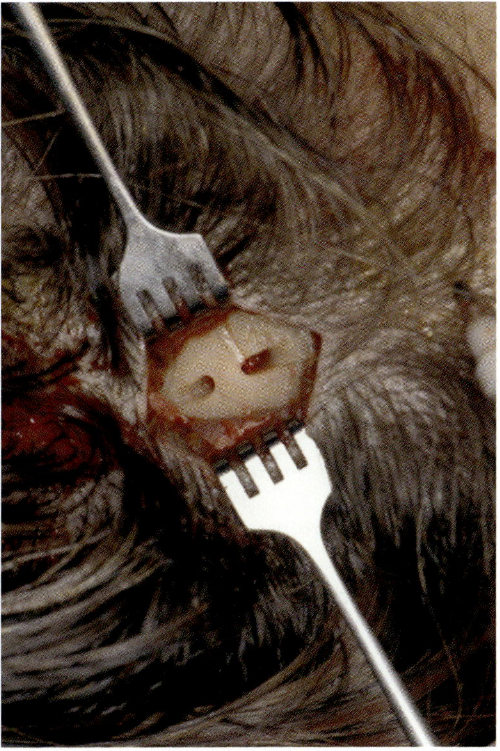

Fig. 13.6. The bone tunnel has been created ready for insertion of the suture

13.9 Simplified Technique of Bone Tunneling

(Fig. 13.5)

Previous studies have shown that the mean calvarial thickness is 6.8–7.7 mm. The outer table of the skull can be drilled to depths of 3–4 mm with safety. After performing the subperiosteal dissection, two holes are drilled opposite each other, approximately 4 mm apart. The distal (closer to the glabella) hole is drilled first with the drill at an angle of 45 degrees and to a depth of approximately 4 mm. We continue to use many different drill types and bits depending upon the surgical suites, but our preferred drill is the Robbins Acrotorque hand Engine dermabrader motor (Urawa Kohgyo Co.). We use a 2-mm cutting burr with a plastic stop at 5 mm from the end. The occurrence of dural perforation, a grave possibility with unprotected drills, is negated by the use of these stops.

The initial hole is made some 10–15 mm dorsal to the anterior aspect of the incision and this allows the drill to be held at the appropriate angle for drilling. The second hole is then drilled 4–5 mm posteriorly with the drill angled at 90 degrees to a depth of 2 mm. The posterior lip is then burred down with the same bit and this then allows the drill to be placed at an angle of some 45 degrees with ease. The two tunnels are connected. When the two holes meet, a give can be felt. A beveling trough is made by drilling away from the bar of bone and with the drill at a much smaller angle (25–30 degrees). It is important to leave 4–5 mm between the holes, as during the drilling at an angle, some of the bony bridge will be destroyed leaving a bridge of 3–4 mm (Fig. 13.6). In menopausal women particularly, bone mineralization may be less than normal. If the drill or suture inadvertently breaks the bone bar, a second tunnel may be created next to the initial attempt, using one of the drill holes and drilling at an angle.

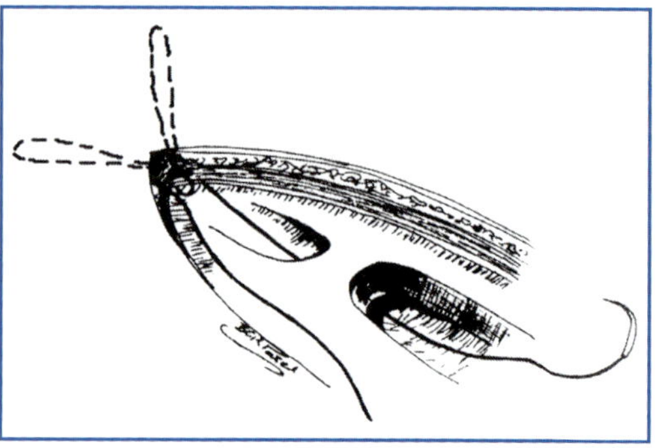

Fig. 13.7. Placement of the fixation suture through the tunnel. A 2-0 Surgidek suture is passed through the periosteum and galea in a figure of eight and then through the tunnel and tied. Note the bevels of the grooves which allow easy passage

13.10 Method of Elevation

We use a 2–0 Surgidek suture, which comes on a half-circle needle and is double armed. Prior to finding this suture, we used free needles to pass a suture through the holes. The beveling of the anterior and posterior parts of the tunnel allows the needle to pass with ease (Fig. 13.7). Although we have described the technique in a stepwise fashion, we perform the drilling on the two sides before suture placement and fixation. With experience, the time to create the tunnels is no more than a few minutes. The needle is passed through the anterior periosteum and galea (as low on the forehead as possible to obtain a good elevation) in a figure of eight to obtain a firm broad purchase and the needle is passed through the bone tunnel (Fig. 13.7). We use one of two methods of passing the needle through the periosteum and frontalis muscle. The first is to hold the needle in a reverse manner on a Webster needle holder: this allows a very firm purchase of the periosteum and subcutaneous tissues (Fig. 13.8). This insertion is done at 45 degrees to the orientation of the paracentral incisions to obtain the figure of eight. The other technique is used when a larger needle is used (certain sutures such as Ticron come on larger needles). The needle is bent into a swan-neck and placed in the needle-holder so as to allow purchase of the forehead tissues lower down than can otherwise be obtained (Fig. 13.9A–D).

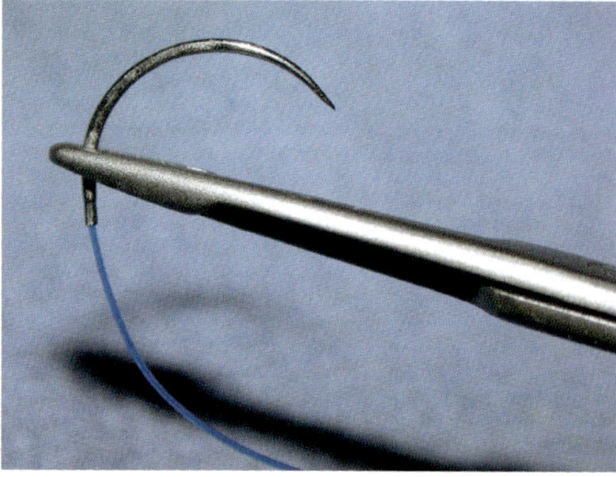

Fig. 13.8. The half-circle needle may be held in reverse as shown and passed through the periosteum and subcutaneous tissues with a better purchase than when the needle is inserted in the traditional method

The forehead is mobilized upwards by an assistant and the suture is tied. As no fixation is performed to the mobile posterior scalp, as is the case with some techniques, slippage is minimized. Furthermore, the exact positioning of the brow may be determined on the table with precision allowing fine-tuning peroperatively. We generally fix the two paramedian points, which have been placed preoperatively to obtain the best vector of elevation. It is also possible to use this technique over a central incision, should it be used, but the sagittal sinus is under this plane and the drill holes must be kept su-

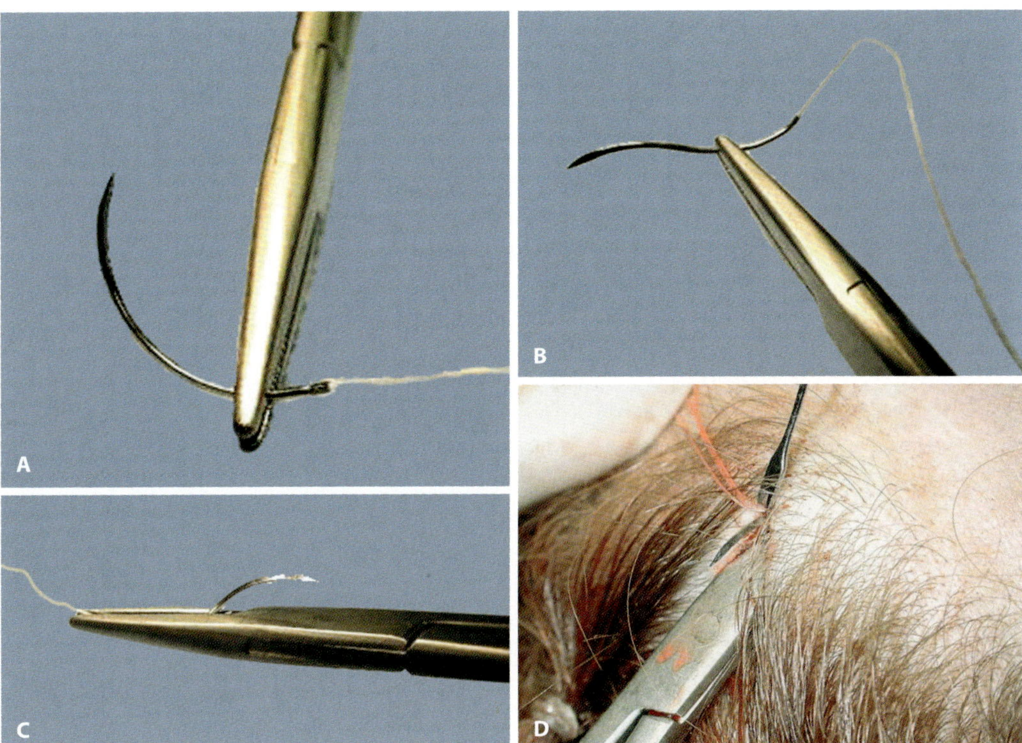

Fig. 13.9 A–D. A larger needle as is found on a Ticron suture may be bent into a swan-neck, mounted in reverse and passed through the tissues giving a lower purchase than can otherwise be obtained

perficial. Emissary veins may be encountered and these are treated with application of bone wax. Disadvantages of this technique include the need for power equipment and slightly wider exposure. The physician must be comfortable with the use of drills. In patients with thin scalps (where the other methods of fixation discussed below are less ideal), we almost routinely use the suture and tunnel method.

13.11 Buried Screw and Suture (Fig. 13.10A–F)

An alternative treatment, which also works very well, involves the use of a permanent screw. These screws can be inserted so that only approximately a millimeter of the head and shaft are above the bone. This is achieved by tightening the screw and then loosening it by two turns. Although electrical drills and microfixation sets can be used, we have found the Synthes Maxillofacial 1.5-mm compact fixation set to be very convenient and portable. No electrical drills are necessary as a manual hand drill allows the creation of the pilot hole for the 1.5-mm-diameter screw. A 4- or a 6-mm screw may be used. A large half-circle needle on a 2–0 Ticron suture is bent in the shape of a swan-neck to allow fixation of the suture to the periosteum several millimeters anterior to the incision. The needle is inserted in a reverse manner. We pass the needle twice, each at 45 degrees to the line of the incision. This allows a figure-of-eight suture support of the forehead. The tension is spread over a larger area than a single suture path and there is less likelihood of a depression of the anterior end of the incision when fixation is carried out. By modifying the angle of the two suture passes, it is possible to achieve a greater or lesser support or lift to the medial or lateral aspect of the forehead on each side.

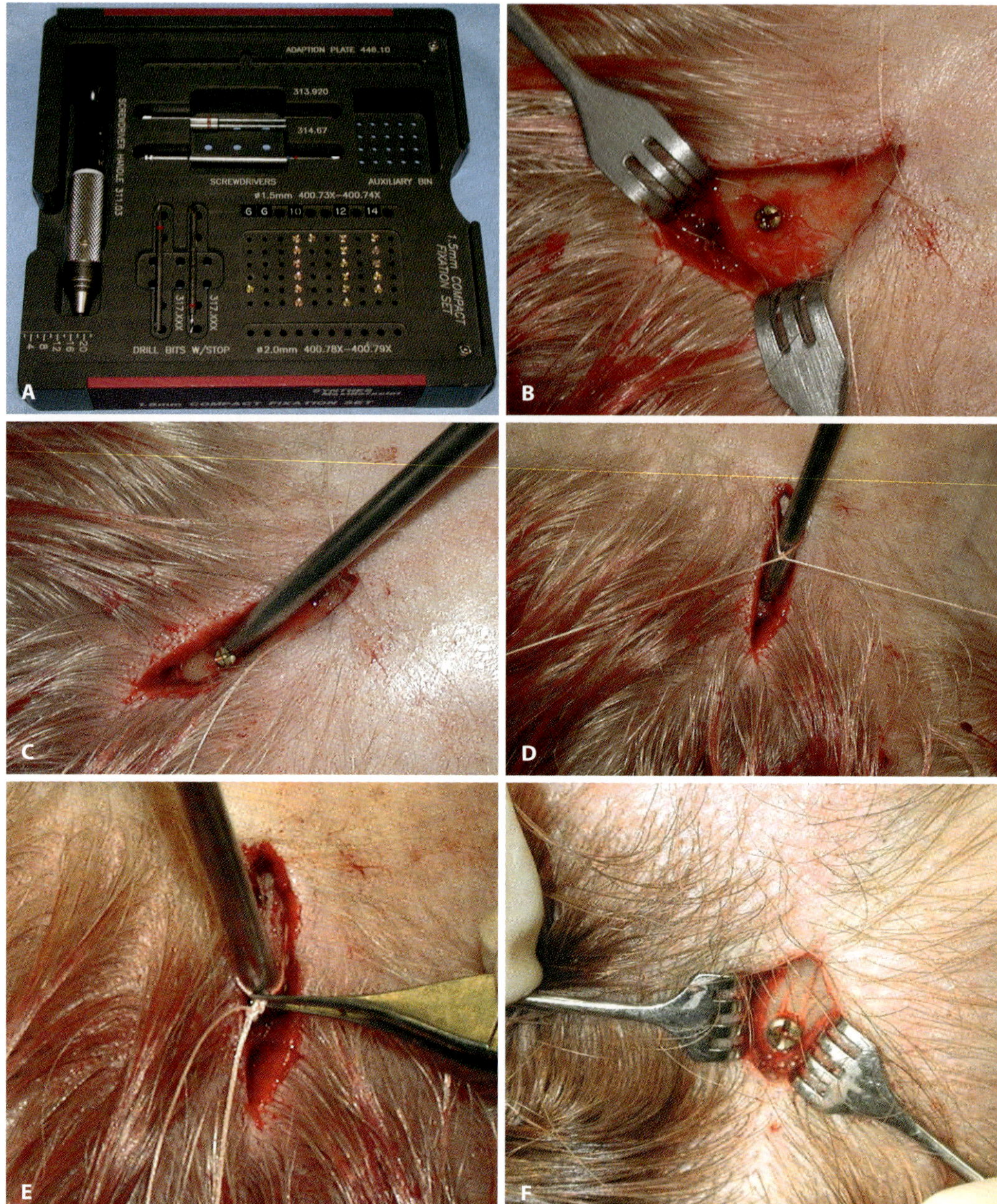

Fig. 13.10. A The Synthes Maxillofacial 1.5-mm Compact fixation set. **B** The 1.5×4-mm screw is inserted and then reversed by two turns. **C** A 12-French suction tip slides over the screw head as it is rotated vertically. **D, E** The suture is tied and slid over the suction tip which is rotated vertically. **F** The suture knot is rotated once the suture is under the screw head

The suture is tied over a 12-gauge suction tip, which is angled anteriorly. The suture is tied with a firmness or looseness depending upon the degree of brow lift desired. A 12-gauge suction tip fits very nicely over the screw head. The suction tip is pivoted posteriorly and the suture is slid down the metal. The suture slides off the suction tip and engages the screw head.

This method allows permanent fixation with a firm anterior support to the forehead periosteum. The degree of elevation of the brow can be judged as the suture is tied over the suction barrel. The screws are not palpable, except in patients with very thin scalps. The microfixation set is self-contained, portable and does not require power equipment. It does, however, introduce a permanent foreign body under each parasagittal incision.

13.12 Endotine Fixation (Fig. 13.11A–G)

The Endotine forehead fixation device (Coapt Systems Inc., Palo Alto, CA) is a triangular bioabsorbable (composed of polylactic and polyglycolic acid derivatives) device, which provides multiple fixation points. The device was designed to provide adequate mechanical strength for implantation and healing and is said to lose 95% strength and 50% mass by 5 months. It is said to absorb in approximately 12 months.

A guarded drill is used at relatively low speeds (less than 1,000 rpm) to drill a fixation hole 3.95 mm deep. An inserter is then used to guide the nub of the Endotine into this hole. When the hole and the post are ideal, a pop is heard or felt when the post is inserted into the hole. The plate is 1.0 mm thick and has a series of five prongs projecting cephalad from the plate. These prongs serve to puncture the periosteum and the galea, providing a secure support to the forehead.

After the plate has been placed in the drill hole, the forehead is elevated by grasping the hair and elevated over the Endotine. Brow and forehead positions may be adjusted throughout the procedure by lifting the periosteum and galea off the Endotine and redraping the forehead over the Endotine.

There will be a small palpable area over the Endotine in some patients, especially those with a thin scalp. Some patients will experience mild to moderate tenderness over the Endotines for up to 6 months. A few patients have reported a popping sound when they comb their hair, up to several months following surgery. If the drill hole is too wide, the post of the Endotine may work loose even during surgery. If a hole is found to be too wide, it is better to drill a second hole a little anterior to the original hole. We have not found the use of bone wax to be useful to anchor the post in a larger drill hole. The commonest cause of too wide a drill hole is using the drill at excessive speeds (greater than 1,000 rpm). Other causes include drilling the same hole more than once and not irrigating while drilling. It is best to drill in one pass, to drill in one continuous motion until the collar-stop is flush with the cranial surface and to irrigate and suction the bone particles out of the hole.

We believe one can get equally effective elevation and fixation using any of these three methods of permanent fixation. Of the three, the bone tunnel is the cheapest and does not introduce a foreign body. The Endotine is the most expensive but may save a few minutes of surgical time. It is probably wise to be proficient in more than one method of fixation as the availability of fixation tools and devices varies from facility to facility.

13.13 Closure

In order to achieve a good balanced temporal brow lift, it is important to insert more than one suture from the superficial to the deep temporal fascia. We generally insert two to three such sutures, which allows one to spread the lifting vector out more broadly, thereby giving a more impressive temporal lift. Also, the chance of slippage of sutures is less likely with such an approach. Another important point to remember is that the lower the fixation of the suture to the superficial temporalis fascia, the better will be the lift and the lower the incidence of postoperative droop of the brow. We therefore make a

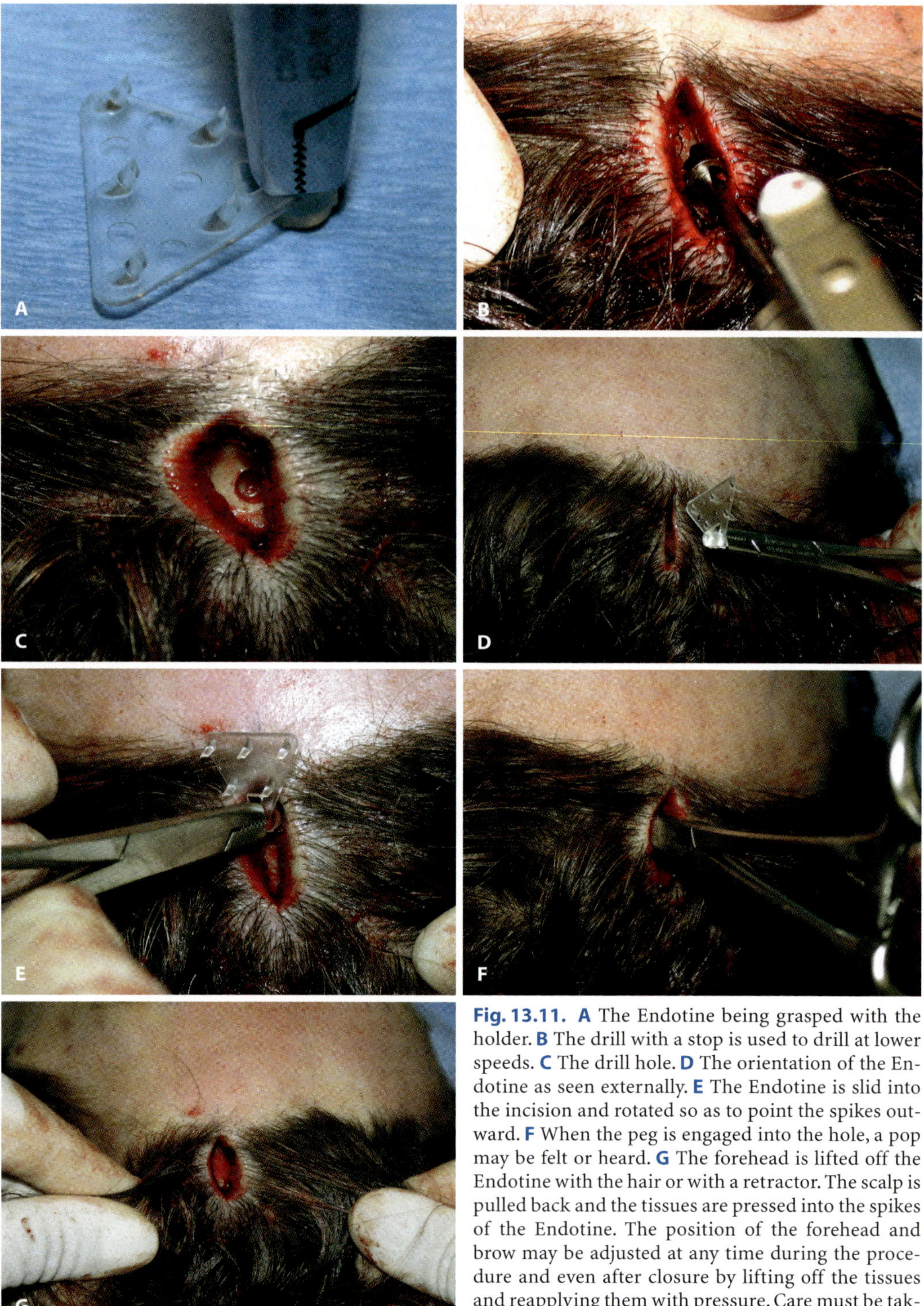

Fig. 13.11. **A** The Endotine being grasped with the holder. **B** The drill with a stop is used to drill at lower speeds. **C** The drill hole. **D** The orientation of the Endotine as seen externally. **E** The Endotine is slid into the incision and rotated so as to point the spikes outward. **F** When the peg is engaged into the hole, a pop may be felt or heard. **G** The forehead is lifted off the Endotine with the hair or with a retractor. The scalp is pulled back and the tissues are pressed into the spikes of the Endotine. The position of the forehead and brow may be adjusted at any time during the procedure and even after closure by lifting off the tissues and reapplying them with pressure. Care must be taken not to disengage the peg from the hole

point of elevating the temporal dissection adequately with retractors to allow an appropriate low placement of the sutures. Some authors advocate resection of the anterior part of the temporal incision and closing with staples without deep sutures. This creates unnecessary tension at the site of closure with a greater risk of hair loss and widened scar. The placement of deep sutures adds little time to the procedure and has the advantages mentioned above.

13.14 Postoperative Care

We do not insert any drains at the end of the procedure. We used to apply a firm forehead dressing but found that patients had less discomfort and less nausea without the pressure of such a dressing. We now apply a soft absorbent dressing, which is removed the next day. Nausea is a common problem following an endoscopic brow lift; we use preoperative scopolamine, intraoperative Decadron, Regulan and Anzemet or Zofran and postoperative Compazine suppositories. Patients are able to shower and shampoo the next day.

13.15 Conclusion

The above nuances have been garnered from multiple modifications and trials and errors over the last 9 years we have been doing endoscopic brow lifts and from over 250 cases. While none of the techniques is profoundly empyrean, they have made our results more redolent of the coronal brow lift, which remains the yardstick by which newer procedures must be measured. With this proviso, results over the last few years have not only proclaimed the acceptance of this procedure, but also justly placed the endoscopic brow and forehead lift at the forefront of the surgeon's armamentarium (Figs. 13.12–13.16) [6–9].

For optimal results, the combination of careful preoperative examination and planning, meticulous dissection with release of the periosteum, appropriate fixation and a premier knowledge of forehead anatomy is a sine qua non. While it is theoretically possible to overcorrect brow positions, it is our experience that undercorrection is more likely. Also, a certain amount of descent in the brow positions is noticed over the first few months even when a rigid fixation technique is used. We therefore aim for an overcorrection at the end of the procedure. To date we have not had an overcorrection that has required release of the brow. Critical assessment also shows that preoperative brow asymmetry will generally persist, albeit to a lesser degree. This may be because many brow asymmetries are secondary to overaction of the frontalis on one side, which cannot be modified by brow elevation.

The Bard noted that 'time delves the parallels in beauty's brow' and today he might have added that the endoscope and laser taketh them away.

Summary for the Clinician

- **A thorough knowledge of forehead anatomy is vital to successful and safe endoscopic forehead elevation**
- **Careful preoperative evaluation of the shape of brows, the desired height and curve and hairline are vital to the planning of endoscopic brow lifts**
- **A subperiosteal dissection is superior to a subgaleal dissection**
- **Adequate release of the periosteum is vital to the outcome of the procedure**
- **The temporal vectors of pull and fixation can be varied according to the desired curve and height of the brows**
- **Permanent fixation methods are superior to temporary fixation**

Acknowledgements. Supported in part by an unrestricted grant from Research to Prevent Blindness, Inc., New York, to the Department of Ophthalmology, University of Utah.

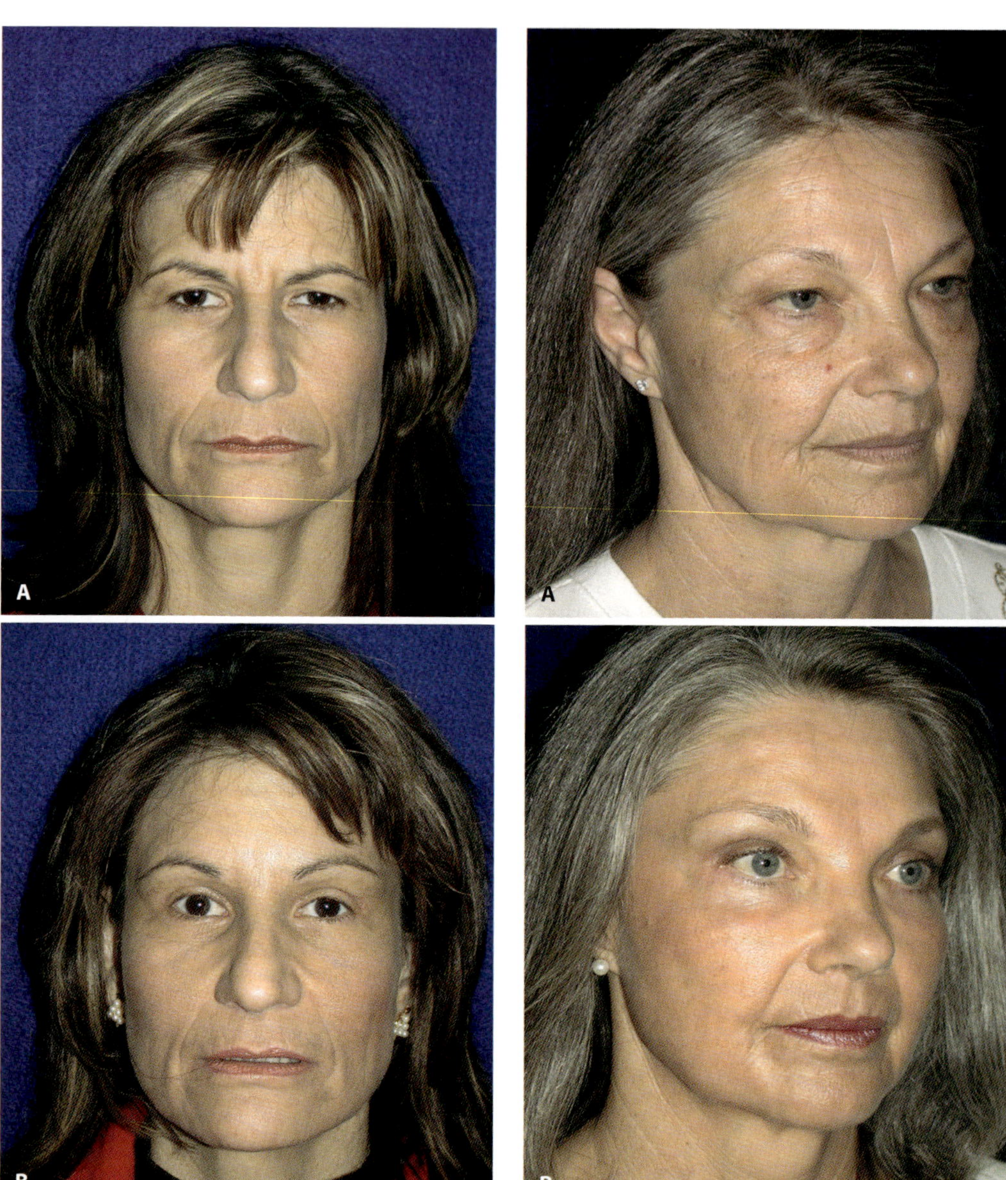

Fig. 13.12. **A** A 42-year-old lady with southern European skin, impressive corrugator and procerus overaction even at rest and marked brow ptosis and secondary dermatochalasis and ptosis was seeking an upper blepharoplasty. **B** Following an extended endoscopic brow lift with an aggressive temporal lift, a good curve of the brow is achieved. Note that in this patient adequate weakening of the procerus and corrugator muscles achieved the separation of the medial brows that rejuvenates the face adequately. An upper blepharoplasty and ptosis repair were also performed

Fig. 13.13. **A** A 58-year-old lady with a tired look was seeking a blepharoplasty. **B** Twelve months following an endoscopic brow lift with a small upper blepharoplasty replaces the patient's well-endowed but formidable brows with elegant arched brows. In square, heavy faces, an effective brow lift will give the illusion of a slimmer face. The patient also underwent a lower blepharoplasty and cheek lifts

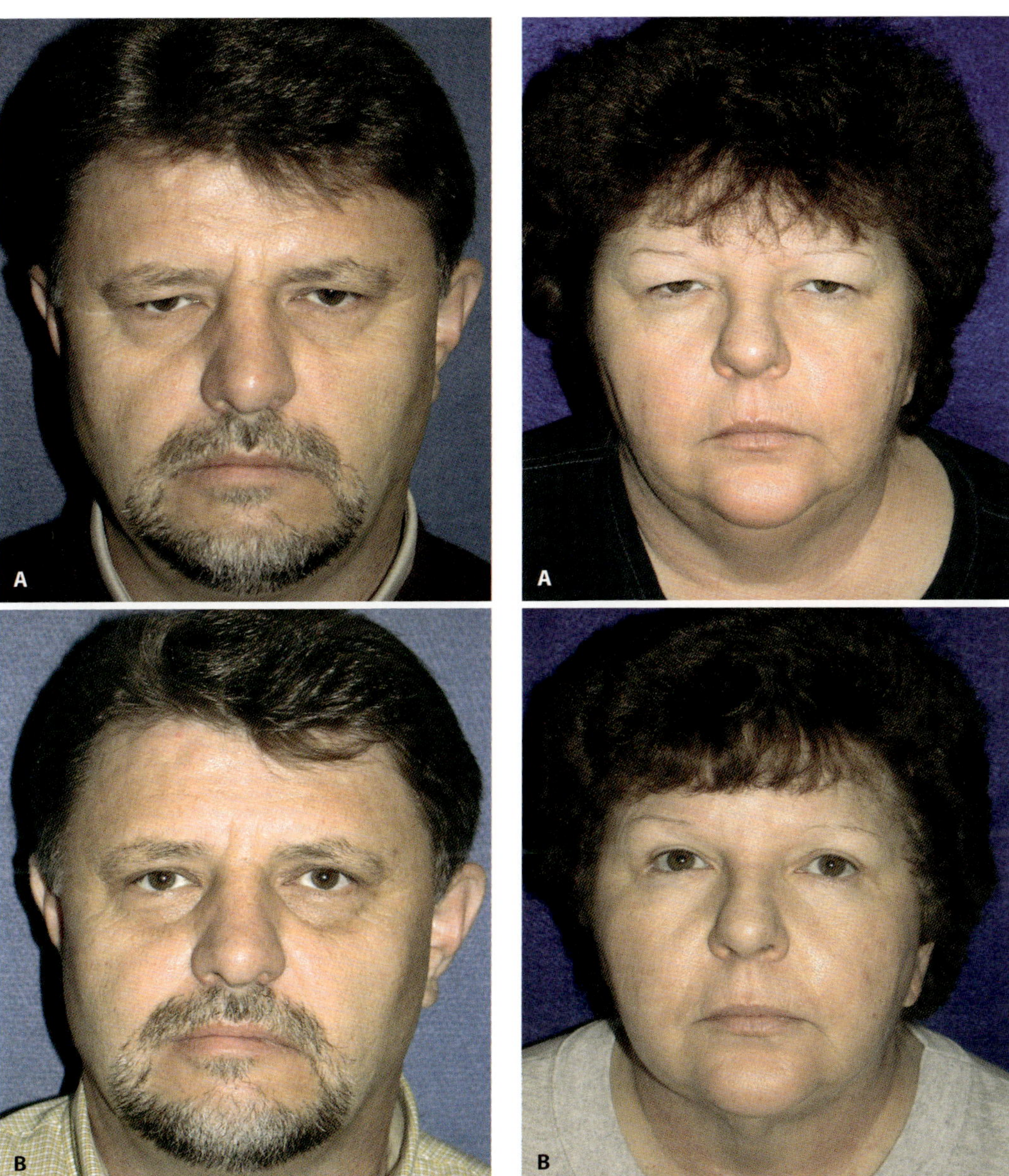

Fig. 13.14. **A** A 46-year-old man complained of difficulty with vision and difficulty with his contact lenses. The thick sebaceous male skin and markedly strong corrugator and procerus muscles make these cases challenging. **B** Nine months following a modified endoscopic brow lift and blepharoplasty with ptosis repair. An attempt was made to create horizontal male-type brows whilst still raising the brows above the superior orbital rim. Note that the patient had a lower right brow and some degree of asymmetry persists following surgery

Fig. 13.15. **A** A 64-year-old lady seeking an improvement in the upper eyelids. Such patients with heavy-set faces can be very challenging. A very aggressive lift and modulation of the corrugator and procerus muscles is required as it is impossible to overcorrect such patients. These patients have a very thick scalp and forehead, making it difficult to manipulate the forehead composite flap efficiently. **B** Twelve months following endoscopic brow lifts with upper blepharoplasty and ptosis repair: a not unreasonable result, under the circumstances

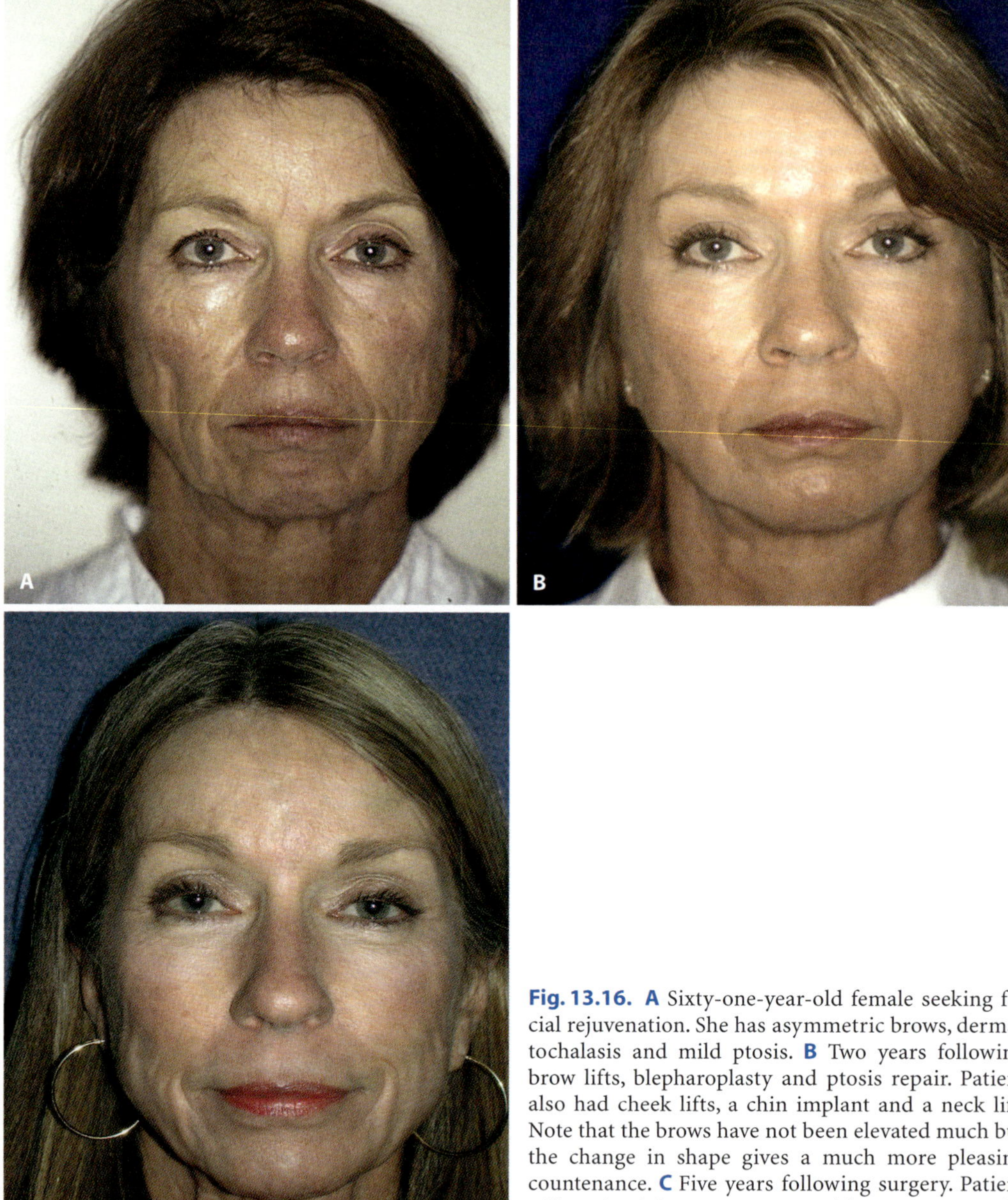

Fig. 13.16. **A** Sixty-one-year-old female seeking facial rejuvenation. She has asymmetric brows, dermatochalasis and mild ptosis. **B** Two years following brow lifts, blepharoplasty and ptosis repair. Patient also had cheek lifts, a chin implant and a neck lift. Note that the brows have not been elevated much but the change in shape gives a much more pleasing countenance. **C** Five years following surgery. Patient still maintaining a very acceptable appearance. She has had right herpes zoster of V1 accounting for forehead scarring

References

1. Beer GM, Putz R, Mager K (1998) Variations of the frontal exit of the supraorbital nerve: an anatomic study. Plast Reconstr Surg 102:334–341
2. Dayan SH, Perkins SW, Vartanian AJ (2001) The forehead lift: endoscopic versus coronal approaches. Aesthetic Plast Surg 25:35–39
3. Nassif PS, Kokoska MS, Homan S (1998) Comparison of subperiosteal vs subgaleal elevation techniques used in forehead lifts. Arch Otolaryngol Head Neck Surg 124:1209–1215
4. Newman JP, LaFerriere KA, Koch RJ (1997) Transcalvarial suture fixation for endoscopic brow and forehead lifts. Arch Otolaryngol Head Neck Surg 123:313–317
5. Dyer WK Jr, Yung RT (2000) Botulinum toxin-assisted brow lift. Facial Plast Surg 8:343–354
6. Ramirez OM (1997) Why I prefer the endoscopic forehead lift. Plast Reconstr Surg 100:1033–1039; discussion 1043–1046
7. Romo T 3rd, Sclafani AP, Yung RT (2000) Endoscopic foreheadplasty: a histologic comparison of periosteal refixation after endoscopic versus bicoronal lift. Plast Reconstr Surg 105:1111–1117; discussion 1118–1119
8. Sullivan MJ (1999) Male brow surgery. Facial Plast Surg 7:421–429
9. Vasconez LO, Core GB, Gamboa-Bobadilla M (1994) Endoscopic techniques in coronal brow lifting. Plast Reconstr Surg 94:788–793

The SOOF Lift in Midface Reconstruction and Rejuvenation

Robert M. Schwarcz, Norman Shorr

Core Messages

- The suborbicularis oculi fat (SOOF) lift, also known as the midface lift, mobilizes the midface structures in a superior fashion and fastens them to the orbital rim
- The outcome of any cosmetic or reconstructive procedure should center around patient satisfaction
- Access routes to the SOOF lift can be achieved in a variety of planes and entry points
- Superiorly the point of entry can be attained transconjunctivally, temporally, or via an infralash incision
- Inferiorly access can be gained by a sublabial approach, and this can be combined with an eyelid, or temporal, incision for a more robust lift
- The SOOF or midface lift provides an excellent tool for approaching midface descent

14.1 Introduction

Midface rejuvenation has long proved a challenge for the esthetic facial surgeon. Recently the role of the midface in rehabilitation of the aging face has been noted. Its position has a direct impact on the lower eyelid position, nasolabial, and nasojugal regions. Gravitational effects of the aging face can result in a profound aged appearance. This is very evident in the three-dimensional loss of the midface.

Standard facelifting techniques from a preauricular approach are designed to lift the descended face laterally and superolaterally. Gravity affecting the midface is most efficiently corrected in a direct superior vector.

The true challenge lies in the anatomical differences between individual patients. Prominent globes with a hypoplastic bony midface prominence display a negative vector. The contrary display of a prominent midface with deeper set globes allows for a positive vector. The hypoplastic bony midface commonly displays early obvious signs of midface descent. To address midface descent, the midface lift provides a form of soft tissue augmentation. Fat atrophy of the lower eyelids with deep nasojugal grooves should ideally be filled with the following options: autologous fat, synthetically fabricated fillers, or lifting the leading edge of the descended midface. In addition, some patients may present with bony concavity to which a malar implant can be utilized to provide anterior projection.

The midface lift has the ability to address cicatricial causes of midface descent, evidenced in unhappy postblepharoplasty, postfracture repair patients, or patients with vertical inadequacy of the lower eyelid lamella.

The suborbicularis oculi fat (SOOF) is lifted vertically to allow for lower eyelid augmentation. The SOOF lift, also known as the midface lift, mobilizes the midface structures in a superior fashion and fastens them to the orbital rim. If necessary, the midface can also be directed in a superotemporal vector.

In this chapter, the authors review midface anatomy and SOOF lifting including its varied surgical approaches.

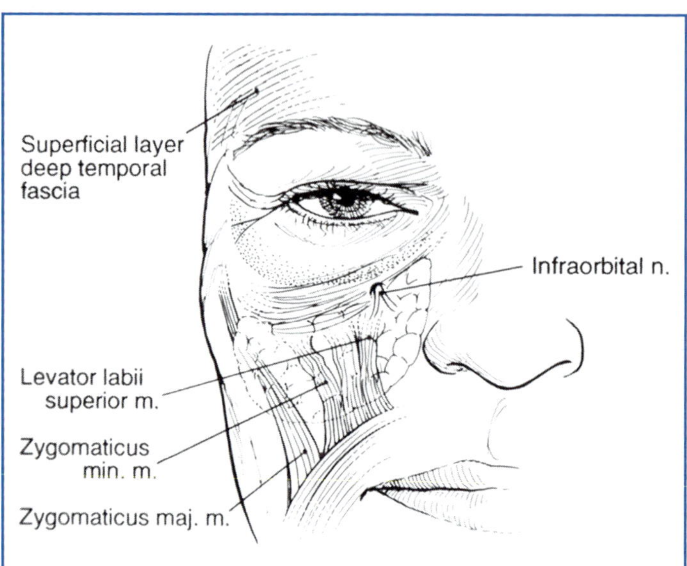

Fig. 14.1. Note the distribution of the muscles within the midface

14.2 Anatomy of the Midface

The midface encompasses the area from the inferior orbital rim to the lateral oral commissure. Its bony components are composed of the maxilla, and the zygoma laterally. From a three-dimensional view, the maxillary bone comprises most of this bony anatomy with significant variations: namely either convex or concave bony prominences. Depending on anatomical variability the infraorbital notch is in line with the supraorbital notch several millimeters to 1 cm inferior to the inferior orbital rim [11]. The zygomaticofacial foramen is found approximately 1 cm inferolateral to the orbital rim in the malar process of the zygoma [1].

The mimetic muscles are the muscles involved in facial expression. The levator labii superioris muscle arises just inferior to the inferior orbital rim often noted superiorly covering the infraorbital neurovascular bundle. The bony origin of this muscle spans from the maxilla to the zygoma, and it inserts inferiorly into the border of the upper lip. This muscle is located superficial to the plane of the facial nerve. Contraction of this muscle raises the upper lip to show the front teeth. The levator labii superioris also plays an integral role in forming the nasolabial fold [12]. The levator labii superioris alaque nasi muscle originates in the frontal process of the maxilla, and divides prior to insertion into the upper lip and the cartilage of the nasal alae [11]. This muscle aids in raising the upper lip as well as flaring the nostril. The zygomaticus minor muscle arises just medial to the zygomaticus major muscle medially and laterally to the zygomaticomaxillary suture respectively. These muscles insert at the upper lip corner drawing the mouth in a superolateral vector [12]. The zygomaticus muscles are found in the plane superficial to the facial nerve as well (Fig. 14.1). Finally, the angularis oris muscle originates just inferior to the infraorbital foramen, inserting by the lateral oral commissure. It contributes to the deepening of the nasolabial fold [12]. The angularis oris muscle is found in the plane deep to the facial nerve.

The mimetic muscles are engulfed in fat, which superiorly begins at the inferior portion of the orbicularis oris muscle and inferiorly is bordered by the inferior orbital rim. The SOOF derives its name from the specific location of this fat. The SOOF is preperiosteal and lies within the zygomaticus muscle system, levator labii superioris and levator labii superioris alaque nasi [13]. The SOOF is further subdivided into anterior and posterior compartments by the malar septum, which has its origins in the arcus marginalis [14]. The zygomaticus muscles and the levator labii superioris muscles forming the nasolabial fold travel through the SOOF and insert onto the dermis underlying the nasolabial fold [1, 14]. The SOOF is continuous with the superficial musculoaponeurotic system (SMAS). With age the SOOF, midfacial musculature, and malar fat pad all descend [10]. The SOOF and all its interrelated structures of the midface can be lifted en bloc to allow for a vertical midface elevation.

14.3 Age Related Changes of the Midface

The orbicularis oculi muscle is attached superiorly to the tarsal plate, and inferiorly to the SOOF/SMAS complex. With the descent of this midface complex the orbicularis muscle is stretched and becomes ptotic, and resulting in loss of elasticity. The new direction of this stretched orbicularis oris muscle is inferolaterally, and the SOOF/SMAS and all its contents tend to shift inferomedially deepening the nasolabial fold and eventually adding to facial jowls noted with aging [14]. In the youthful midface the indentation made by the inferior tarsal edge bowing into the continuous mound of midfacial tissue represents a single convexity. Aging causes the lower eyelid to present with postseptal fat herniation secondary to orbital septal laxity, or fat deflation producing a second convexity [1]. The double convex deformity or the 'double bubble sign' is apparent with a profile lateral view of a patient (Fig. 14.2).

In the past, lower eyelid blepharoplasty has been noted as a fat removal procedure. More recently the literature supports ideas of fat deflation and midface augmentation, especially in midfaces with significant preoperative bony concavity. Whether this augmentation entails bony implants, soft tissue filling with fat or other substances, filling the area of concavity created by the aged midface becomes a main goal. The midface lift has consistently addressed this issue by vertical augmentation. This can be used as a cosmetic

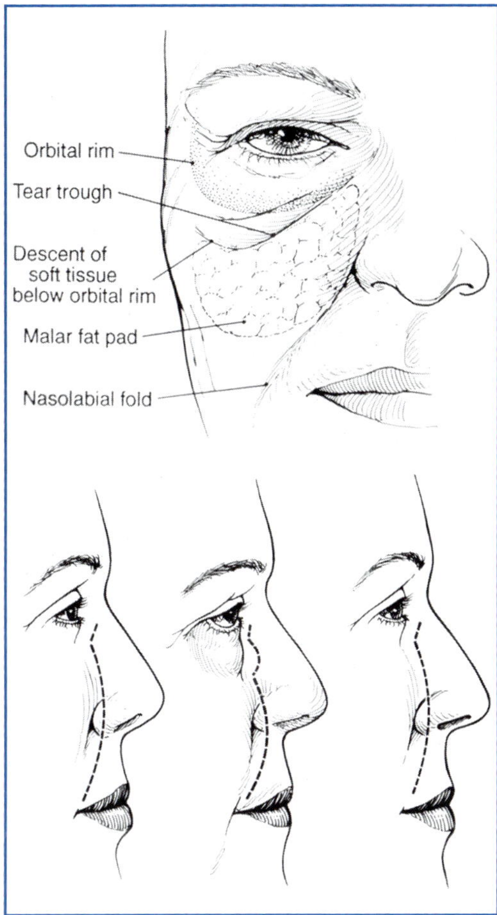

Fig. 14.2. The youthful face has a single convexity; with aging a double convexity develops secondary to atrophy and tissue descent

adjunct to many other procedures, or to address issues of lower eyelid vertical inadequacy noted in the unhappy postblepharoplasty patient, or other reconstructive efforts to lift the midface [16].

14.4 Patient Selection

The outcome of any cosmetic or reconstructive procedure should center around patient satisfaction. During the selection process a clear and mutual understanding of the patients' goals and expectations must be delineated. A detailed evaluation must entail, but should not be limited to, bony facial anatomy including pre-existing asymmetry. One should also observe the condition of the skin: laxity, solar changes, and deep tissue descent. Attention to preoperative position of the eyelids, including a forced upward traction test of the lower eyelid, should be performed. Position of the brows and cheeks, and evaluation of the jowls and depth of the nasolabial fold, should also be noted. Fat atrophy, SOOF descent, and tear trough deformities are also discussed with the patient. A focused ophthalmological examination including cornea, glaucoma status, dry eye evaluation, and orbicularis strength with a focus on eyelid closure, and pre-existing lagophthalmos, or any facial nerve weakness is of importance.

A complete medical history should be taken with a note made of any blood dyscrasias, aspirin, or blood thinner usage including vitamin E, or herbal remedies. Any significant past medical history or patients over the age of 60 years should be referred for a full medical workup and preoperative evaluation.

Preoperative photographs should be taken to document the status of the facial changes. Photographs are taken in the standard surgical series format: full face, periocular region, 45 degrees, and 90 degrees. Photos should also highlight any considerate preoperative problems such as lagophthalmos. These photographs should be displayed at eye level during the surgery in the operating room for easy access for the surgeon. Patients should be encouraged to bring old photographs of themselves in order to demonstrate anatomical and aging differences.

As described below there are many approaches in approaching the midface lift. Each patient should be viewed independently and approach should be guided by the presentation of their respective interrelationship of anatomy and aging changes.

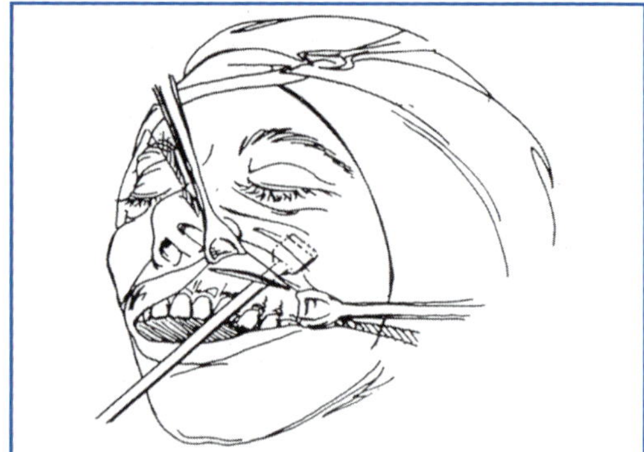

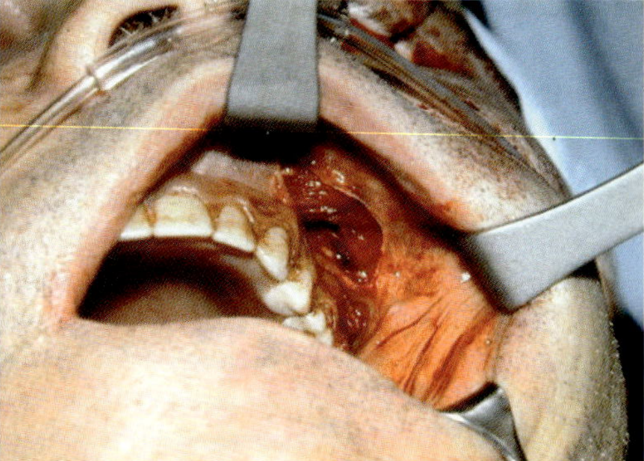

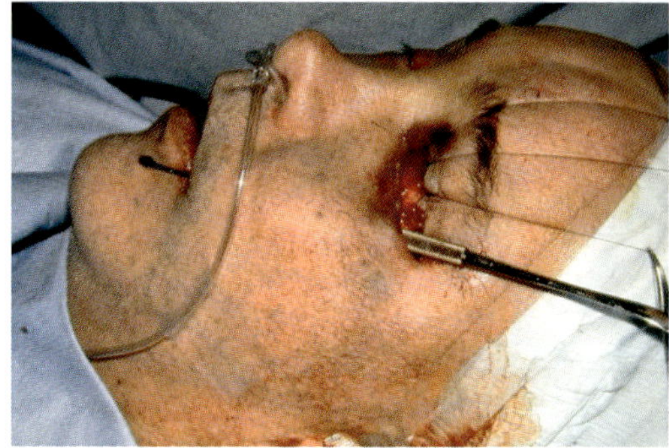

Fig. 14.3. Sublabial incision, full release with a transconjunctival approach (*right*)

14.5 Surgical Technique

Access routes to the SOOF lift could be achieved in a variety of planes and entry points. Superiorly the point of entry could be attained transconjunctivally, temporally, or via an infralash incision. Inferiorly access could be gained by a sublabial approach, and this could be combined with an eyelid, or temporal incision for a more robust lift (Fig. 14.3). The dissection could be achieved in either a subperiosteal or a preperiosteal plane (Fig. 14.4).

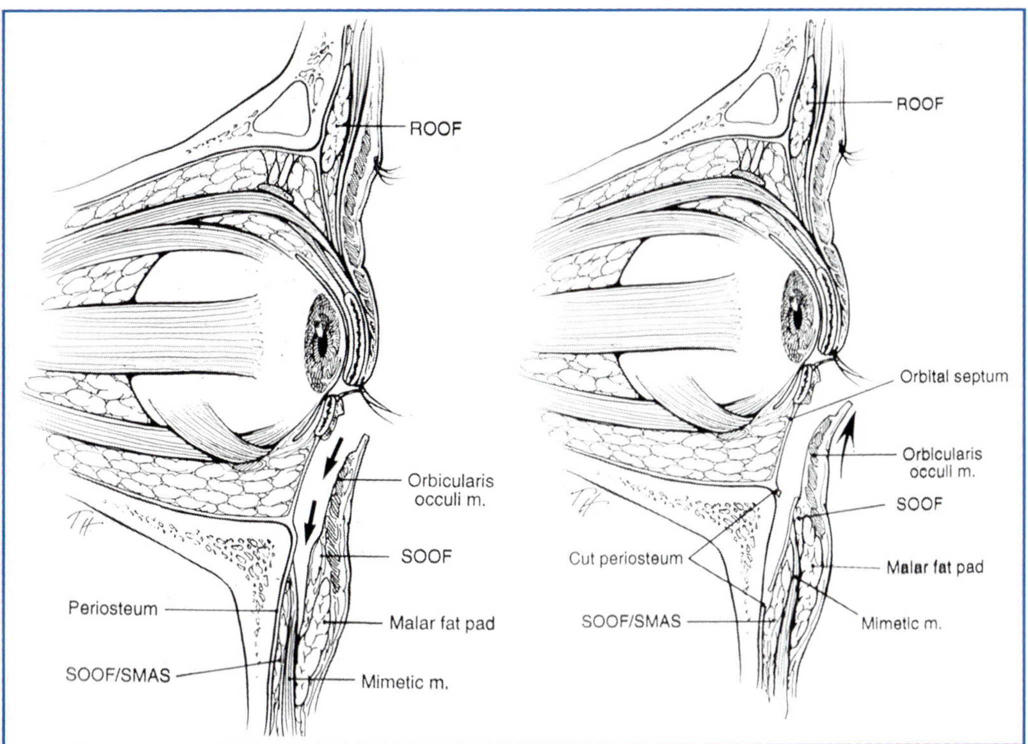

Fig. 14.4. Preperiosteal (*left*) and subperiosteal (*right*) dissection

14.5.1 Transconjunctival Approach

14.5.1.1 Subperiosteal Dissection

The lower eyelid and midface are infiltrated with 2% lidocaine with 1:100,000 adrenaline. After several minutes are allowed for the vasconstrictive properties of the adrenaline to begin, the patient is cleaned and draped in a sterile manner. A lateral cantholysis is performed, and the lower eyelid is retracted with a lacrimal rake or a Desmarres retractor. Using a Colorado tip, cutting cautery is utilized to make a transconjunctival incision halfway between the lower edge of the tarsus and the inferior fornix [1]. The incision spans from lateral canthus to 1 mm lateral to the caruncle. The orbital fat contained in its septa is noted and pushed posteriorly using an eyelid plate or malleable retractor. Blunt dissection is continued down to the level of the orbital rim. Orbicularis muscle is noted at the rise of the bony orbital rim. Once over the rim and on the face of the maxillary bone the SOOF is visible. At this point a pre- or subperiosteal route could be achieved. Using either a number 15 blade or a Colorado tip cutting cautery, an incision is made in the periosteum several millimeters inferior to the edge of the orbital rim, thus leaving a cuff of arcus marginalis for later suspension of the midface structures. An elevator is then used to elevate the periosteum off the face of the maxilla, thus creating a subperiosteal plane. Continuing inferiorly, the levator labii superioris muscle is noted, and its disinsertion should be performed with caution because the infraorbital neurovascular bundle lies immediately inferior to it. With direct visualization using a Parks midface retractor, this dissection is continued until the desired area of the inferior aspect of the midface is reached. The level of the nasal alae is usually

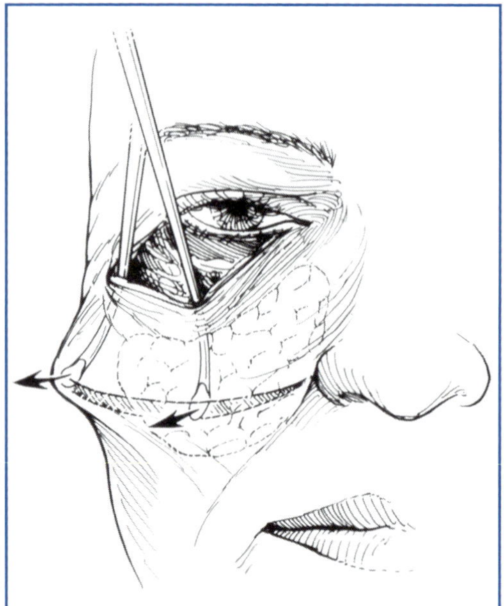

Fig. 14.5. The periosteum is incised to allow for the appropriate release

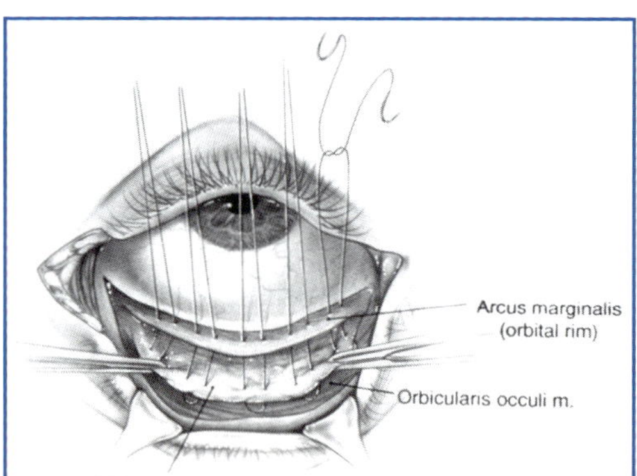

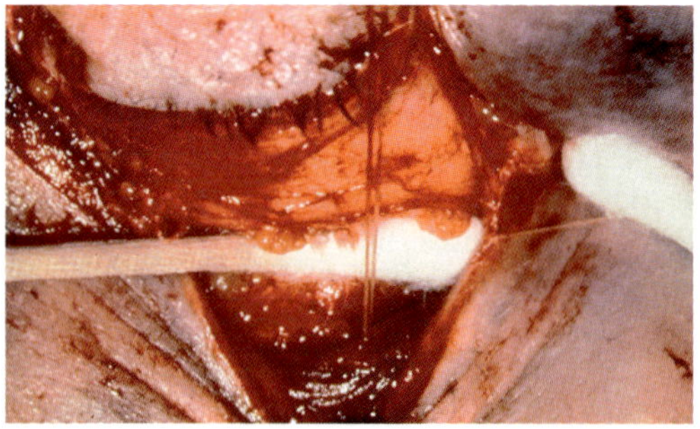

Fig. 14.6. Sutures passed through the arcus marginalis securing the newly lifted SOOF

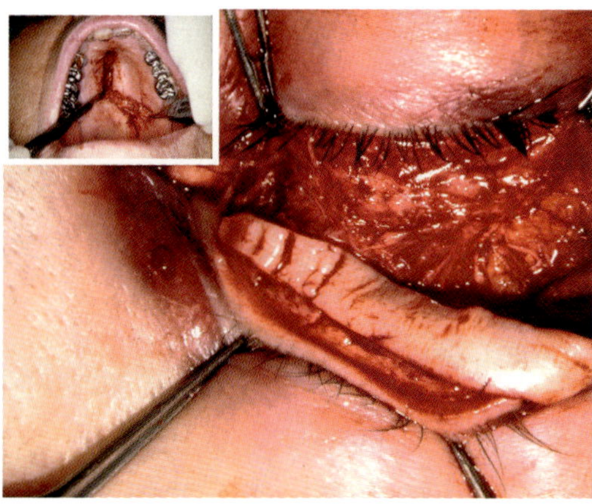

Fig. 14.7. Harvesting and placement of a hard palate graft as a posterior lamella spacer graft used in addressing posterior vertical inadequacy of lower eyelid

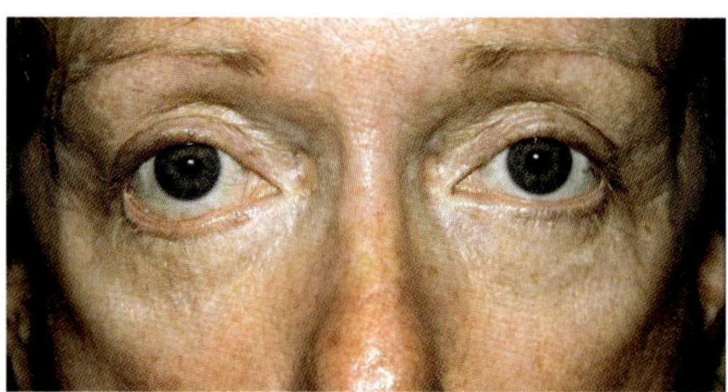

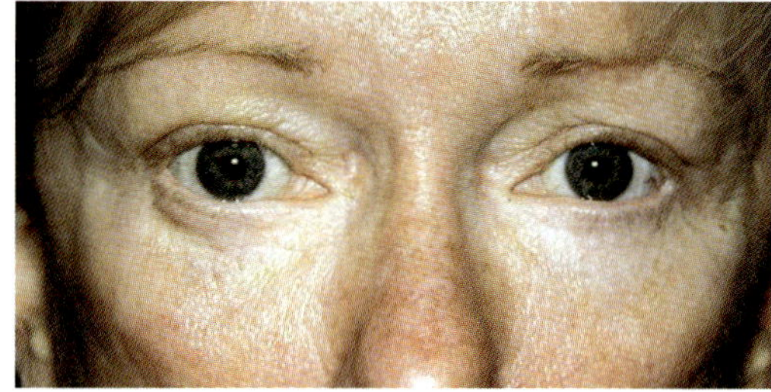

Fig. 14.8. Forty-seven-year-old female before and after transconjunctival subperiosteal midface lift with hard palate graft

adequate, but the dissection may be continued to the lateral oral commissure if desired. The distal periosteum is next released by incising it with a cut cautery at the inferiormost border of the lifted midface (Fig. 14.5). The periosteum is next stretched using a reverse endoscopic elevator.

Four midface purchases are secured using 4-0 Prolene suture in a horizontal mattress type fashion beginning with a purchase at the arcus

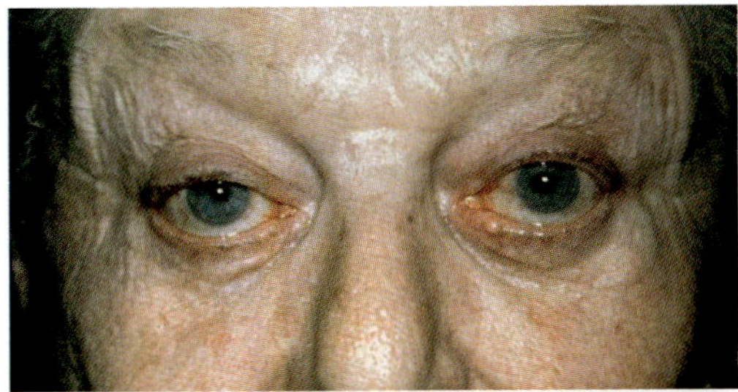

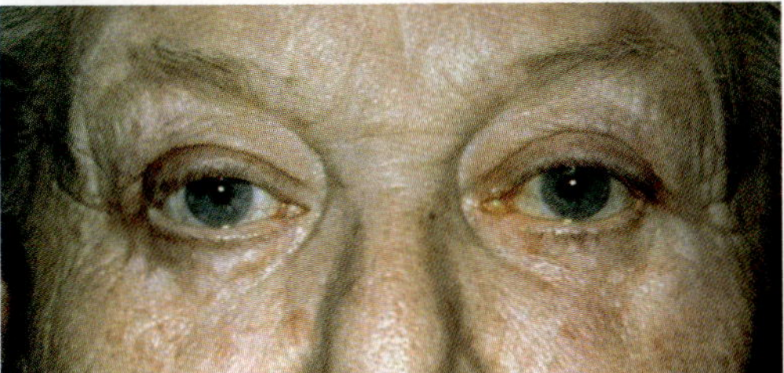

Fig. 14.9. Sixty-two-year-old female before and after transconjunctival subperiosteal midface lift with hard palate graft and excision of left lower eyelid meibomian gland cyst

marginalis cuff, next incorporating the SOOF, testing the lift by providing traction to the suture and finally returning to the arcus marginalis to be tied securely (Fig. 14.6). The lateral canthus is then reconstructed in the standard fashion.

When used for reconstructive efforts, the posterior lamella of the eyelid is often augmented with the aid of a spacer graft, as described by Shorr, and a hard palate graft could be harvested and used for posterior lamella vertical augmentation in conjunction with the above mentioned subperiosteal SOOF lift (Fig. 14.7 a) [16].

Two examples of the transconjunctival subperiosteal midface lift with hard palate graft are shown in Figs. 14.8 and 14.9.

14.5.1.2 Preperiosteal Dissection

Once a transconjunctival incision is achieved, a No. 15 blade is used to make a SOOF incision horizontally. A Stevens tenotomy scissor and a Brown-Adson forceps are used to perform blunt dissection in this plane inferiorly for 1 cm. The forceps are used to grasp the SOOF and, using a 4–0 Prolene suture in a horizontal mattress fashion, the SOOF is secured to the arcus marginalis. The cut edges of the conjunctiva are closed in running type fashion using 6–0 fast gut, and the lateral canthus is reconstructed in a standard fashion.

14.5.2 Sublabial Approach

The sublabial approach should be combined with a temporal endoscopic approach, or a transconjunctival incision. This approach allows for a more robust dissection, and easier access for placement of submalar implants if desired.

The midface, lower eyelid and gingivobuccal sulcus are infiltrated with 2% lidocaine with 1:100,000 adrenaline, and 0.5% Marcain is used for infraorbital blocks. With the use of monopolar cutting cautery with a Colorado needle, an incision is made from the first molar to the lateral incisor in the gingivobuccal sulcus (Fig. 14.3). Attention should be given to avoid injuring Stenson's duct. Periosteal elevators are used to allow for a superiorly directed subperiosteal dissection on the maxillary bone. The infraorbital bundle is identified and care is taken not to injure this structure. If combined with a transconjunctival incision, the dissection is carried superiorly to this previously established entry site.

When combined with a temporal incision superiorly, the dissection is then carried laterally to the fibers of the masseteric muscle. Caution is advised in the area of the masseteric fibers as the facial nerve lies in the superficialmost aspect of the masseteric fibers. Attention is now turned to the temporal approach under endoscopic guidance. The temporal incision is carried down to the level of the deep temporalis fascia and then continuing inferiorly to Yassergil's fat pad, where the dissection is directed in the plane between the fascia and Yassergil's fat pad, over the medial aspect of the zygomatic arch until meeting the area previously dissected with the superiormost aspect of the sublabial approach. Two 4–0 Goretex sutures are placed through the sublabial incision in a mattress type fashion through the periosteum, then retrieved via the temporal incision with the guidance of an endoscopic needle holder, then secured with a free needle to the deep temporalis fascia. The sutures are adjusted until the desired amount of lift is achieved. The temporal incision is closed with skin staples, and the sublabial incision is closed with interrupted 4–0 chromic sutures.

14.5.3 Closed Cable Lift

A closed meloplication technique as described by Sasaki [17] can be utilized as a closed SOOF lift. Anesthesia is achieved by injection of a tumescent solution of 0.1% lidocaine and 1:1,000,000 adrenaline. Sutures consisting of 4–0 Goretex with 3–0 Vicryl (to be removed) are passed from the nasolabial fold after making a stab incision with an 11 blade, and a 6-in. Keith needle is introduced in a superolateral vector. The needle travels immediately above the level of the SMAS and exits superiorly piercing through the deep temporalis fascia. At the inferior entry site, the nasolabial fold, the Keith needle is again introduced through the same stab incision site completing the loop towards the deep temporalis fascia. A 3×3-mm square of Goretex is passed over the Keith needle onto the Goretex and Vicryl sutures. Upon tightening these sutures to achieve the desired lift, dimpling of the skin is addressed by utilizing the sawing motion with the braided Vicryl suture. When the desired lift is achieved, the Vicryl suture can be removed, and the remaining suture is tied at the level of the deep temporalis fascia over another Goretex patch (Fig. 14.10).

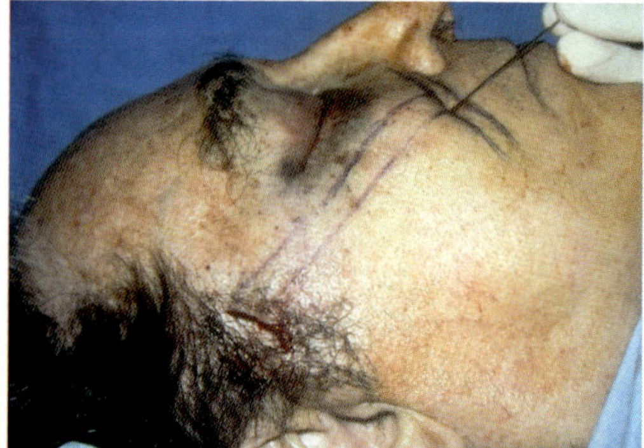

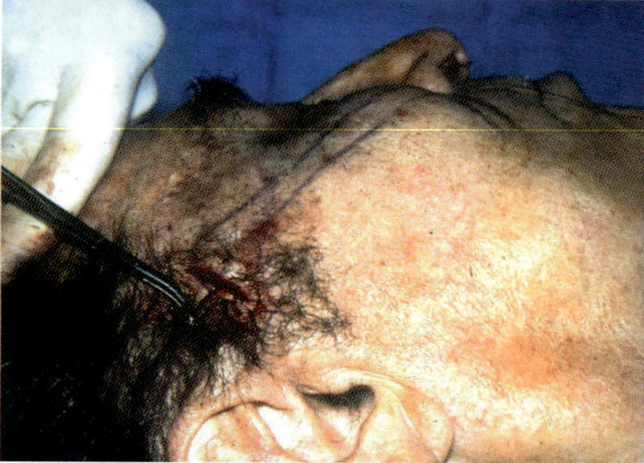

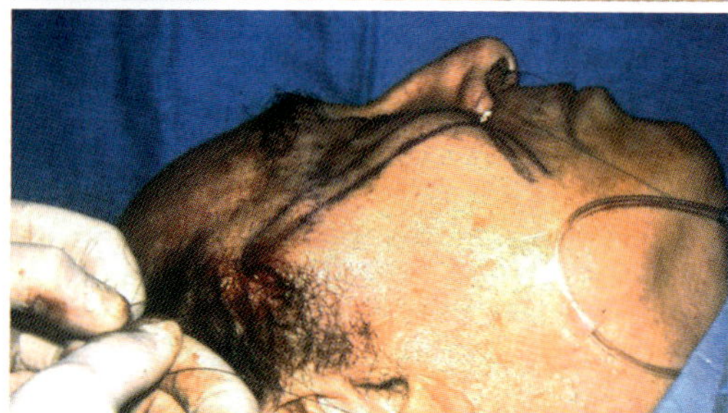

Fig. 14.10. Introduction of Keith needle into the stab incision made in the nasolabial fold. Keith needle exiting out of deep temporalis fascia. Tightening of the cables displaying a midface lift

Summary for the Clinician

- Complications to note are injuries to buccal, temporal and zygomatic branches of the facial nerve
- To avoid future vertical inadequacy of the lower eyelid, the lower eyelid should be placed on a Frost suture, and patch casting the eyelid up on stretch for 1 week should be performed postoperatively
- The SOOF lift should be considered in conjunction with other facial rejuvenation procedures. It is also a necessary tool in the surgeon's armamentarium when addressing situations involving vertical lamella inadequacy of the lower eyelid, management of cicatricial, or paralytic, ectropion, or other instances where midface recruitment in a superior vector is necessary for rehabilitation purposes
- Described above are various techniques for midface lifting. The authors' experience

shows that the more robust subperiosteal dissections with release allow for a longer duration of lift. A cable suspension lift, although much less invasive, provides only temporary results. The preperiosteal approaches provide a greater anterior projection of lift as well

- The SOOF or midface lift provides an excellent tool for approaching midface descent
- The approach is tailored to the structural facial anatomy as well as the needs of each presenting patient

References

1. Hoenig JA, Shorr N, Shorr J (1997) The suborbicularis oculi fat in aesthetic and reconstructive surgery. Int Ophthalmol Clin 37:179–191
2. Hoenig JA, Shorr N, Goldberg RA (1998) The versatile SOOF lift in oculoplastic surgery. Facial Plast Surg Clin North Am 6:205–219
3. Freeman MS (2003) Rejuvenation of the midface. Arch Facial Plast Surg 19:223–236
4. Quatela VC, Jacono AA (2003) The extended centrolateral endoscopic midface lift. Arch Facial Plast Surg 19:199–207
5. Horlock N, Sancers R, Harrison DH (2002) The SOOF lift: its role in correcting midfacial and lower facial asymmetry in patients with partial facial palsy. Plast Reconstr Surg 109:839–849
6. Turk JB, Goldman A (2001) SOOF lift and lateral retinacular canthoplasty. Facial Plast Surg 17:37–48
7. Alford EL (2000) The SOOF lift as an adjunct in rehabilitation of facial paralysis: help or hype? Facial Plast Surg 16:345–349
8. Olver JM (2000) Raising the suborbicularis oculi fat (SOOF): its role in chronic facial palsy. Br J Ophthalmol 84:1401–1406
9. Freeman MS (2000) Transconjunctival sub-orbicularis oculi fat (SOOF) pad lift blepharoplasty: a new technique for the effacement of nasojugal deformity. Arch Facial Plast Surg 2:16–21
10. Shorr N, Edelstein C, Balch K C, et al. (2000) Post-blepharoplasty transeyelid subperiosteal mid-facelift. In: Mauriello J (ed) Unfavorable results of eyelid and lacrimal surgery. Butterworth-Henneman, Woburn, MA, pp 99–132
11. Williams PL, et al. (eds) Gray's anatomy, 37th edn. Churchill Livingstone, Edinburgh
12. Pessa JE, Brown F (1992) Independent effect of various facial mimetic muscles on the nasolabial fold. Aesthetic Plast Surg 16:167–171
13. Aiche A, Ramirez OH (1995) The suborbicularis oculi fat pads: an anatomic and clinical study. Plast Reconstr Surg 95:37–42
14. Furnas DW (1993) Festoons, mounds, and bags of the eyelids and cheek. Clin Plast Surg 20:2
15. Hamra S (1993) Composite rhytidectomy. Quality Medical Publishing, St. Louis
16. Shorr N (1995) Madame Butterfly procedure: total lower eyelid reconstruction in three layers utilizing a hard palate graft: management of the unhappy postblepharoplasty patient with round eye and scleral show. Int J Aesthetic Restorative Surg 3:3–26
17. Sasaki GH, Cohen AT (2002) Meloplication of the malar fat pads by percutaneous cable-suture technique for midface rejuvenation: outcome study (392 cases, 6 years' experience). Plast Reconstruct Surg 10:635–654

Facial Paralysis: A Comprehensive Approach to Current Management

15

Roberta E. Gausas

Core Messages

- The causes of facial paralysis are myriad, but the most common etiologies are idiopathic, infectious, traumatic, or neoplastic
- A thorough patient history including onset, duration, and associated symptoms is essential in establishing the correct etiology
- The facial nerve is a mixed nerve carrying motor, sensory, and parasympathetic information
- Anatomically, the facial nerve runs a complex course divided into four segments: the supranuclear, nuclear, fascicular, and peripheral nerve
- Patients with facial paralysis suffer both functional and esthetic deficits, and both may lead to altered self-image and social handicap
- Examination of the face is simplified by subdividing the face into four functional units; the brow complex, the periorbital complex, the midface complex, and the lower face/oral complex. Each unit has specific functional and esthetic considerations
- Reversible facial paralysis is managed with supportive care consisting of lubrication and enhancement of corneal coverage
- Irreversible facial paralysis is managed surgically and tailored to the individual functional and esthetic desires of each patient and each of his or her facial functional units. These procedures are generally categorized as those aimed at dynamic reanimation, which involve repair or grafting of the nerve, or muscle grafting, and those aimed at static rehabilitation, which involve repositioning and resuspension of soft tissues

15.1 Introduction

Facial nerve palsy may arise from a myriad of conditions, some benign and some potentially life-threatening. Depending on the etiology, the paralysis and facial disfigurement may be temporary or permanent. Often a multidisciplinary team approach is needed for patient care. The oculoplastic surgeon plays a crucial role in the evaluation and rehabilitation of patients with facial palsy. Immediate attention must be aimed at corneal protection and maintenance of vision; however, long-term management of facial disfigurement, epiphora, and secondary effects of aberrant regeneration are significant elements in patient care. Use of a systematic and methodical approach to evaluation and management of facial paralysis, as described in this review, provides the oculoplastic surgeon with the ability to coordinate care for patients with this complex condition.

15.2 Diagnosis

The most common cause of facial nerve weakness is Bell's palsy, named after the British neurologist, Sir Charles Bell. This unilateral, lower motor neuron facial palsy of acute onset occurs with an incidence of 15–40 per 100,000 and a recurrence rate of up to 10% [1]. Bell's palsy is a diagnosis of exclusion, however, and should only be proposed after all other possible causes have been reviewed and eliminated. The possible causes of facial palsy are numerous, but the three most common categories of etiology after

Table 15.1. Causes of facial palsy

Causes of facial palsy
Idiopathic
Bell's palsy
Melkerson-Rosenthal syndrome
Infectious
Herpes zoster oticus (Ramsay-Hunt syndrome)
Varicella virus
Otitis media
Mastoiditis
Lyme disease
Tuberculosis
HIV/AIDS
Poliomyelitis
Mumps
Mononucleosis
Leprosy
Syphilis
Cat scratch
Botulism
Influenza
Neoplastic
Parotid gland tumor
Facial nerve schwannoma
Glomus jugulare tumor
Nasopharyngeal carcinoma
Perineural invasion of skin cancer
Metastatic cancer
Traumatic
Blunt and penetrating craniofacial trauma
Scuba diving
Lightning
Birth/congenital
Birth trauma
Moebius syndrome
Dysgenesis of infratemporal facial nerve
Iatrogenic
Postimmunization
Postsurgical sequelae of removal of brain tumor or parotid gland tumor
Inflammatory
Sarcoidosis
Heerfordt's disease (uveoparotid fever)
Infiltrative
Amyloidosis
Neurologic
Guillain-Barré syndrome
Myasthenia gravis
Metabolic
Pregnancy
Diabetes mellitus
Hypertension

idiopathic are infection, trauma, and neoplasm, or the sequelae of its treatment (Table 15.1).

15.2.1 Patient History

A meticulous history can be critical in uncovering the cause of facial palsy. A patient may not volunteer pertinent historical information unless appropriately questioned. The onset and the duration of the palsy should be established. Associated symptoms such as pain or facial numbness should be recorded. The patient should be asked about changes in hearing, taste, or tearing. Hyperacusis results from impairment of the stapedius muscle. Decreased sense of taste may occur with distal lesions. Excessive tearing is a complex issue and may have more than one cause. Tearing may result from dryness secondary to poor tear production or corneal exposure, from poor outflow secondary to ectropion or tear pump mechanism loss, or from gustatory reflex tearing secondary to aberrant regeneration. A history of a rash or vesicles may suggest certain diagnoses, such as Lyme disease or Ramsay-Hunt syndrome. It is important to elicit a full history of previous skin cancer or head and neck cancer, and any surgical intervention for cancer. An immunization history is pertinent since recent immunizations for influenza or polio have also been linked to facial palsy (Table 15.2).

A carefully obtained history aids tremendously in determining the cause and location of a palsy. For example, a 6-month history of nonresolving facial paralysis that was preceded by facial numbness in a patient with distant history of facial skin cancer, despite lack of a recurrent cutaneous component, suggests perineural invasion of skin cancer, rather than Bell's palsy, and warrants further work-up (Fig. 15.1).

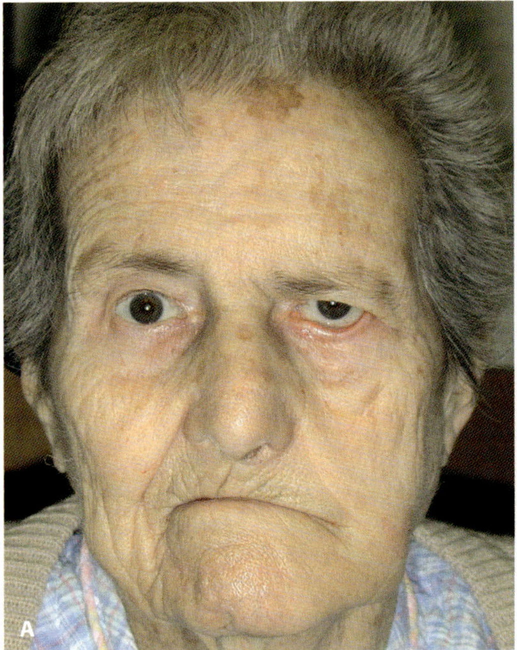

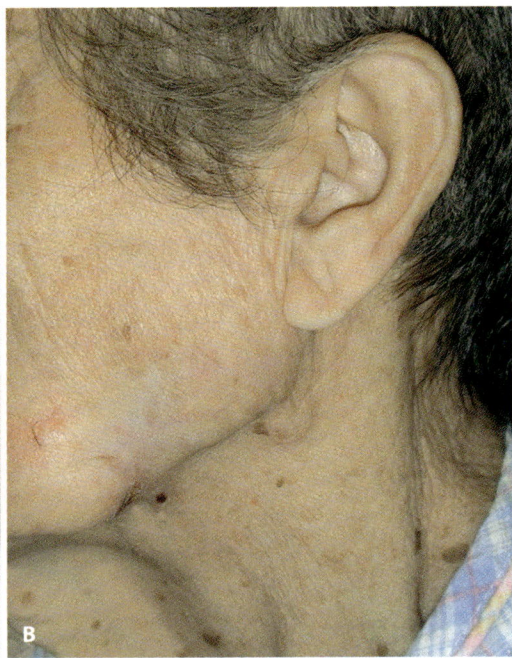

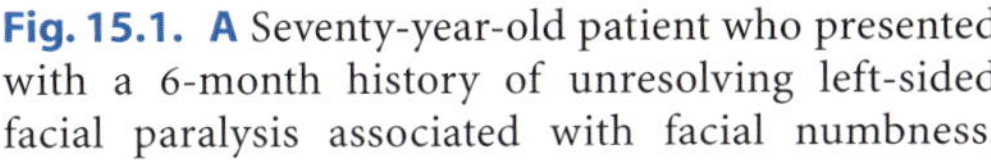

Fig. 15.1. A Seventy-year-old patient who presented with a 6-month history of unresolving left-sided facial paralysis associated with facial numbness. **B** Physical examination revealed old scar and subcutaneous mass along left jawline. Biopsy of site revealed squamous cell carcinoma with perineural invasion

Table 15.2. Pertinent patient history for facial palsy

1. *Onset and duration of palsy:* rapid vs. gradual
2. *Status of palsy:* resolving, persistent, worsening
3. *Associated symptoms:* facial numbness, pain, change in hearing, loss of taste, epiphora
4. *Associated physical findings:* vesicles, rash, swollen lymph node
5. *Past medical and surgical history:* previous skin cancer, previous head and neck cancer, surgical treatment for cancer, recent immunizations

15.2.2 Anatomy and Function

Ability to perform a thorough physical examination of facial paralysis is facilitated by an understanding of the anatomy and function of the facial nerve. This knowledge is also critical in developing a surgical plan for facial rehabilitation.

15.2.2.1 Facial Nerve Pathophysiology

The facial nerve is a mixed nerve in that it carries motor, sensory, and parasympathetic information. It serves a predominantly motor function, however, and is responsible for all facial motion except mastication. Of its approximately 10,000 neurons, 7,000 fibers innervate muscles of facial expression. For the oculofacial surgeon, muscles of particular importance innervated by the facial nerve are the frontalis, which lifts the eyebrows and forehead; the orbicularis oculi, which closes the eyes; and the orbicularis oris, which closes the lips.

The remaining 3,000 fibers of the facial nerve form the nervus intermedius, which conveys sensory and parasympathetic fibers. The sensory fibers carry taste from the anterior two-thirds of the tongue. The parasympathetic secretomotor fibers innervate the lacrimal, parotid and salivary glands. Facial nerve injury affects non-motor function by producing abnormalities not only in taste and hearing, but also in lacrimation, most important for the ophthalmologist. Facial nerve lesions above the geniculate ganglion may cause decreased lacrimal secretion with subsequent epiphora from dry eye. Central lesions may result in aberrant regeneration with gustatory reflex tearing.

15.2.2.2 Facial Nerve Anatomy

In its complex course through the posterior fossa, temporal bone, and parotid gland, the facial nerve is vulnerable to many neoplastic, traumatic, and infectious disorders. It may be divided into four anatomic segments: supranuclear, nuclear, fascicular, and peripheral nerve.

Supranuclear Pathway

Neural activity within the facial motor area of the frontal lobe initiates voluntary movement of the face. The supranuclear neurons that innervate the facial nerve nucleus lie in the precentral gyrus of the frontal lobe. Upon leaving the precentral gyrus, these axons coalesce to become part of the corticobulbar tracts that descend through the internal capsule towards the cerebral peduncle [2]. It is just below this level that most of the supranuclear fibers cross over to the opposite side of the pons to innervate the facial nerve nucleus. Some fibers, however, do not cross over and synapse in the ipsilateral facial nerve nucleus. This anatomic feature explains why the upper face is supplied with innervation from both cerebral hemispheres and why supranuclear lesions involving the descending motor pathways cause palsy of the contralateral lower face only.

Pons

The motor nucleus of the facial nerve lies within the reticular formation of the pons. It may be subdivided into four cell groups, one of which, the intermediate cells, innervates the frontalis, orbicularis oculi, and corrugator muscles. Motor axons constituting the facial nerve exit the facial nucleus, travel towards the fourth ventricle, bend around the sixth nerve nucleus, and exit the pons.

The parasympathetic component of the facial nerve arises in the superior salivatory nucleus, above the facial motor nucleus. The parasympathetic component of the facial nerve supplies secretomotor fibers to the lacrimal, sublingual and submandibular glands.

The nervus intermedius consists of both these parasympathetic fibers and sensory fibers. The sensory fibers subserve taste to the anterior two-thirds of the tongue, and somatic sensation to the external auditory meatus and postauricular region. Afferent fibers to the facial nucleus also derive from the trigeminal nucleus as part of the corneal reflex, and the acoustic pathways as part of the stapedius reflex.

Cerebellopontine Angle

The facial motor root and nervus intermedius exit the brain stem along with the vestibular acoustic nerve at the cerebellopontine angle. The facial nerve then travels through the temporal bone via the internal auditory canal with the nervus intermedius and auditory nerve.

Fallopian Canal

The facial nerve separates from the acoustic nerve to enter its own canal, the fallopian, or facial, canal. It then winds its way along an approximately 30-mm path through the labyrinthine, tympanic, and mastoid segments. The labyrinthine segment contains the geniculate ganglion and the first branch of the facial nerve, the greater petrosal nerve. This nerve carries secretomotor fibers to innervate the lacrimal gland and nasopalatine glands after synapsing in the sphenopalatine ganglion. The mastoid segment is where the nerve to the stapedius originates and the chorda tympani nerve branches off. The chorda tympani nerve carries taste fibers from the anterior two-thirds of the tongue, parasympathetic fibers to the sublingual and submaxillary glands, and somatic sensation from the external auditory meatus.

Extracranial Course

The motor branches of the facial nerve exit the fallopian canal at the skull base via the stylomastoid foramen. The facial nerve then penetrates the parotid gland and divides into superi-

Table 15.3. Facial functional units

Facial unit	Physical findings	Functional, esthetic and social impairment
1. Brow complex	Brow ptosis	Impaired superior visual field
		Heavy upper eyelid
		Brow asymmetry
2. Periorbital complex	Upper lid retraction	Epiphora
	Lower lid retraction	Photophobia
	Paralytic lagophthalmos	Eye pain
	Lower lid/punctal ectropion	Blurred vision
	Decreased blink	Lid asymmetry
	Exposure keratitis	
3. Midface complex	Descent of malar eminence	Facial asymmetry
	Loss of nasolabial fold	Impaired breathing
	Collapse of nostril	
4. Perioral complex	Ptosis (lengthening) of lip	Impaired eating/drinking
	Inferomedial rotation of oral commissure	Impaired speech
	Jowling	Oral incompetence/drooling
		Inability to smile

or (temporofacial) and inferior (cervicofacial) divisions. These divisions may be further subdivided from top to bottom into the temporal, zygomatic, buccal, mandibular, and cervical branches [3]. The branching patterns of these five subdivisions vary among individuals and extensive interconnections exist among the branches. This accounts for the variety of aberrant regeneration phenomena that may occur following recovery from facial nerve palsy. Such phenomena include gustatory reflex tearing (crocodile tears) where salivary gland nerve fibers are redirected towards the lacrimal gland and involuntary tearing occurs with salivation while eating.

Summary for the Clinician

- **A thorough patient history is crucial in establishing an accurate diagnosis and should include associated symptoms such as facial pain or numbness, and changes in hearing, taste, or tearing**
- **Motor, sensory and parasympathetic fibers constitute the facial nerve. The nervus intermedius carries facial nerve sensory and parasympathetic information and is responsible for tearing, salivation, and taste**

15.3 Facial Nerve: Physical Examination

Patients with facial paralysis suffer both functional and esthetic deficits. The degree of deficit will depend on the amount of facial weakness, which can vary from mild paresis to complete paralysis, and the patient's age. Younger patients with greater tissue tone and support may experience a lesser degree of functional abnormality, whereas older patients with the same medical condition but weaker tissue tone will experience more significant dysfunction. However, problems encountered by these patients are not just limited to physical findings, but also include altered self-image and social handicap. Patients experience chronic eye pain and tearing, difficulty breathing, impaired speech, difficulty eating and drinking, and drooling. Additionally, there is the obvious facial asymmetry which is made worse during facial animation and laughter. These problems may lead the patient to feel stigmatized and to avoid social contact. Therefore, the surgeon responding to the needs of the facial paralysis patient must be cognizant of both the desire for functional rehabilitation and the desire for esthetic restoration, and include the patient's concern about their social handicap in the evaluation.

Detection of subtle weakness and aberrant regeneration requires careful observation, whereas severe paralysis is obvious from a distance. The surgeon should observe the patient's entire face both during rest and during conversation throughout the examination, noting voluntary and involuntary facial movements. Certain grading systems have been described to quantify facial paralysis, such as the House-Brackman classification of facial nerve dysfunction. The House grading system is used to document the degree of paralysis in late stages of the process and the Brackman modification attempts to include early stages of paralysis [4].

The physical examination can be simplified by subdividing the face into four functional units. These units are the brow complex, the periorbital complex, the midface complex, and the lower face/oral complex. Each unit has specific functional and esthetic considerations (Table 15.3).

15.3.1 Brow Complex

Evaluation of the face should begin with determination of whether the facial palsy is central or peripheral. Therefore frontalis muscle function should be tested first, by asking the patient to look up. If frontalis muscle function is intact bilaterally, the palsy is central. If frontalis muscle function is unilaterally impaired, the palsy is peripheral.

The physical findings of the brow complex observed in patients with frontalis muscle impairment include: loss of forehead rhytids, lengthening of the forehead, and brow ptosis. These features combine to apply weight to the upper eyelid and may accentuate pre-existing upper lid dermatochalasis (Fig. 15.2 A). The patient may complain of superior visual field impairment and heaviness of the eyelid, making it difficult to open the eye or sustain activities such as reading or driving. Esthetically, facial asymmetry is noticeable both in the resting and in the animated position.

Brow ptosis is measured by manually elevating the brow to the desired level, and measuring the amount of descent in millimeters after releasing the brow. Attention should be paid to the degree of both medial and lateral droop, as well as the ultimate brow shape desired, keeping in mind that a male brow tends towards a flat arch compared to the more curved arch of a female brow. The amount of brow ptosis can be documented photographically. The degree of superior visual impairment can be documented with formal visual field testing.

15.3.2 Periorbital Complex

Patients with facial paralysis often complain of pain, burning, photophobia, epiphora, and lid asymmetry. These complaints are directly related to loss of orbicularis muscle tone, and are attributable to excessive corneal exposure. Exposure keratitis is a serious sequela of facial paralysis, and will dictate the urgency of treatment. Several physical findings may contribute to corneal exposure.

Retraction is the most common finding in the upper eyelid. With loss of the usual protractor function of the orbicularis oculi muscle, the action of the levator palpebrae muscle is unopposed, and therefore the lid elevates. Lid retraction may be partially masked by significant dermatochalasis and brow ptosis, becoming evident only when the brow is manually elevated. Functionally, upper eyelid retraction increases corneal surface exposure and contributes to lagophthalmos. Esthetically, it creates an unnatural and asymmetrical facial appearance.

Eyelid position is measured by recording the distance from the corneal light reflex to the lid margin with the patient's face in the frontal plane and a light directed at the cornea. This is referred to as the marginal reflex distance, or MRD. The position of the upper lid relative to the corneal light reflex is designated as MRD_1, whereas the position of the lower eyelid is designated as MRD_2.

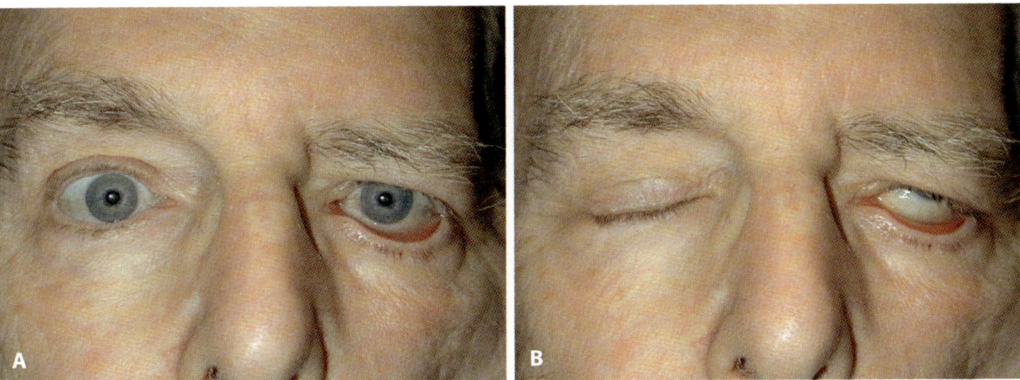

Fig. 15.2 A, B. Physical findings of brow and periorbital functional units include brow ptosis, paralytic lagophthalmos, and ectropion

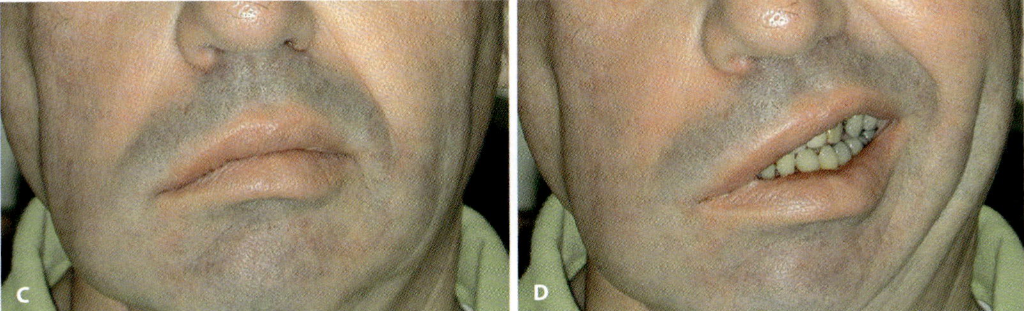

Fig. 15.2 C, D. Physical findings of perioral and lower face functional units include loss of nasolabial fold, lengthening of lip, and rotation of nose and mouth. These findings are exaggerated with facial animation

Lower eyelid physical findings include: retraction, ectropion, and punctal eversion. Ectropion describes an outward turning of the eyelid margin, separating it from the globe. This may occur along the entire length of the eyelid, or medially affecting only the punctum. Both ectropion and punctal eversion lead to impaired tear drainage and accumulation of tear debris, resulting in epiphora and irritation. The degree of ectropion will be related to the amount of pre-existing lower lid laxity, which is dependent on the patient's age.

Loss of orbicularis oculi muscle tone leads not only to eyelid retraction, but also to paralytic lagophthalmos and incomplete blink reflex (Fig. 15.2 B). Paralytic lagophthalmos is measured in millimeters as the vertical interpalpebral distance during gentle eyelid closure. The presence or absence of a Bell's phenomenon should be noted by gently lifting the eyelids during forced closure. A poor Bell's phenomenon worsens the usual risk of corneal exposure during sleep.

Examination of the eye should include corneal sensation. Decreased corneal sensitivity can be seen in facial nerve palsy, but when coexistent with hypoesthesia of adjacent eyelid skin, fifth cranial nerve involvement should be suspected.

15.3.3 Midface and Perioral Complex

The midface complex is closely related to the lower eyelid and affects lower eyelid position and function. Physical findings in this region include: descent of the malar tissues with loss of the malar eminence, loss or flattening of the nasolabial fold, and inferomedial rotation of the nasal ala (Fig. 15.2 C). This leads to collapse of the nostril and interference with normal breathing.

Malar descent can be evaluated by manually elevating the midface to the desired level to match the opposite side, and noting the amount of vertical shift in millimeters. The distance from the nasolabial fold to the vermilion border of the upper lip on the unaffected side should be measured in order to appropriately plan for suspension of the nasolabial fold on the affected side. Older patients with paralysis are particularly prone to jowling of the lower face. If left unaddressed, the persistent downward pull of the weight of the lower face will diminish the long-term effect of any midface or nasolabial fold suspension.

Physical findings of the perioral complex include lip ptosis, which is lengthening of the upper lip with inferior and medial rotation of the oral commissure (Fig. 15.2 C). Loss of orbicularis oris muscle tone leaves the effect of gravity unopposed, resulting in inferior displacement. This muscle weakness also leaves the contraction of the opposite orbicularis oris muscle unopposed, resulting in medial displacement of the lips. These forces combine to create a twisting or rotation of facial structures which is evident at rest and exaggerated during speech (Fig. 15.2 D). Patients may complain of drooling, difficulty eating, and difficulty speaking. This may lead to social handicap.

Summary for the Clinician

- **Examination of facial paralysis is simplified by subdividing the face into four functional units, each with distinct findings producing physical, esthetic, and social impairment**
- **The brow complex will exhibit brow ptosis impairing the superior visual field**
- **The periorbital complex will be characterized by paralytic lagophthalmos causing discomfort and epiphora due to exposure keratitis**
- **The midface complex will exhibit effacement of the nasolabial fold and impaired breathing due to collapse of the nostril**
- **The lower face/oral complex will be characterized by ptosis and rotation of the mouth causing impairment of speech and eating**

15.4 Treatment Strategies (Table 15.4)

Normal facial tone exists in the presence of a delicate balance between vertical and horizontal forces, between gravitational pull and muscular contraction. Clearly understanding the orientation and function of each facial muscle and the orientation of the forces acting upon it leads to a full understanding of the affects of facial paralysis. The physical results of facial paralysis represent a disruption of the balancing act between vertical and horizontal forces that normally exists.

15.4.1 Supportive Care

Facial paralysis can be categorized as reversible or irreversible. Patients with reversible facial palsy can be treated with supportive care, while those with irreversible palsy are candidates for surgical intervention. In either situation, corneal decompensation dictates the urgency of intervention. Therefore, testing for corneal sensation cannot be emphasized enough.

Initial supportive therapy consists of frequent ocular lubrication. This is achieved through the use of artificial tears, usually a minimum of four times a day and as frequently as every hour while awake, and lubricant gel or ointment at night. Additionally, a moisture chamber can be created at night by fashioning a circular piece of cellophane wrap over the orbital rim, use of an eye patch over the cellophane, or use of a pre-manufactured moisture bubble.

Temporary interventions can be considered in situations in which the cornea requires short-term added protection. External lid weights (Meddev Co., Palo Alto, CA) fixed to the upper eyelid pretarsal skin aid in lid closure. A temporary suture tarsorraphy is useful for acute situations of corneal decompensation or for patients who are unable to instill lubricating drops or gel.

Table 15.4. Treatment strategy by involved facial functional unit

Facial unit	Treatment strategy
1. Brow complex	Brow lift: – Direct approach: suprabrow, midforehead, pretricheal – Endoscopic approach – Coronal approach – Browpexy
2. Periorbital complex	Lubrication Tarsorraphy: – Temporary: suture – Permanent: lateral intermarginal adhesion Correction of upper lid retraction/lagophthalmos: – Gold weight placement – Lid spring placement Correction of lower lid/punctual ectropion: – Horizontal lid shortening: lateral tarsal strip, medial canthal placation – Punctal inversion: excision conjunctival diamond, cauterization Correction of lower lid retraction: – Placement of spacer graft: hard palate, tarsus, banked sclera, Alloderm
3. Midface complex	Reanimation procedures: – Facial nerve repair, nerve grafting, nerve transfer – Temporalis muscle transfer – Microvascular free flap transfer Static support procedures: – Midface lift: Subperiosteal or supraperiosteal suspension sutures – Lateral rotation of nasal ala – Recreation of nasolabial fold: Suspension sutures Direct lift
4. Perioral complex	Oral commissure lift: – Suspension sutures – Wedge resection

15.4.2 Surgical Strategies

For patients with irreversible facial palsy, such as those who have lost facial nerve function after resection of a head and neck cancer, surgical rehabilitation should be considered. Each individual patient will have a unique situation in which either some or all of the facial units are involved and either some or all of the facial units are causing symptoms. The surgical plan must be tailored to each individual patient, and take into consideration the patient's needs and desires for both functional and social rehabilitation.

The following is an outline of the surgical strategies available for each facial unit. The goals of facial rehabilitation can be aimed at either reanimation or static resuspension. Procedures that have the goal of facial reanimation include direct or indirect hypoglossal-facial nerve anastomosis, facial nerve grafts, cross-face seventh nerve grafts, and temporalis muscle transfers. This chapter focuses on surgical procedures with the goal of static facial suspension (Fig. 15.3 A, B). Proper coordination between the orbitofacial surgeon and other disciplines, including neurosurgery, head and neck surgery, and plastic surgery, is needed to provide affected patients with the optimal surgical plan and care.

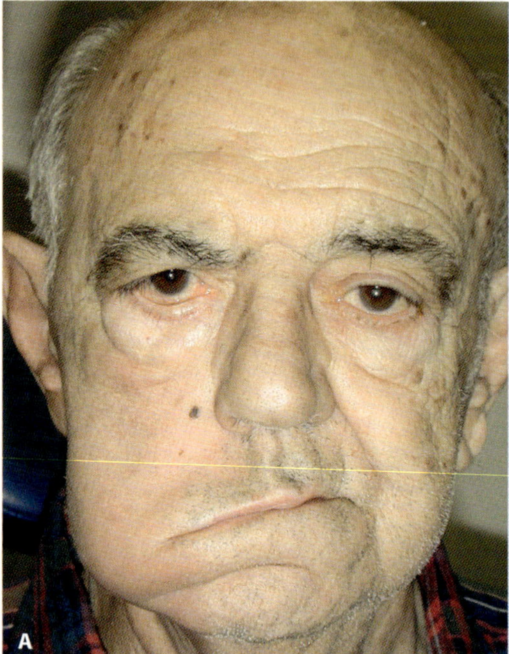

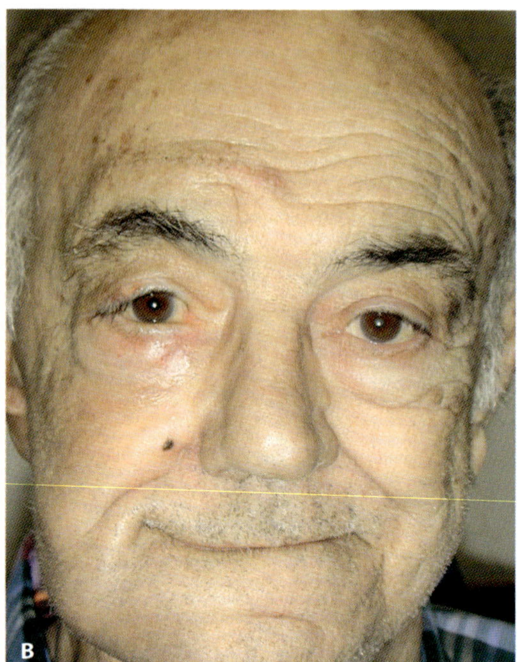

Fig. 15.3. A Preoperative view of irreversible right-sided facial paralysis. **B** Postoperative view following static facial rehabilitation consisting of direct brow lift, upper lid gold weight placement, lower lid horizontal shortening, midface suspension, and repair of nasolabial fold

15.4.2.1
Surgical Strategies: Brow Complex

Of the number of surgical techniques which are available to obtain a brow lift in the paralyzed brow, some are more effective than others. Each of them is a compromise between esthetic and functional outcome. The advantages and disadvantages of each technique should be reviewed with the patient. Esthetically, an endoscopic brow lift, or browpexy, avoids a visible scar, but in the paralyzed brow tends not to provide a robust or durable elevation. The most effective means of elevating the weight of a paralysed brow is through a direct approach, which carries the risk of some form of scar. A unilateral direct brow lift via a suprabrow, midforehead, or pretricheal incision provides significant and durable elevation with minimal scar if closed in multiple layers with attention to detail (Fig. 15.4 A, B).

15.4.2.2
Surgical Strategies: Periorbital Complex

The goal of rehabilitation of the periorbital complex is to provide corneal coverage and eliminate lagophthalmos. Lateral tarsorraphy has been a traditional approach to this problem; however, this procedure creates peripheral field loss, often does not entirely alleviate medial and central lagophthalmos, and is esthetically unappealing.

Upper eyelid retraction is best addressed with placement of a lid weight in order to overcome unopposed levator muscle action. The most common method used is placement of a gold weight (Meddev Co., Palo Alto, CA) [5, 6]. In a patient with gold allergy, a platinum weight is an alternative [7]. The size of the weight is tested preoperatively incrementally with the patient in the sitting position. With each size of weight tested, the amount of lagophthalmos and induced ptosis should be

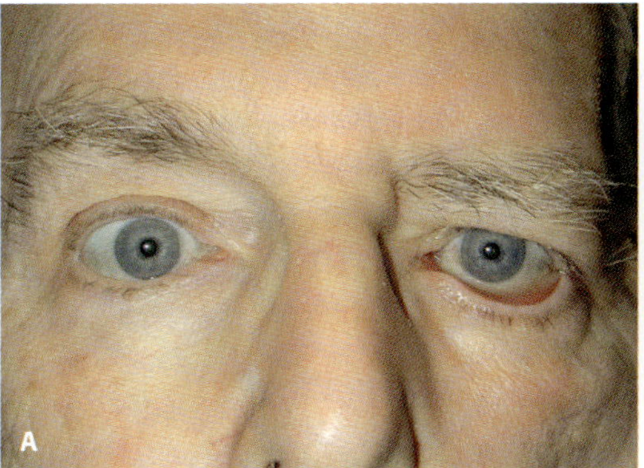

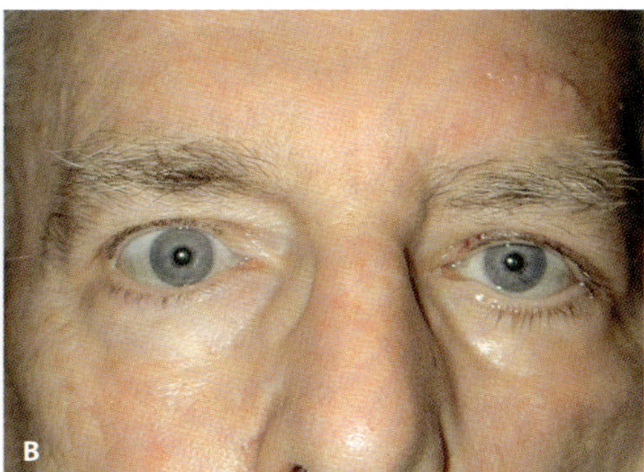

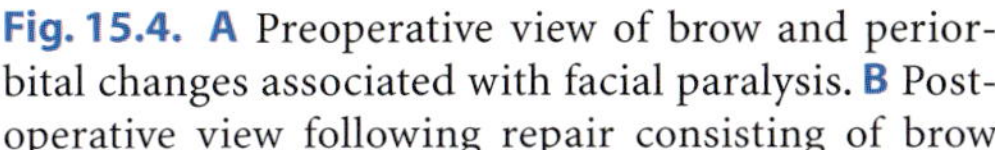

Fig. 15.4. A Preoperative view of brow and periorbital changes associated with facial paralysis. **B** Postoperative view following repair consisting of brow lift, upper lid retraction repair, and lower lid lateral tarsal strip

recorded. The selected weight should be the one that achieves the greatest closure with the least ptosis.

Some surgeons advocate a stainless steel palpebral spring to reanimate the eyelid. Advantages of a spring include a more natural blink process and the esthetically appealing low profile of the implant. Disadvantages of this technique include the need for postoperative spring tension adjustment, and the risk of spring fatigue or extrusion.

The goals of repair for the lower eyelid are threefold: (1) horizontal shortening to correct ectropion or retraction, (2) central support to alleviate lagophthalmos, and (3) inversion of the punctum to improve epiphora (Fig. 15.4 A, B). A short lateral intermarginal tarsorraphy can enhance these steps and not impede peripheral vision. The amount of surgery needed will depend on the degree of lid laxity present, which in turn is dependent upon the patient's age.

Horizontal lower eyelid shortening is best achieved through a lateral tarsal strip procedure [8–10]. This is performed via a lateral canthotomy and inferior cantholysis. A lateral strip of tarsus is fashioned, appropriately shortened, and anchored to the periosteum of the lateral orbital rim as a substitute tendon. If medial canthal laxity is present, it must be corrected first to avoid significant lateral displacement of the punctum which interferes with tear outflow [11, 12]. The punctum must be in contact with the tear lake to allow tear outflow. Subtle vertical orientation of the punctum or frank eversion of the punctum will inhibit outflow even in the presence of an adequately tightened lower eyelid [7, 8]. Punctal inversion can be achieved surgically via excision of a small tarsoconjunctival diamond or via laser or cautery conjunctivoplasty [13, 14].

Lower eyelid shortening alone may not correct the central lid sagging often seen in facial paralysis. Such lower eyelid retraction is due to loss of vertical support from loss of orbicularis tone. In these cases, a spacer graft is required to bolster the central lower lid position upward, which will help relieve lagophthalmos. A great variety of spacer material is available. The surgeon must decide between autogenous, donor, or alloplastic material. Selection of the material will be influenced by any alterations in the host bed tissue, such as irradiation, previous surgery, or the disease process. Autogenous materials include hard palate graft, tarsal graft, ear cartilage graft or septal graft [15–18]. Donor materials include banked sclera or Alloderm (Life Cell Co., Brauchburg, NJ) [19, 20]. Alloplastic materials include a lid spacer implant consisting of Medpor (Porex Surgical Inc., Newman, GA) [21, 22]. Donor materials avoid the morbidity associated with harvesting tissue, but are susceptible to contraction [23]. Of these choices, hard palate has been shown to be an effective and durable graft material [24–26].

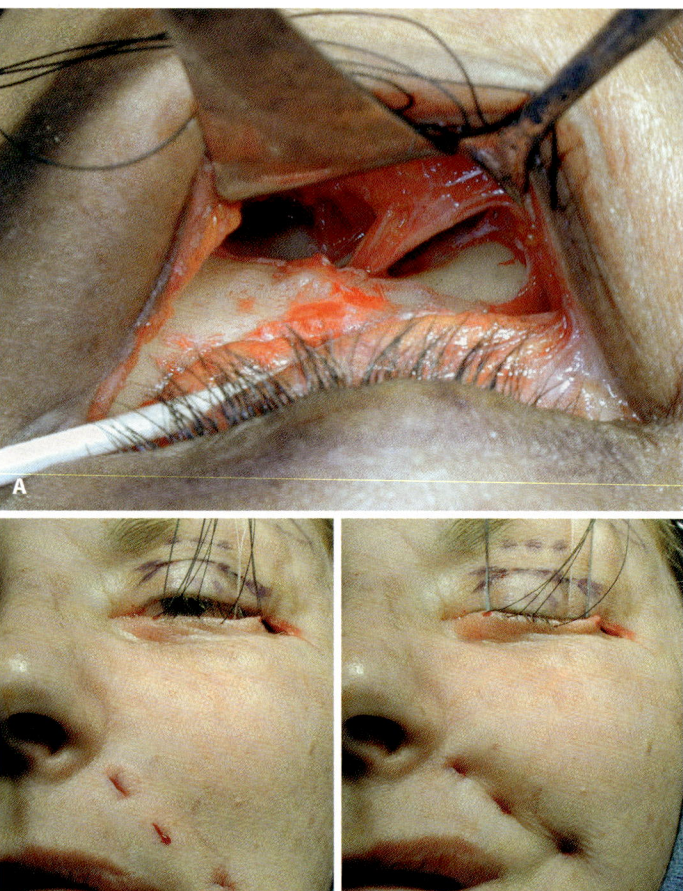

Fig. 15.5. A Intraoperative view of subperiosteal dissection with sparing of infraorbital nerve during static midface suspension. **B, C** Intraoperative view of pre- and postelevation of nasolabial fold and midfacial soft tissues via suspension sutures anchored at inferior orbital rim.

The surgeon must remember that the lower eyelid is a continuum of the midface and is influenced by and subject to forces acting on midface position. Long-term success of correcting lower eyelid position and function greatly depends upon correction of midface position.

15.4.2.3 Surgical Strategies: Midface and Perioral Complex

The treatment of midface and perioral paralysis is challenging, with many techniques available. The surgeon may select from reanimation procedures that aim to provide some degree of voluntary facial movement, or those that aim to provide static facial support. Both the extent and level of nerve injury will determine the appropriate procedure for each patient.

To achieve dynamic reanimation, the choice of procedures includes facial nerve repair, facial nerve repair with nerve grafting, hypoglossal nerve transfer, temporalis muscle transfer, or a microvascular functional muscle transfer, such as gracilis, latissmus dorsi, or inferior rectus abdominus free flap transfer [27–30].

Static rehabilitation is achieved through methods which resuspend soft tissues to fixed structures. The specific areas of the midface, nasolabial fold, and oral commissure can be addressed via a direct lift or via suspension sutures. Techniques which resuspend a paralysed face parallel those used for facial rejuvenation. The goals of elevation and anchoring of soft tissues are the same as in surgery aimed at rejuvenation; however, the weight of the tissues and the effects of gravity in the paralyzed face are often more difficult to overcome. Several techniques of static suspension are available, each varying in approach to incision, suspension material, and anchoring device and location [31–35] (Fig. 15.5 A). The orbital rim is an ideal location for fixation via either an anchoring device or suspension sutures passed through drill holes. Important aspects of midface elevation include emphasis on vertical lift over lateral lift to avoid joker-like facies [36]. Important aspects of nasolabial fold elevation include adequate outward suspension of the nostril to improve breathing, and adequate elevation of the upper lip to improve speech and ability to eat (Fig. 15.5 B, C).

Summary for the Clinician

- **The need for corneal protection dictates the urgency of management. Whether the facial palsy is temporary or permanent guides the method of management**
- **The brow complex is surgically managed by a brow lift**
- **Paralytic lagophthalmos is commonly surgically managed by gold weight placement in the upper lid and horizontal shortening of the lower lid, with or without a spacer graft**
- **Mid- and lower-face paralytic descent may be addressed via dynamic reanimation procedures or via static resuspension of facial tissue to overcome mouth ptosis**

15.5 Aberrant Regeneration

Aberrant regeneration as a late effect of facial paralysis may occur in two forms: gustatory hyperlacrimation (crocodile tears) and synkinetic facial movements [37]. Aberrant innervation of the lacrimal gland results from misrouting of postganglionic parasympathetic secretomotor fibers and produces hypersecretion of tears during mastication. Facial synkinetic movements similar to hemifacial spasm result from misrouting of fibers of the orbicularis oris and orbicularis oculi muscles. Both forms of aberrant regeneration respond to botulinum toxin injection [38–40]. Neuromuscular facial retraining via biofeedback has also been shown to be effective treatment for synkinesis after facial palsy [41, 42].

Summary for the Clinician

- **Gustatory reflex tearing and synkinetic facial movements are two late effects of facial paralysis secondary to aberrant regeneration. Both respond well to botulinum toxin injection**

References

1. Papazian MR, Campbell JH, Nabi S (1993) Management of Bell's palsy. J Oral Maxillofac Surg 51:661–665
2. Crosby EC, Dejonge BR (1963) Experimental and clinical studies of the central connections and central relations of the facial nerve. Ann Otol Rhinol Laryngol 72:735–755
3. Davis RA, Anson BJ, Budinger JM, Kurth LR (1956) Surgical anatomy of the facial nerve and parotid gland based upon a study of 350 cervicofacial halves. Surg Gynecol Obstet 102:385–412
4. Smith IM, Murray JA, Cull RE, Slattery J (1992) A comparison of facial grading systems. Clin Otolaryngol 17:303–307
5. Caesar RH, Friebel J, McNab AA (2004) Upper lid loading with gold weights in paralytic lagophthalmos: a modified technique to maximize the long-term functional and cosmetic success. Orbit 23:27–32
6. Tower RN, Dailey RA (2004) Gold weight implantation: a better way? Ophthal Plast Reconstr Surg 20:202–206
7. Berghaus A, Neumann K, Schrom T (2003) The platinum chain: a new upper-lid implant for facial palsy. Arch Facial Plast Surg 5:166–170
8. Anderson RL, Gordy DD (1979) The tarsal strip procedure. Arch Ophthalmol 97:2192–2196
9. Anderson RL (1981) Tarsal strip procedure for correction of eyelid laxity and canthal malposition in the anophthalmic socket. Ophthalmology 88:895–903
10. Vick VL, Holds JB, Hartstein ME, Massry GG (2004) Tarsal strip procedure for the correction of tearing. Ophthal Plast Reconstr Surg 20:37–39
11. Jordan DR, Anderson RL, Thiese SM (1990) The medial tarsal strip. Arch Ophthalmol 108:120–124
12. O'Donnell FE Jr (1986) Medial ectropion: association with lower lacrimal obstruction and combined management. Ophthalmic Surg 17:573–576

13. Hurwitz JJ (1978) Investigation and treatment of epiphora due to lid laxity. Trans Ophthalmol Soc U K 98:69–70
14. Nainiwal S, Kumar H, Kumar A (2003) Laser conjunctivoplasty: a new technique for correction of mild medial ectropion. Orbit 22:199–201
15. Stephenson CM, Brown BZ (1985) The use of tarsus as a free autogenous graft in eyelid surgery. Ophthal Plast Reconstr Surg 1:43–50
16. Brown BZ (1985) The use of homologous tarsus as a donor graft in lid surgery. Ophthal Plast Reconstr Surg 1:91–95
17. Inigo F, Chapa P, Jimenez Y, Arroyo O (1996) Surgical treatment of lagophthalmos in facial palsy: ear cartilage graft for elongating the levator palpebrae muscle. Br J Plast Surg 49:452–456
18. Harashina T, Wakamatsu K, Kitazawa T (1996) How to harvest a septal chondromucosal graft. Ann Plast Surg 37:676–677
19. Olver JM, Rose GE, Khaw PT, Collin JR (1998) Correction of lower eyelid retraction in thyroid eye disease: a randomised controlled trial of retractor tenotomy with adjuvant antimetabolite versus scleral graft. Br J Ophthalmol 82:174–180
20. Shorr N, Perry JD, Goldberg RA, et al. (2000) The safety and applications of acellular human dermal allograft in ophthalmic plastic and reconstructive surgery: a preliminary report. Ophthal Plast Reconstr Surg 16:223–230
21. Tan J, Olver J, Wright M, et al. (2004) The use of porous polyethylene (Medpor) lower eyelid spacers in lid heightening and stabilisation. Br J Ophthalmol 88:1197–1200
22. Kinney SE, Seeley BM, Seeley MZ, Foster JA (2000) Oculoplastic surgical techniques for protection of the eye in facial nerve paralysis. Am J Otol 21:275–283
23. Sullivan SA, Dailey RA (2003) Graft contraction: a comparison of acellular dermis versus hard palate mucosa in lower eyelid surgery. Ophthal Plast Reconstr Surg 19:14–24
24. Patipa M, Patel BC, McLeish W, Anderson RL (1996) Use of hard palate grafts for treatment of postsurgical lower eyelid retraction: a technical overview. J Craniomaxillofac Trauma 2:18–28
25. Beatty RL, Harris G, Bauman GR, Mills MP (1993) Intraoral palatal mucosal graft harvest. Ophthal Plast Reconstr Surg 9:120–124
26. Reiser GM, Bruno JF, Mahan PE, Larkin LH (1996) The subepithelial connective tissue graft palatal donor site: anatomic considerations for surgeons. Int J Periodontics Restorative Dent 16:130–137
27. Takushima A, Harii K, Asato H, et al. (2004) Neurovascular free-muscle transfer for the treatment of established facial paralysis following ablative surgery in the parotid region. Plast Reconstr Surg 113:1563–1572
28. Chuang DC, Mardini S, Lin SH, Chen HC (2004) Free proximal gracilis muscle and its skin paddle compound flap transplantation for complex facial paralysis. Plast Reconstr Surg 113:126–132; discussion 33–35
29. Doi K, Hattori Y, Tan SH, Dhawan V (2002) Basic science behind functioning free muscle transplantation. Clin Plast Surg 29:483–495, v–vi
30. Harrison DH (2002) The treatment of unilateral and bilateral facial palsy using free muscle transfers. Clin Plast Surg 29:539–549, vi
31. Anderson RD, Lo MW (1998) Endoscopic malar/midface suspension procedure. Plast Reconstr Surg 102:2196–2208
32. Hagerty RC (1995) Central suspension technique of the midface. Plast Reconstr Surg 96:728–730
33. Ramirez OM (2002) Three-dimensional endoscopic midface enhancement: a personal quest for the ideal cheek rejuvenation. Plast Reconstr Surg 109:329–340; discussion 41–49
34. Yousif NJ, Matloub MD, Summers AN (2002) The midface sling: a new technique to rejuvenate the midface. Plast Reconstr Surg 110:1541–1553; discussion 54–57
35. Douglas RS, Gausas RE (2003) A systematic comprehensive approach to management of irreversible facial paralysis. Facial Plast Surg 19:107–112
36. Hamilton JM (1998) Serial plication facelift. Aesthetic Plast Surg 22:304–308
37. Valls-Sole J, Montero J (2003) Movement disorders in patients with peripheral facial palsy. Mov Disord 18:1424–1435
38. Borodic GE, Pearce LB, Cheney M, et al. (1993) Botulinum A toxin for treatment of aberrant facial nerve regeneration. Plast Reconstr Surg 91:1042–1045
39. Montoya FJ, Riddell CE, Caesar R, Hague S (2002) Treatment of gustatory hyperlacrimation (crocodile tears) with injection of botulinum toxin into the lacrimal gland. Eye 16:705–709
40. Keegan DJ, Geerling G, Lee JP, et al. (2002) Botulinum toxin treatment for hyperlacrimation secondary to aberrant regenerated seventh nerve palsy or salivary gland transplantation. Br J Ophthalmol 86:43–46
41. Nakamura K, Toda N, Sakamaki K, et al. (2003) Biofeedback rehabilitation for prevention of synkinesis after facial palsy. Otolaryngol Head Neck Surg 128:539–543
42. Cronin GW, Steenerson RL (2003) The effectiveness of neuromuscular facial retraining combined with electromyography in facial paralysis rehabilitation. Otolaryngol Head Neck Surg 128:534–538

Self-Inflating Hydrogel Expanders for the Treatment of Congenital Anophthalmos

16

Michael P. Schittkowski, James A. Katowitz, Karsten K.H. Gundlach, Rudolf F. Guthoff

Core Messages

- Clinical congenital anophthalmos is the absence of any visible globe
- Tissue expansion is necessary to insert a regular prosthesis in order to achieve a more normal appearance
- Congenital anophthalmos is very rare; estimated prevalence is 1–4/100,000 births
- The relationship with a variety of syndromes and anomalies makes it important to routinely undergo genetic evaluation
- Due to the variety of symptoms an individual treatment plan is needed for each patient
- The current preferred option is the use of non-expanding conformers
- In cases of severe anophthalmos with extreme underdeveloped cul-de-sacs, success with conformers is often limited
- Silicone balloon expanders, mucous membrane grafts, dermis fat grafts or even craniofacial surgery are not methods of first choice. They are reserved for those patients who have failed to achieve adequate expansion or facial symmetry despite aggressive conformer or expander therapy
- Hydrogel expanders can be recommended for congenital anophthalmic patients as a method with good results and minimal surgical trauma
- Hydrogel expanders may permit an earlier ability to wear a prosthesis than standard serial conformer expansion

16.1 Introduction

16.1.1 Clinical Features

Children born with clinical anophthalmos – true anophthalmos or extreme microphthalmos – present with a shortened eyelid fissure (Fig. 16.1). When opening the lids a small, reduced mucosal socket becomes visible (Fig. 16.2). Under such circumstances it is often not possible to insert a regular prosthesis in order to stimulate the growth of the surrounding tissues to normal proportions. Tissue expansion is necessary to stimulate growth of the bony orbit in order to prevent or to reduce midface asymmetry. In cases of untreated unilateral anophthalmos disturbing asymmetry will usually result.

The disfiguring appearance is distressing to the family, and on occasion parents may have difficulty accepting the child. Social integration of these children may be severely endangered unless a more normal appearance can be achieved.

16.1.2 Epidemiology

Congenital anophthalmos is rare. Prevalence is reported at 1.1/100,000 for Bohemia [41], 2/100,000 for France [22], 2.7/100,000 for Sweden [22], 3.1/100,000 for California [22], 3.3/100,000 for northern Italy [8] and 4/100,000 for Spain [3]. There are obvious regional variations. The other reason for these differences is that some papers include some degree of microphthalmos and others do not (see below).

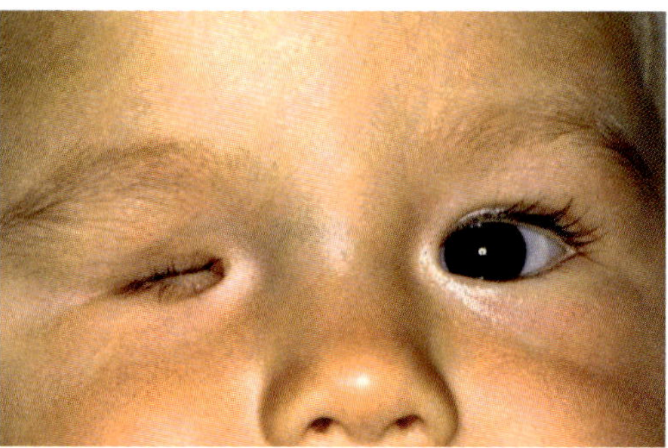

Fig. 16.1. Nine-month-old girl with unilateral clinical anophthalmos, reduced horizontal lid length, and epicanthus

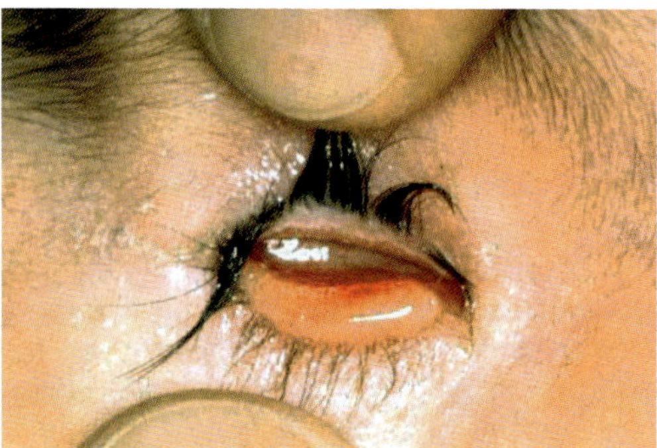

Fig. 16.2. Clinical anophthalmos: reduced mucosal socket, nearly no cul-de-sacs developed

16.1.3 Definition of Terms

Severe microphthalmos is difficult to differentiate from true anophthalmos, which can only be confirmed radiologically or histologically [33]. Therefore, the term "clinical anophthalmos" has been recommended for the absence of any visible globe [13]. An acquired anophthalmos (early enucleation, e.g. because of retinoblastoma, trauma) is usually treated differently (e.g. primary implant or dermis fat graft). Therefore the disease entity discussed here will be referred to as "congenital clinical anophthalmos".

Embryological considerations [27]:

1. Primary anophthalmos: Evagination of the frontal brain fails to develop and an optic vesicle is not formed. The histogenetic determination period falls into the time of the emergence of the optic vesicle in the first 2 weeks of gestation.
2. Secondary anophthalmos: Disturbance of the front end of the neural crest is present. This disease is not compatible with life.
3. Consecutive anophthalmos: Degeneration or atrophy of the already formed optic vesicle is the reason. This can be produced by endo- or exogenous damage in all phases of gestation.

16.1.4 Aetiology

Warburg [44] gives an overview of the role of genetics in the etiology of the disease. Patients with autosomal-dominant [39], autosomal-recessive [21, 32] or recessive X-linked [5] transmission have been reported. Also a deletion at chromosome 14 has been described [15]. Handler et al. [17] gave an overview of an assumed infectious genesis. The influence of different, usually toxic environmental factors is controversial. Most cases, however, seem to develop sporadically. Numerous reports describe associated systemic changes (e.g. [6, 8, 31, 43]).

The relationship of congenital anophthalmos and microphthalmos to a variety of syndromes and anomalies identifying a genetic link makes it important for such patients routinely to undergo genetic evaluation. This will also facilitate better epidemiological reporting so that any relationship between environmental factors and a specific etiologic cause for these disorders can be elucidated [18].

16.1.5 Treatment

The time and type of treatment are primarily determined by the type and severity of the conjunctival, eyelid and orbital changes. Children with clinical anophthalmos require prolonged and complicated socket management. A patient with a visible microphthalmic eye often requires only minimal therapy to produce an acceptable cosmetic appearance. Because of the wide variations, it is nearly impossible to set a

Table 16.1. Used expanders (Osmed GmbH, Germany)

	Socket expander 0.9 ml	Orbit expander 2 ml	Orbit expander 3 ml	Orbit expander 4 ml	Orbit expander 5 ml
Shape	Hemisphere	Sphere	Sphere	Sphere	Sphere
Volume (dry)	0.12±0.02 ml	0.3±0.03 ml	0.3±0.03 ml	0.43±0.03 ml	0.43±0.03 ml
Diameter (dry)	6±0.1 mm	8±0.2 mm	8±0.2 mm	9±0.2 mm	9±0.2 mm
Volume after swelling[a]	1±0.2 ml	2±0.3 ml	3±0.3 ml	4±0.3 ml	5.5±0.5 ml
Diameter after swelling[a]	12.4±0.8 mm	15.5±0.5 mm	18±0.5 mm	19.75±0.5 mm	21.8±0.6 mm
Swelling capacity	8.3	6.7	10	9.3	12.8

aIn vitro results in 0.9% NaCl.

uniform timetable as to the specific steps in treatment necessary for rehabilitating each child; each individual situation must be carefully assessed in order to plan appropriate treatment [17].

There are several methods for the treatment of congenital clinical anophthalmos. Most frequently, rigid plastic shells, so-called conformers, are used. They have to be changed frequently to a larger size in order to expand the lid fissure and to achieve the therapeutic goal of retaining a suitable prosthesis. Less frequently inflatable silicone expanders which must be refilled regularly with a saline solution have been used. In extreme cases, direct surgical craniofacial reconstruction of the bony orbit may be necessary.

The goals of treatment are to enlarge conjunctival space, to promote normal development of the lid margins and lashes and to increase bony orbital volume. The guiding principle is to avoid surgery wherever possible, particularly to the lids and conjunctival cul-de-sacs, in order to prevent any form of potential contractive scar formation. In the present chapter, our current experience with high-hydrophilic self-inflating hydrogel expanders is reported.

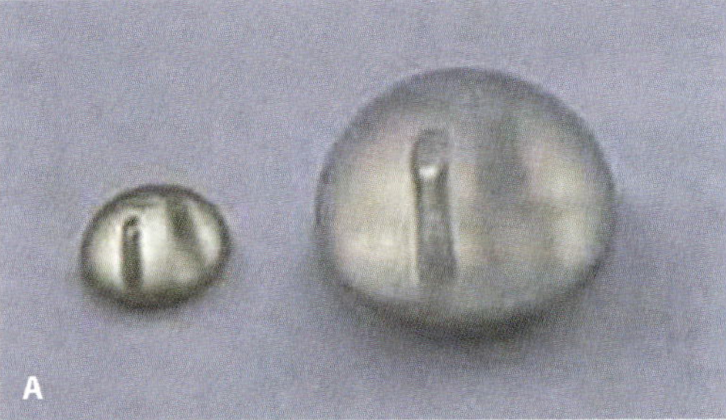

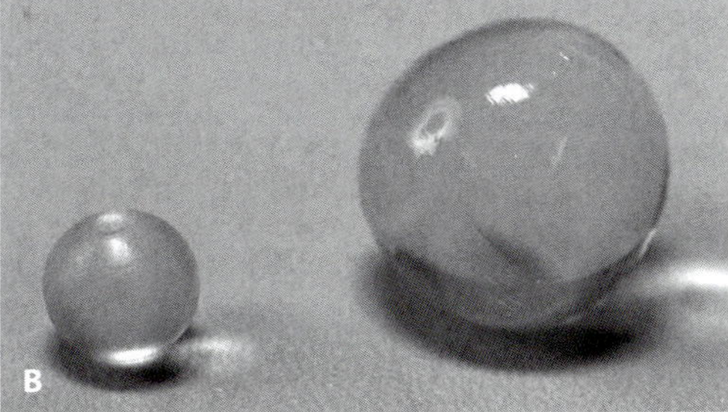

Fig. 16.3. Hydrogel expander as hemisphere for the socket (**A**) and as sphere for the orbit (**B**), dry and completely hydrated

16.2 Patients and Method

16.2.1 Osmotic Expanders

Since Wiese's studies [45, 46, 47, 48], hydrophilic gel expanders with high swelling factors have been available. These expanders deliver a continuous pressure and volume increase. The an-

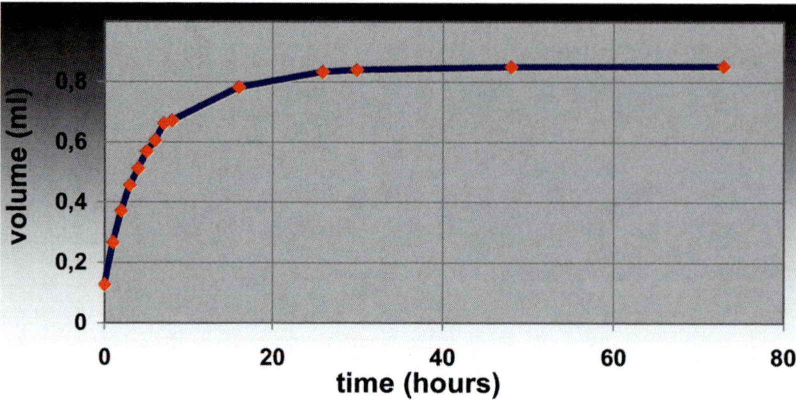

Fig. 16.4. In vitro swelling curve for a socket expander (data from Osmed GmbH Ilmenau, Germany, with permission)

hydrous expander is a solid body consisting of an interlaced, physiologically well tolerated hydraulic gel (copolymer on the basis of methylmethacrylate and vinyl pyrrolidone – MMA-VP). The material allows the manufacture of expander devices in any shape and size (Table 16.1, Fig. 16.3). After implantation, water (tears, intercellular fluid) is absorbed. An automatic volume increase takes place. The swelling degree, i.e. the extent of the volume increase over the time or the quotient of anhydrous expander volume and swollen volume, is adjustable by chemical modification of the ionization degree between 3 and 50 [26, 48]. The time in which the final volume is reached is constantly given (Fig. 16.4). Material pore size is 10 nm, which makes it impervious to cells and tissue and is biologically inert [48].

16.2.2 Patients

We report the clinical analysis of 30 congenital anophthalmic patients, 17 unilateral and 13 bilateral (43 orbits), who were treated at least once with hydrogel expanders. Patient age was 1–78 months (average 10 months) at the time of first expander implantation. The observation period thus far has extended to a maximum of 83 months (average 26.9 months).

Patients referred for treatment were evaluated by a team consisting of a craniofacial surgeon, an ocularist and an oculoplastic surgeon. Informed consent was obtained before beginning treatment. Each patient was photo-documented at each visit in the office and pre- /postoperatively. The following data were obtained:

- The horizontal length of each eyelid fissure was determined, i.e. the distance from the medial to the lateral canthus [42]
- Number of operations needed
- Number of complications
- Time course until an ocular prosthesis could be permanently worn (related to patient's age and to treatment period)

The data and the measured parameters were recorded in an Excel table. Considering the small number of patients, no further statistical analysis was performed.

Summary for the Clinician

- **Self-inflating high hydrophilic hydrogel expanders developed by Wiese are a new option for tissue expansion**
- **This type of expander material was modified for use in ophthalmology**
- **Forty-three orbits in 30 congenital anophthalmic patients were treated**

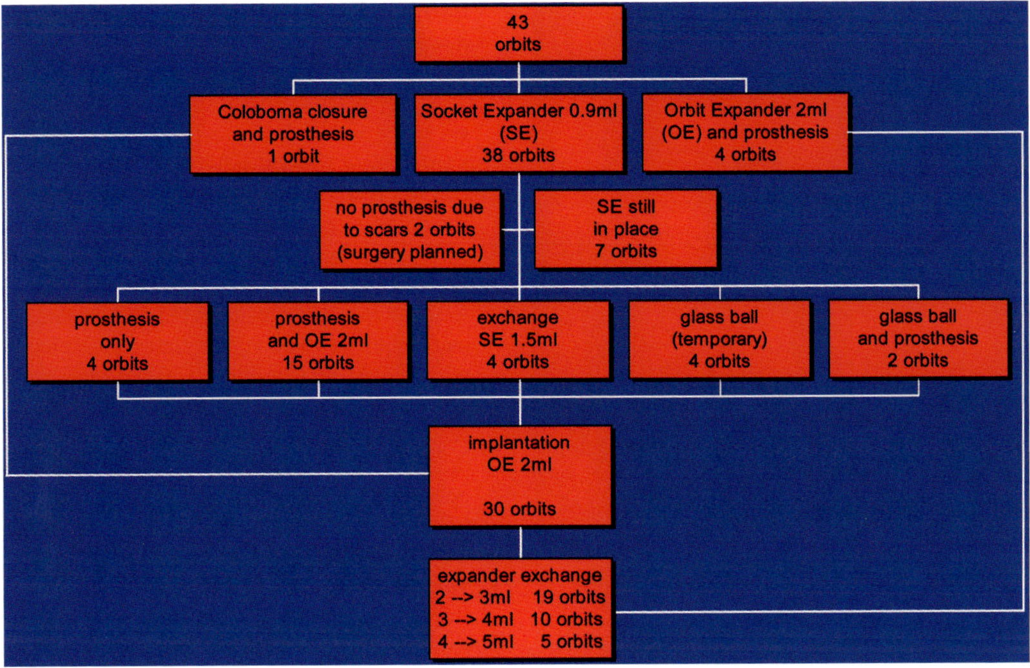

Fig. 16.5. Treatment course (schematic) and number of orbits treated

16.3 Results

16.3.1 Treatment Course (see Fig. 16.5)

16.3.1.1 Socket Expansion

A hemispherical socket expander (Table 16.1) was implanted in the reduced conjunctival sac in 27 out of 30 patients as early as possible. This was done between 1 and 15 months of age (average 4.8 months) as a first step procedure and between 13 and 78 months of age (average 10 months) in children previously treated elsewhere. The average age with the first socket expander was 10 months.

Placement of the expander was initiated with the patient under general anesthesia. The implant was fastened with a non-absorbable suture at the back of the socket in the conjunctival tissue (Fig. 16.6). A complete tarsorrhaphy was

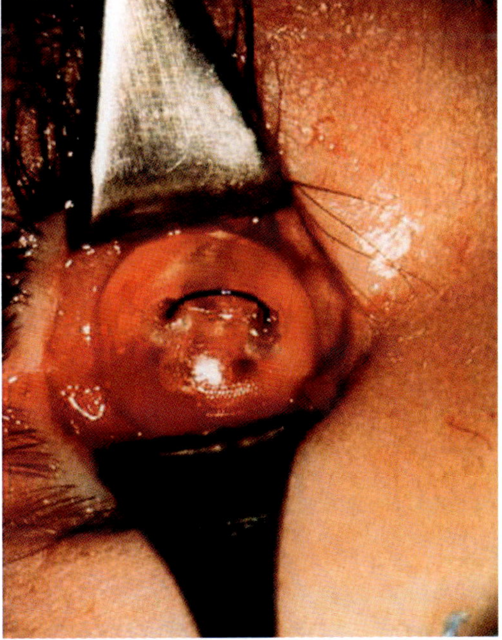

Fig. 16.6. Hemisphere socket expander sutured on the conjunctiva

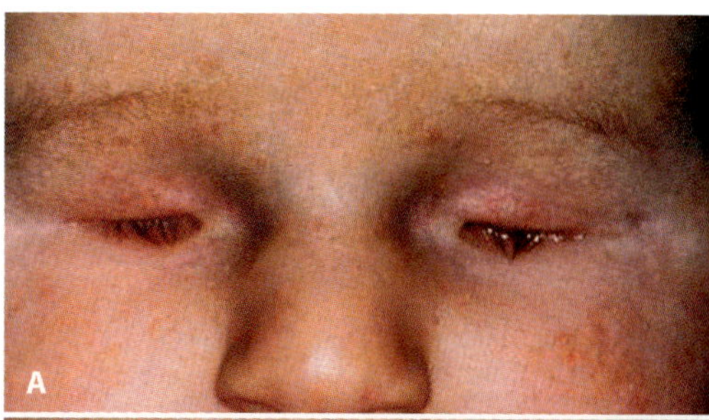

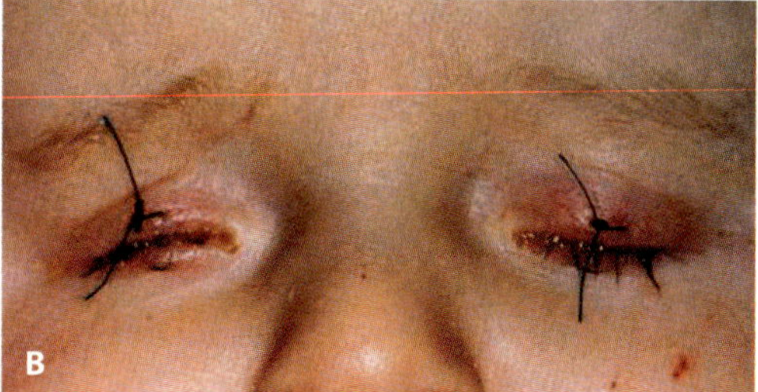

Fig. 16.7. Eight-week-old boy with bilateral clinical anophthalmos before (**A**) and 2 days after surgery (**B**) with well shaped lids

done, using a temporary suture technique, to distribute uniform pressure to the eyelids and the conjunctival fornices and to limit the potential for extrusion of the expander.

The final volume of the expander was reached with the eyelid structures already better formed out within 2–3 days (Fig. 16.7). The tarsorrhaphy was released to remove the expander after 1–9 months (average 2.9 months). In three patients the hemisphere expander is still in place and will be removed in the future. Treatment was continued individually as follows (Fig. 16.5):

- **Variant A**
  In three patients, a properly sized, double-walled glass prosthesis was fitted. After 2–3 months an orbit expander was implanted (see below). In most patients the socket space created by the expander was too large to stabilize a prosthesis alone. Therefore additional volume replacement was needed in the orbit.
- **Variant B**
  With the first three patients treated a glass ball only was inserted temporarily in the expanded socket after removing the socket expander to allow conjunctival tissue to reform. Over the past 5 years glass balls have no longer been needed.
- **Variant C**
  Together with a prosthesis in the conjunctival space a glass ball was inserted in two patients. Glass was initially preferred to avoid conjunctival irritation. After 6 weeks to 4 months, the glass balls were removed and orbital expanders were implanted.
- **Variant D**
  In three patients a more extended expansion was required even if the first hemispheres with 0.9 ml final volume worked very well. Therefore larger hemispheres with a final volume of 1.5 ml were implanted. This procedure led to better lid expansion in all but in one socket, where due to induced conjunctival scarring an additional socket expander was needed.
- **Variant E** (see Sect. 16.3.1.2 below)
  In 3 of 30 patients (5 orbits) no socket expansion was needed (see Fig. 16.5). With an orbital expander implanted (see below) and surgical closure of a lower lid coloboma (1 orbit) they were then able to maintain an artificial eye.

16.3.1.2 Orbit Expansion

Orbit Expander Implantation

After completion of socket expansion and successful prosthetic fitting, further orbital volume expansion or substitution is then performed: Socket expander therapy improves transconjunctival access to soft orbital tissue by increasing the eyelid fissure width. The expanded palpebral fissure facilitates the subsequent step of expanding the tissues of the deep orbit with a spherical expander. This was performed in 13 patients immediately after explanting the socket expander and later in the remaining patients, who were treated with variants A–D in between.

A spherical implant of 2 ml final volume (Table 16.1) is inserted via a central conjunctival (Fig. 16.8) or an inner subtarsal lower lid approach using an incision directly below the tarsal plate and through the lower lid retractors. Through the opening, blunt dissection with

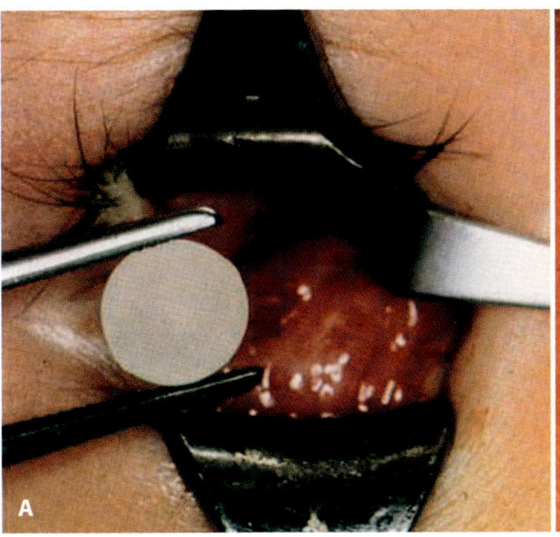

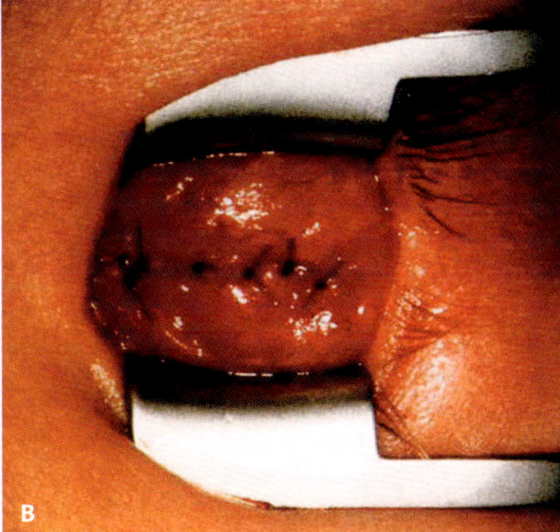

Fig. 16.8. Sphere orbital expander before transconjunctival implantation (**A**) and incision sutured in two layers (**B**)

Stevens' scissors allows access to the deep orbit in order to create an extensive space in the muscle cone. A visible adhesion between the posterior end of the socket and the orbital apex, which is present in most cases, has to be dissected via the same approach. Otherwise the space for expander inflation is limited and dislocation or extrusion can occur. The dry sphere is inserted and positioned as deep as possible in the orbital apex. Care is taken that sufficient soft tissue spontaneously covers the implant. The incision for the spherical expander is closed in two layers with absorbable sutures.

A glass prosthesis was shaped to fit snugly into the conjunctival fornices. A temporary tarsorrhaphy for 1–3 weeks was used to help prevent extrusion of the expander. The ball-shaped expander also achieves its final size within 2 days. The presence of scar tissue is limited and the socket is well formed to receive a prosthesis. The orbit expander helps to stabilize the prosthesis and permits a thinner shell which can more easily be enlarged to continue serial expansion of the horizontal lid fissure length.

Prosthetic Fitting

The prosthesis is enlarged as necessary every 3–6 months (Fig. 16.9). Frequent communication with the ocularist is necessary to monitor the treatment plan and to gauge progress. This has to be continued in unilateral cases until symmetry is reached and in bilateral cases until acceptable cosmesis results.

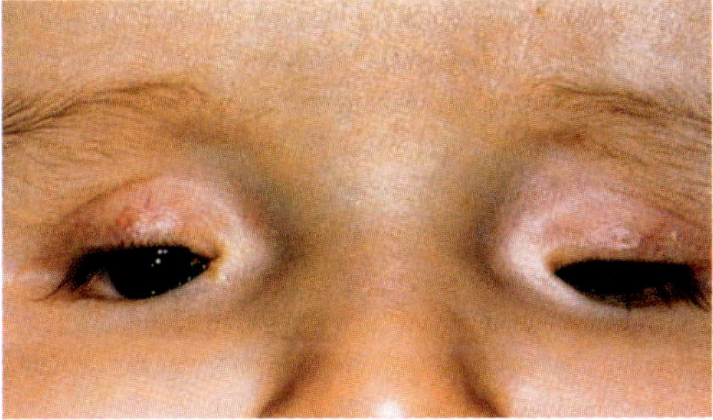

Fig. 16.9. Patient from Fig. 16.6, socket expander removed, orbital expander (2 ml) implanted and first glass prosthesis fitted

Exchange of Orbital Expander

Whenever clinical impression dictated, the orbit expander was replaced with a consecutively 1 ml larger sphere. This was done in the case of reduced prominence of the lids even with a larger prosthesis or if the ocularists were no longer able to fit a larger one because the lid fissure was too small to place a larger prosthesis. In these cases the 2-ml expander was replaced by a 3-ml one. The next steps were to place 4-ml and 5-ml expanders respectively.

When exchanging the orbital implant a similar access and surgical technique is used. The material in place is easily fragmented and delivered out via an equally small incision as mentioned above. One must be sure to dissect the capsule surrounding the previous expander, to allow the larger implant to expand properly.

16.3.2 Expander Failures/Complication

16.3.2.1 Socket Expanders

There were 11 failures in 38 treated orbits:

- Four expander losses resulted from too high a swelling capacity in the preliminary group of patients. Therefore this factor was reduced to 8.3, which is now available.
- Three expander losses occurred due to manipulations by the child after tarsorrhaphy removal. If possible, sutures should be kept in place until the expander is removed to avoid access to the hydrated, soft expander.
- Three expander losses were due to conjunctival scarring which might have been caused by previous operations such as dermis-fat graft [2] or osteotomy combined with conjunctival surgery [1]
- One case was conjunctival scarring without expander loss in a 5-year-old girl who needed additional surgery

All failures could be successfully treated with new socket expanders and/or conjunctival surgery.

16.3.2.2 Orbit Expander Implantation

There were 15 failures/complications in 30 orbits:

- Six expander losses were due to insufficient wound closure in the first group of treated patients. After changing technique to suturing two layers no further expander loss was observed.
- Two expander extrusions were due to an incorrect size/swelling capacity in the first group of treated patients (Fig. 16.10).

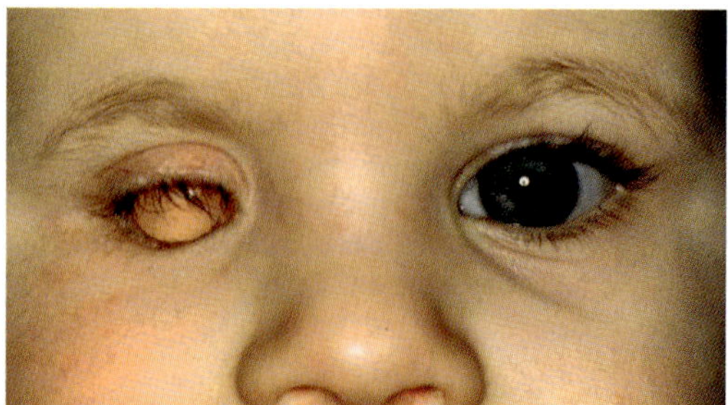

Fig. 16.10. Orbit expander extrusion in a girl with unilateral congenital anophthalmos; after reimplantation a prosthesis was fitted, and no new complications occurred

- Two expander extrusions were due to insufficient preparation; thus space for expansion was too small.
- Five cases of conjunctival scarring were due to inflammation or excessive intraoperative manipulations.

All failures were resolved with new orbit expanders and/or conjunctival surgery.

16.3.2.3 Orbit Expander Exchange

There were 10 failures/complications in 34 orbits:

- Five expander losses due to insufficient opening of the capsule which had formed around the previous expander. Therefore too much pressure on the suture resulted.
- Four expander extrusions occurred months after surgery from unknown causes (i.e. without inflammation)
- One "exophthalmos" due to incomplete removal of the old expander

All failures were resolved with additional surgery/new orbit expanders.

16.3.3 Number of Operations

In Table 16.2 the number of planned operations and the number of operations due to complications are presented per completed treatment year.

Table 16.2. Treatment data

Year completion of treatment	Number of patients	Time with prosthesis (months)	Planned operations	Operations due to complications
1	22	6.3±3.2 (0–12)	1–4 (2.7±0.8)	0–4 (1.3±1.3)
2	16	10.9±1.7 (6–12)	0–2 (0.5±0.6)	0–4 (0.8±1.1)
3	11	11.6±0.7 (11–12)	0–2 (0.9±0.6)	0–2 (0.4±0.7)
4	10	10.3±3.5 (2–12)	0–2 (0.5±0.6)	0–2 (0.6±0.8)
5	8	10.6±3.2 (3–12)	0–1 (0.2±0.4)	0–7 (0.8±2)
6	2	12	1–2 (1.5±0.5)	0
7	2	12	0–1 (0.5±0.5)	0

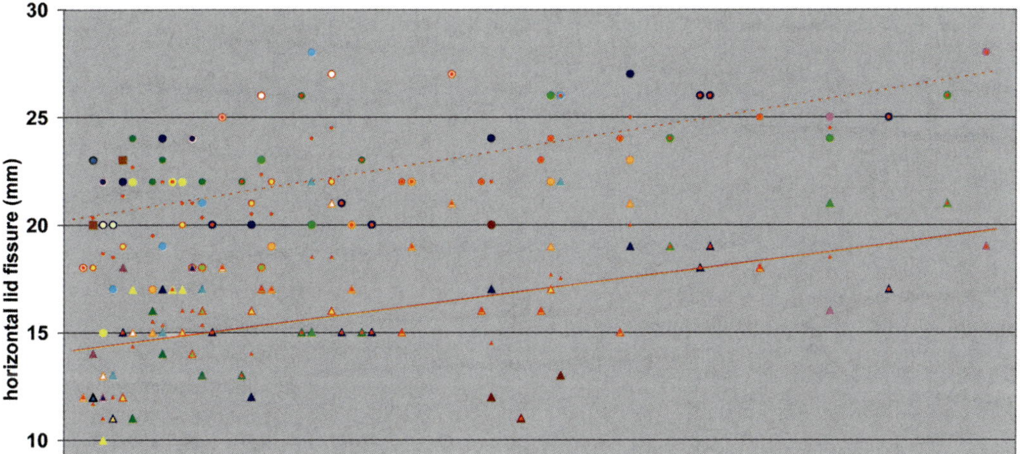

Fig. 16.11. Horizontal lid fissure development in unilateral anophthalmos with age (*lines* trend estimation for mean value, *dotted line* healthy side, *continuous line* anophthalmic side – one color for each individual case, *solid circles* healthy eye, *solid triangles* anophthalmic orbit)

16.3.4 Treatment Results

16.3.4.1 Prosthesis

Patients could wear a regular double-walled glass prosthesis at an average of 2.8 months after treatment was started. Table 16.2 demonstrates how many months per year patients could wear a prosthesis or in other words how long they had to go without a prosthesis due to planned surgery and/or complications. Note that this value became very stable by the 2nd year of treatment.

16.3.4.2 Lid Fissure Development

Unilateral Anophthalmos

Figure 16.11 presents the development of the horizontal lid fissure during the follow-up period. In Fig. 16.12 the anophthalmic/healthy side ratio is calculated to see if there is any progress towards symmetry. The range of preoperative eyelid length deficit in the unilateral cases was mildly reduced during treatment.

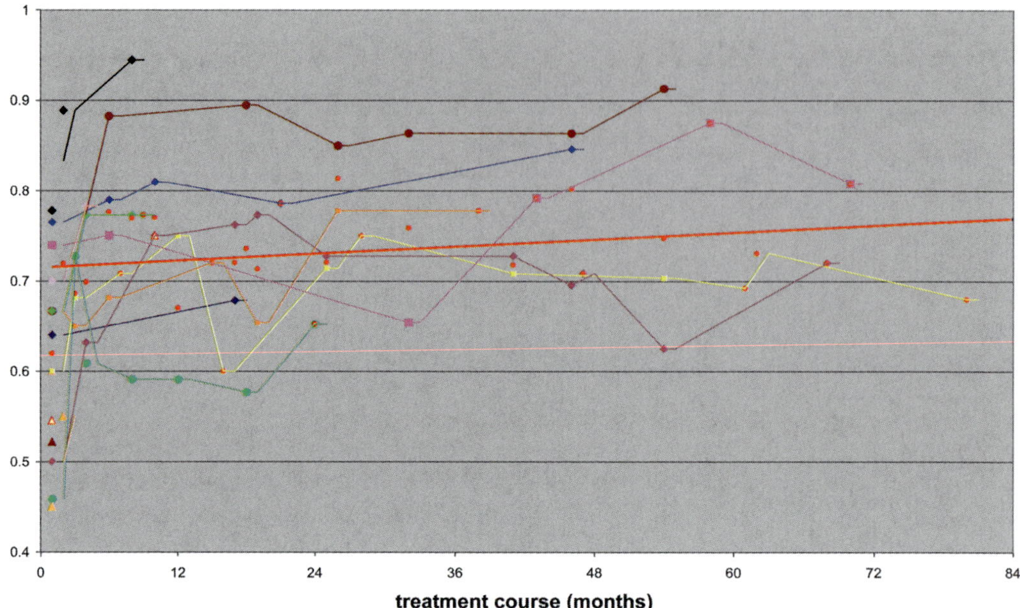

Fig. 16.12. Horizontal lid fissure development in unilateral anophthalmos with treatment course (*0* treatment started), calculated anophthalmic/healthy side ratio (*1* symmetry), individual lines and trend estimation for mean value

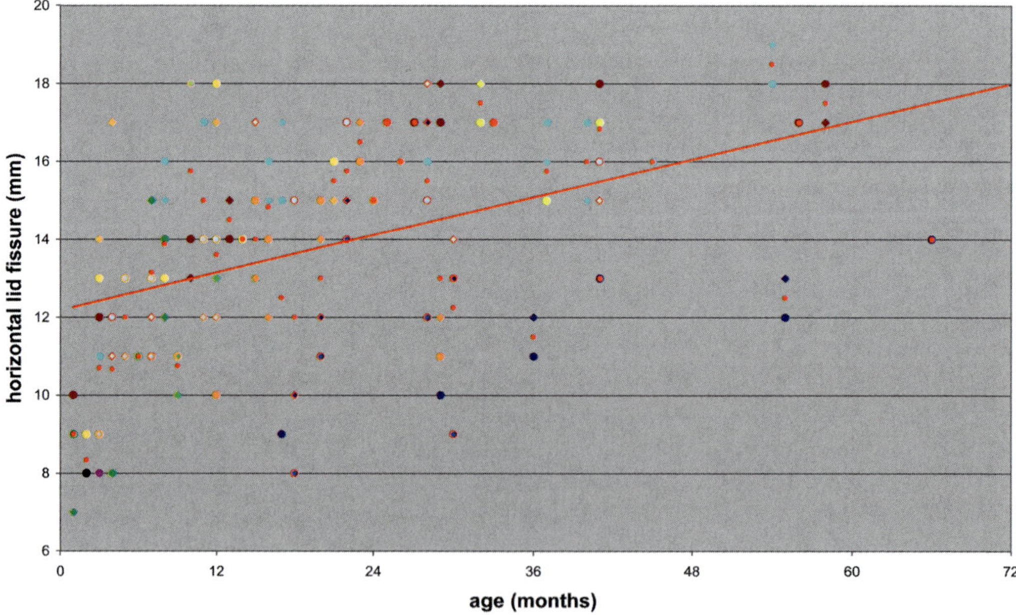

Fig. 16.13. Horizontal lid fissure development in bilateral anophthalmos with age (*solid circles* right eye, *solid triangles* left eye – one color for each individual case, *line* trend estimation for mean value)

Bilateral Anophthalmos

The bilateral cases demonstrated an increase during treatment (Fig. 16.13), but it is almost impossible to calculate further estimations due to huge variations between individual patients. Compared to unilateral cases the mean value for bilateral patients starts from a lower value (12.3 vs. 14.2) but reaches nearly the same level of 18 mm after 72 months.

16.3.5 Acceptance

The treatment is mostly well accepted by parents. Especially in bilateral cases the most often mentioned benefit is that it allows the fitting of a properly sized prosthesis so early in life: "Today my child looked at me for the first time". This may help parents to accept their child better, but we do not understand exactly what happens. As a result, we have recently initiated a study on the psychosocial problems for these patients and their parents.

We feel that it is especially critical to obtain an acceptable cosmetic result in the unilateral cases because of the previously discussed problems of asymmetry.

Summary for the Clinician

- **First step: a hemisphere expander of 0.9 ml final volume is used for socket expansion**
- **Second step: the socket expander is removed and replaced by a custom-made glass prosthesis**
- **Third step: orbital volume expansion or substitution is performed: spherical expander (2 ml) implantation is made into deep soft orbital tissue**
- **Whenever clinical impression is dictated, the orbit expander is replaced with a consecutively 1 ml larger sphere until 5 ml is reached**
- **All expander failures (which happened mainly with the first patients treated) could be successfully managed with new expanders and/or conjunctival surgery**

16.4 Discussion

16.4.1 Introduction

Congenital clinical anophthalmos is a very rare disorder with a prevalence in Europe of between 1/100,000 [24] and 1/10,000 [8, 22, 40] live births. The data are not clear due to the partial inclusion of patients with microphthalmos, whose severity is usually not clearly defined [10].

Anophthalmos presents both functional and cosmetic problems. The missing growth stimulus of an eye leads – even more than after early enucleation – to a considerably smaller orbit [7, 16]. The cosmetic aspect is particularly problematic with unilateral anophthalmos due to the glaring contrast of the hypoplastic eyelids and orbit on one side as compared to the normal opposite side.

16.4.2 Pathogenesis

The eye represents the main growth stimulus for the intrauterine physiological formation of the orbit and eyelid structures [14]. Several papers prove that congenital anophthalmos is associated with a substantially smaller orbit [7, 16]. This has to be differentiated clearly from the situation after early enucleation. Hintschich [20] demonstrated that enucleation leads to a measurable reduction of the orbital volume. The difference between the enucleated and normal side has been shown to be maximally 7%. This is less than is usually accepted and there was also no visible facial asymmetry. The extent of the volume difference is more strongly correlated with the temporal interval to enucleation rather than with the age at enucleation. This can be interpreted to indicate that there is an adaptation process which is, interestingly, not dependent on the use of an orbital implant. There is even no genuine growth delay. This leads, in our opinion, also to an essential point of criticism for all animal experiments. The intrauterine absence of an eye seems to represent a substantial growth stimulus factor in the retarded orbital development. There may be, however, other genetic or growth factors that can affect orbital bone growth. These may be represented by the small group of patients that do not respond to internal volume expansion and require craniofacial surgical expansion.

16.4.3 Existing Therapy Concepts – Pros and Cons

So far no agreement exists over the most effective concept for the treatment of congenital anophthalmos. This is not surprising considering the extremely small number of patients compared with other ophthalmologic diseases. Many reports are anecdotal or consist of a series of a few patients. There are three general approaches to the treatment of anophthalmos.

16.4.3.1 Conformer

The most commonly selected option is the use of non-expanding conformers, which is the current preferred method [17, 23]. A conformer must be replaced regularly by a larger model, in order to obtain the necessary stretch effect [11]. This requires repeated manipulations and may in some cases require general anesthesia for the conformer exchange [42]. This is not the usual experience – almost all exchanges can be done in the ocularist's office.

Frequent communication with the ocularist is necessary to monitor the treatment plan and to gauge progress [18]. The ocularist is therefore an important and critical member of the medical team treating these patients.

Conformers require cul-de-sacs which are well enough developed to maintain the conformer – a condition which was often not found in our patients, which demonstrates the limitations.

16.4.3.2 Socket Surgery

Silicone Balloon Expanders

Balloon expanders require a difficult surgical procedure, usually utilizing a coronal approach. Spherical expanders can be implanted intraconally or as C-shaped devices subperiosteally [18, 25]. The inflation tube is then passed through an osteotomy in the lateral orbital wall and connected to an injection port placed subcutaneously above the ear [14]. A regular refilling of the depot with saline solution is necessary [7, 16].

For a satisfying result regarding eyelid development, the procedure by itself is not suitable [14]. O'Keefe reports [31]: Despite the combination of balloon expander and other surgical therapy, 6 of 14 patients could not wear a prosthesis, and 4 of the patients needed repeated eyelid surgery, which ended with scars. Only four patients had a satisfying cosmetic result, the patients without eyelid surgery and at the beginning of treatment in the 1st year of life.

In an effort to reduce the surgical complexity, orbital tissue expansion within the cul-de-sac with an anterior self-sealing system has been attempted [18]. In several orbits there appeared to be positive changes. Horizontal lid fissure length was also improved. Difficulties were similar to those reported with intraorbital expanders [4, 34].

Mucous Membrane Graft

The grafting of oral mucous membrane is an attempt significantly to improve deficiencies in the conjunctival lining [29]. It is not the method of first choice [18], but is sometimes needed for patients with a reduced conjunctival surface related to extensive scarring due to prior unsuccessful surgery or inflammation.

Dermis Fat Graft

Another treatment option for pediatric anophthalmic and microphthalmic socket rehabilitation is an autogenous dermis fat graft [18]. When placed in the orbits of young children it appears to grow after implantation. Unlike adults, fat atrophy with this implant is rare in children. In fact, when implanted below age 3 years, the graft sometimes requires some debulking to reduce later proptosis of the prosthesis. This growth of the implant may help to stimulate orbital growth, potentially leading to more symmetry between the involved and uninvolved sites [19]. Another advantage is that this implant delivers more surface and helps to increase the conjunctival sac significantly. Not only is the deficit orbital volume enhanced but it may help the socket to better maintain a conformer or prosthetic shell.

The unique ability to grow makes the dermis fat graft an extremely useful alternative in those situations where the orbit is still growing and where a fixed diameter sphere will be less than ideal for providing volume over time. Although this implant is not entirely without complications, it may come close to resembling the "ideal" implant for very young children [19]. It should not, however, be placed unless there is sufficient space both to insert and to place it through the lid fissure. A lateral canthotomy should be avoided if at all possible.

16.4.3.3 Craniofacial Surgery

Direct surgical craniofacial reconstruction of the orbit is a very complex procedure [30]. Pathogenetically the stimulus for further orbital growth is still missing, so that the operation is usually performed after growth of the skull is finished, in order to avoid another repeated operation [28]. The main goal of therapy, to allow prosthetic fitting, is not obtained [16], so that further lid and socket surgical efforts are often necessary. These procedures can be considered for older patients who had a late beginning in therapy and with pronounced face asymmetry. It is not the method of first choice but is reserved for those patients who have failed to achieve adequate expansion or facial symmetry despite aggressive conformer or other forms of expansion therapy [18, 23].

16.4.3.4 Hydrophilic Expanders as an Alternative Concept

Tissue Expansion

In plastic surgery a gradual, continuous and thus careful pressure development is demanded for skin expansion and induction of skin growth. Conventional silicone balloon expanders, which must be refilled regularly with a liquid, correspond to these requirements only conditionally.

Low Hydrophilic Expanders

The idea of using hydrophilic, soft contact lens polymer (HEMA) was reported in 1982 [9]. Downes et al. [12] and Tucker et al. [42] reported their experiences with HEMA having an expansion capacity of only 1.2. The minimal expansion properties of the HEMA hydrophilic expanders limited the use to cases of extreme contracted sockets to allow a following conformer therapy. The use of HEMA as an expansion material did gain wide acceptance as reported by Bennett [2] in a historical overview of the development of tissue expansion.

High Hydrophilic Expanders

Wiese introduced a new concept of an osmotically driven expander in 1993 [45]. The objective was to create a method which offers the advantages of the inflatable silicone expanders, but does not include the complex surgical procedures otherwise required. This was achieved through the development of an expanding copolymer without the potentially tissue-damaging effect of hyperosmolar solutions. The feasibility of the concept was demonstrated in several investigations [45–48].

Hydrogels in Ophthalmology

In 1997 we first used the material in the therapy of clinical congenital anophthalmos ([1, 47], Fig. 16.14). Thus far 30 patients (16 unilateral, 14 bilateral anophthalmos) have been treated. Significant enlargement of both the eyelids and the

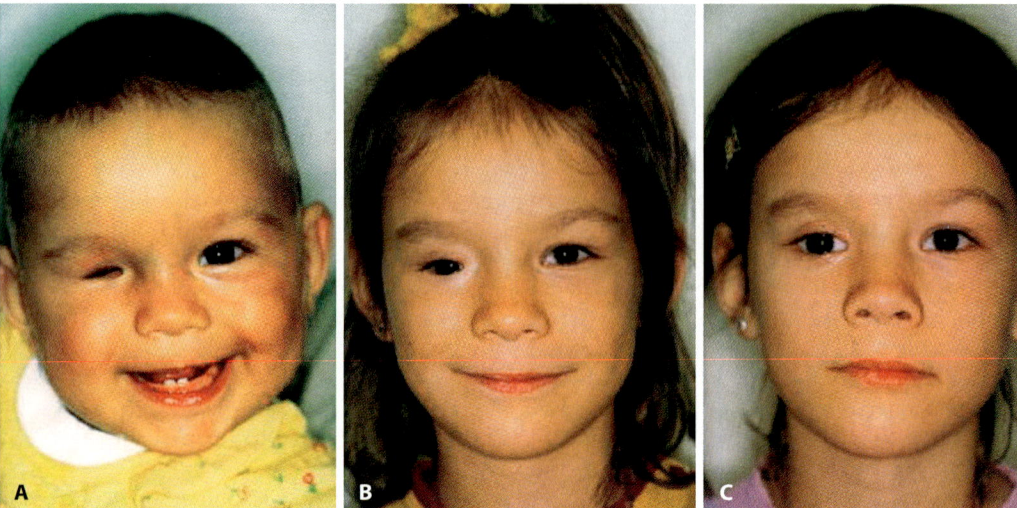

Fig. 16.14. Unilateral anophthalmos in a girl, 11 months old before treatment started (**A**), 6 years old with orbital expander and glass prosthesis (**B**), 7 years old with expander enlarged to 5 ml and epicanthus corrected (**C**), similar horizontal lid length on both sides

socket has been achieved in all cases. Expansion of the conjunctival socket and lengthening of the eyelid fissures, both horizontally and vertically, have improved the cosmetic result and thus achieved the major goal of the therapy. Osmotic expansion therapy enabled the ocularists to accommodate properly sized prostheses in all cases but one. In this case, where previous operations had led to cicatricial socket closure, hydrogel expanders were successful only partly; mucosal grafting will be needed.

More recently larger hemispherical expanders (1.5 ml) have been manufactured to induce greater socket expansion for the insertion of subsequently larger prostheses. In our experience there are very few indications for these expanders because of the risk of induced scarring when treatment becomes too aggressive.

The expansion of the socket with the osmotically active expander can be regarded as a relatively simple and very effective procedure, compared to existing therapies. In primarily treated patients, as has been previously discussed [36, 38], no additional lid surgery or grafting was needed in this series. Because of the great capacity for swelling, the implant often does not require serial exchanges to achieve increased volume. However, several sizes are available.

Prosthetics

A certain influence on eyelid development also results from the continuous wearing of a prosthesis as well as the size adjustment. It is difficult to assess the respective effects of the expander and/or the prosthesis. Continuous treatment is necessary, however, in order to avoid a renewed contraction of the socket and loss of the ability to retain a prosthesis. Another advantage of the procedure is that there is usually no need for extensive eyelid-surgical procedures, which often lead to significant scarring particularly in the young child.

Our treated patients were able to maintain a prosthesis 2.8 months after therapy started. When a socket expander was implanted within 3 months of age, these infants could receive an artificial eye within at least 6 months. This is much earlier than has previously been reported with any other treatment option. Even when continuing therapy, including all the complications patients did not have to go without a prosthesis for more than 1–2 months in any year.

Orbit Expansion

The existing preliminary data are not significant enough to quantify the degree of expansion of the bony orbit [37]. With a longer follow-up and larger number of patients it may be possible to calculate the MRI-measured volumetric effects of orbital hydrogel expanders.

The orbital implant compensates for volume deficiency and helps to stabilize the prosthesis. Sufficient posterior stability must be achieved in order to deliver anterior pressure to the lids to achieve better horizontal and vertical lid growth.

Complications

Complications occurred in a few cases due to the loss or early removal of the expander material. The hydrogel material becomes increasingly softer and more friable as it expands. Mechanical irritation such as rubbing the eyes may fragment and dislodge the device.

The expander strength depends on the swelling capacity. The implants are now produced with a lower swelling ratio and are less fragile. On the other hand, the tarsorrhaphy is now left in place until the expander can be removed and replaced by the custom-made prosthesis. In each case of loss of the socket, expander shrinking of the socket could be prevented by immediate insertion of a prosthesis or a simple glass shell, in order to preserve the expansion achieved and improve the outcome. Parents should be advised to notify the surgeon and/or ocularist immediately if the expander is inadvertently removed.

Extrusion of the orbit expander can be caused by a disproportion between selected expander size and orbital volume. MRI can be a decision-making aid. How much resistance the orbital soft tissue supplies is also difficult to measure. In the case of a too large pressure build-up, the only possibility for relaxation is wound rupture and extrusion of the material. This can be prevented by selecting the appropriate-sized implant and by consistently using a two-layered wound closure utilizing the orbit approach mentioned above.

Even though the number of complications appears large, most complications actually occurred in the first 2–3 years after developing this treatment model. Several general anesthesia sessions are still necessary because of the need for multiple operations and control MRI studies. The number of complications have already been remarkably reduced by the standardization of the expander sizes, their swelling factors and revised surgical techniques.

Outlook

The expander final volume is almost completely achieved within 2 days. The expansion speed cannot be modified chemically [26]. A slower and thus surely more preserving expansion speed would be very useful in addition to the range of sizes now available. Complications by expander extrusion could be decreased or better avoided. Also, primary expanders with a larger final volume could then be used, thus decreasing the expander exchange frequency, which when compared to other techniques is already very low. The number of general anesthesias required could also be decreased. At the moment, our approach is to explore physical modifications of the implants in order to increase the expansion time. Preliminary results [35] show that this may be a possible solution, but we need to continue our measurements for a more conclusive statement.

Summary for the Clinician

- **The guiding principle for congenital anophthalmic patients is conservative therapy, avoiding surgery if at all possible**
- **If conformer treatment fails or is too slow to progress, hydrogel expanders are a useful alternative method with good results and minimal surgical trauma**
  Based on our experience as described above, we now recommend the following therapeutic concepts:
- ***Blind microphthalmos:* If the fornices are reasonably developed, usually scleral shells of increasing size or in the case of constricted fornices a hemisphere hydrogel socket expander can help to fit a prosthesis**

- ***Clinical congenital anophthalmos:* (1) Hemisphere expander for the conjunctival sac; (2) sphere expander placed in orbital soft tissue, which will compensate for volume deficiency, help to stabilize a prosthesis and may stimulate bony growth; (3) orbit expander exchange 1 ml/year until 5 ml is reached**
- ***Children >5 years* (or patients operated on previously who present with constricted conjunctival sac due to scarring): An individual combination must be found of mucosal graft/dermis-fat graft/expander or even surgical osteotomies to approach a reasonable midface symmetry and prosthetic appearance**

References

1. Bacskulin A, Vogel M, Wiese KG, Gundlach K, Hingst V, Guthoff R (2000) New osmotically active hydrogel expander for enlargement of the contracted anophthalmic socket. Graefes Arch Clin Exp Ophthalmol 238:24–27
2. Bennett RG, Hirt M (1993) A history of tissue expansion. Concepts, controversies, and complications. J Dermatol Surg Oncol 19:1066–1073
3. Bermejo E, Martinez-Frias ML (1998) Congenital eye malformations: clinical-epidemiological analysis of 1,124,654 consecutive births in Spain. Am J Med Genet 75:497–504
4. Berry FD (1991) A modified tissue expander for socket enlargement in clinical anophthalmos. Ophthal Plast Reconstr Surg 7:41–47
5. Brunquell PJ, Papale JH, Horton JC, Williams RS, Zgrabik MJ, Albert DM, Hedley-Whyte ET (1984) Sex-linked hereditary bilateral anophthalmos. Pathologic and radiologic correlation. Arch Ophthalmol 102:108–113
6. Busby A, Dolk H, Collin R, Jones RB, Winter R (1998) Compiling a national register of babies born with anophthalmia/microphthalmia in England 1988–94. Arch Dis Child Fetal Neonatal Ed 79:168–173
7. Cepela MA, Nunery WR, Martin RT (1992) Stimulation of orbital growth by the use of expandable implants in the anophthalmic cat orbit. Ophthal Plast Reconstr Surg 8:157–167; discussion 168–169
8. Clementi M, Turolla L, Mammi I, Tenconi R (1992) Clinical anophthalmia: an epidemiological study in northeast Italy based on 368,256 consecutive births. Teratology 46:551–553
9. Collin JR, Moriarty PA (1982) Management of the contracted socket. Trans Ophthalmol Soc U K 102:93–97
10. Dolk H, Busby A, Armstrong BG, Walls PH (1998) Geographical variation in anophthalmia and microphthalmia in England, 1988–94. BMJ 317:905–909; discussion 910
11. Dootz GL (1992) The ocularists' management of congenital microphthalmos and anophthalmos. Adv Ophthalmic Plast Reconstr Surg 9:41–56
12. Downes R, Lavin M, Collin R (1992) Hydrophilic expanders for the congenital anophthalmic socket. Adv Ophthalmic Plast Reconstr Surg 9:57–61
13. Duke-Elder S (1964) Anophthalmos and extreme microphthalmos. In: Duke-Elder S (ed) System of ophthalmology, vol III. Mosby, St. Louis, pp 416–29
14. Dunaway DJ, David DJ (1996) Intraorbital tissue expansion in the management of congenital anophthalmos. Br J Plast Surg 49:529–535
15. Elliott J, Maltby EL, Reynolds B (1993) A case of deletion 14(q22.1→q22.3) associated with anophthalmia and pituitary abnormalities. J Med Genet 30:251–252
16. Eppley BL, Holley S, Sadove AM (1993) Experimental effects of intraorbital tissue expansion on orbitomaxillary growth in anophthalmos. Ann Plast Surg 31:19–26; discussion 26–27
17. Handler LF, Heher KL, Katowitz JA (1994) Congenital and acquired anophthalmia. Curr Opin Ophthalmol 5:84–90
18. Handler LF, Heher KL, Katowitz JA (2002) Management of the microphthalmic orbit. In: Katowitz JA (2002) Pediatric oculoplastic surgery. Springer, New York, Berlin, Heidelberg, pp 559–583
19. Heher KL, Katowitz JA, Low JE (1998) Unilateral dermis-fat graft implantation in the pediatric orbit. Ophthal Plast Reconstr Surg 14:81–88
20. Hintschich C, Zonneveld F, Baldeschi L, Bunce C, Koornneef L (2001) Bony orbital development after early enucleation in humans. Br J Ophthalmol 85:205–208
21. Hornby SJ, Dandona L, Foster A, Jones RB, Gilbert CE (2001) Clinical findings, consanguinity, and pedigrees in children with anophthalmos in southern India. Dev Med Child Neurol 43:392–398
22. Kallen B, Robert E, Harris J (1996) The descriptive epidemiology of anophthalmia and microphthalmia. Int J Epidemiol 25:1009–1016
23. Krastinova D, Kelly MB, Mihaylova M (2001) Surgical management of the anophthalmic orbit, part 1: congenital. Plast Reconstr Surg 108:817–826

24. Lang GE, Apple DJ, Naumann GOH (1997) Mißbildungen und Anomalien des ganzen Auges. In: Naumann GOH (1997) Pathologie des Auges, vol I, 2nd edn. Springer, Berlin Heidelberg New York, pp 99–105
25. Lo AK, Colcleugh RG, Allen L, Van Wyck L, Bite U (1990) The role of tissue expanders in an anophthalmic animal model. Plast Reconstr Surg 86:399–408; discussion 409–410
26. Lohse P (Osmed GmbH, Ilmenau, Germany): personal communication
27. Mann I (1964) Congenital anomalies. In: Mann I (1964) The development of the human eye, 3rd edn. Butler and Tanner, Frome, pp 276–281
28. Marchac D, Cophignon J, Achard E, Dufourmentel C (1977) Orbital expansion for anophthalmia and micro-orbitism. Plast Reconstr Surg 59:486–491
29. Molgat YM, Hurwitz JJ, Webb MC (1993) Buccal mucous membrane-fat graft in the management of the contracted socket. Ophthal Plast Reconstr Surg 9:267–272
30. Morax S, Hurbli T (1992) Orbito-palpebral reconstruction in anophthalmos and severe congenital microphthalmos. Adv Ophthalmic Plast Reconstr Surg 9:67–80
31. O'Keefe M, Webb M, Pashby RC, Wagman RD (1987) Clinical anophthalmos. Br J Ophthalmol 71:635–638
32. Pearce WG, Nigam S, Rootman J (1974) Primary anophthalmos – histological and genetic features. Can J Ophthalmol 9:141–145
33. Pritikin RI (1980) The rarity of true congenital bilateral anophthalmos. Metab Pediatr Ophthalmol 4:165–167
34. Rodallec A (1996) Orbit and eyelid expansion: intraorbital expander prosthesis. In: van der Mullen JC, Gruss JS (1996) Ocular plastic surgery. Mosby-Wolfe, London, pp 55–59
35. Schittkowski M, Gundlach K, Hingst V, Behrend D, Guthoff R (2002) Self-inflating hydrogel expanders for treatment of congenital anophthalmos – clinical outcome, therapy failure and first biomechanical modifications. In: Abstracts of the 20th Meeting of the European Society of Ophthalmic Plastic and Reconstructive Surgery, 19–21 September 2002, Münster 2002
36. Schittkowski MP, Gundlach KK, Guthoff RF (2003) [Treatment of congenital clinical anophthalmos with high hydrophilic hydrogel expanders]. Ophthalmologe 100:525–534
37. Schittkowski M, Hingst V, Knaape A, Gundlach K, Fichter N, Guthoff R (2004) [Orbital volume in congenital clinical anophthalmos]. Klin Monatsbl Augenheilkd 221:898–903
38. Schittkowski MP, Gundlach KK, Guthoff RF (2004) 6 years experience with self-inflating hydrogel expanders for treatment of congenital anophthalmos. Abstracts of the 22nd Meeting of the ESOPRS 2004
39. Sjörgen T, Larsson T (1949) Microphthalmos and anophthalmos with or without coincident oligophrenia: clinical and genetic statistical study. Acta Psychiatr Neurol Suppl 56:1–103
40. Spagnolo A, Bianchi F, Calabro A, Calzolari E, Clementi M (1994) Mastroiacovo P, Meli P, Petrelli G, Tenconi R (1994) Anophthalmia and benomyl in Italy: a multicenter study based on 940,615 newborns. Reprod Toxicol 8:397–403
41. Srsen S (1974) Congenital anophthalmos in two siblings. Acta Univ Carol Med Monogr 56:136–139
42. Tucker SM, Sapp N, Collin R (1995) Orbital expansion of the congenitally anophthalmic socket. Br J Ophthalmol 79:667–671
43. Tucker S, Jones B, Collin R (1996) Systemic anomalies in 77 patients with congenital anophthalmos or microphthalmos. Eye 10:310–314
44. Warburg M (1981) Genetics of microphthalmos. Int Ophthalmol 4:45–65
45. Wiese KG (1993) Osmotically induced tissue expansion with hydrogels: a new dimension in tissue expansion? A preliminary report. J Craniomaxillofac Surg 21:309–313
46. Wiese KG (1998) Gewebedehnung mit osmotisch-aktiven Hydrogelsystemen. Habilitationsschrift. Quintessenz, Berlin
47. Wiese KG, Vogel M, Guthoff R, Gundlach KK (1999) Treatment of congenital anophthalmos with self-inflating polymer expanders: a new method. J Craniomaxillofac Surg 27:72–76
48. Wiese KG, Heinemann DE, Ostermeier D, Peters JH (2001) Biomaterial properties and biocompatibility in cell culture of a novel self-inflating hydrogel tissue expander. J Biomed Mater Res 54: 179–188

Methods to Improve Prosthesis Motility in Enucleation Surgery Without Pegging and With Emphasis on Muscle Pedunculated Flaps

17

Rudolf F. Guthoff, Michael P. Schittkowski, Artur Klett

Core Messages

- Implant wrapping is not necessary to obtain optimal prosthesis motility
- Full thickness or lamellar muscle pedunculated scleral flaps are suitable to cover the anterior implant surface
- The less soft tissue material is needed to cover the anterior implant surface, the better motility transmission to the artificial eye works
- The deeper the inferior and superior fornix is configured, the better prosthesis motility can be achieved
- Composite implants with solid silicone for the posterior and porous hydroxyapatite for the anterior part may improve prosthesis motility and maintain it as a permanent joint-like structure in Tenon's capsule

17.1 Introduction

Function is irreversibly lost, organ preservation is impossible, and esthetic demands are high. This is the dilemma we are faced with when enucleation or evisceration is inevitable. As Callahan mentioned in his introduction on surgical reconstruction in the anophthalmic socket: "To lose an eye is to suffer one of life's greatest tragedies" [1].

The person who has to undergo this procedure not only loses an organ with an important sensory function, but is also faced with a cosmetic deformity due to the absence of the eyeball. Distress over the loss of sight is generally accompanied by serious anxiety about the facial appearance. This anxiety will further increase if enucleation is recommended due to an intraocular malignancy. The latter recommendation was actually regarded as a contraindication for any orbital implant surgery by some authors up to the 1980s.

For many years it has been a common attitude for ophthalmologists to feel mainly responsible for maintaining or restoring vision. Enucleation surgery was often regarded as a straightforward and simple procedure, and was often performed as the surgical training exercise for young ophthalmologists. This has changed since orbital implant surgery has been proven to be a safe and effective procedure in the hands of specially trained eye surgeons.

17.2 Short History of Alloplastic Implants

It was Mules who first described in 1885 the use of an orbital implant to achieve better cosmetic results. He used a volume replacement of 6–7 ml resulting from the removal of the eye and inserted a spherical hollow glass implant in the scleral cavity after evisceration [2]. It was William Frost in 1886 who first buried a similar implant within Tenon's capsule, covering the glass sphere by suturing the horizontal and vertical recti muscles separately in front of the implant [3].

Most volume replacement strategies suitable for enucleation and evisceration can be regarded as being over 125 years old. Even the application of biocolonizable implants is about 100 years old: reports of Mules and Frost about their early and late complications led to trials of a wide variety of different implant materials, including the mineral matrix of cancellous bone (of bovine origin) introduced by Schmidt in 1906 [4]. He prepared his spheres by heating the cancellous bone in order to destroy all organic material leaving the calcium phosphate mineral framework [5]. This material was subsequently shown to consist predominantly of hydroxyapatite crystals with small amounts of calcium carbonate [6, 7]. Schmidt inserted the first implant in 1899 and reported the follow-up and subsequent cases at regular intervals until 1930 [4, 5, 8]. This concept, which was also recommended by Aust and Guist in 1926 [9], stimulated Molteno to combine the Allen implant buried in muscle [10] with Schmidt's original idea. He designed spherical biocolonizable implants of various sizes with good clinical results, recently summarized by Suter et al. [11].

Ruedemann in 1941 described a "plastic eye implant": This device was inserted into the orbit after enucleation and all recti muscles were directly attached using tantalum wires [12].

Motility improvement by an open contact of prosthesis and implant via an intentionally produced conjunctival defect was first proposed by Cutler in 1946 [13].

In the following decades many modifications of this implant were introduced where transmission of motility from the implant to the prosthesis was made by direct contact through a peg implanted secondarily or by means of pins primarily incorporated into the implant penetrating the conjunctiva [14–19].

Gradually the exposed or semiburied implants in conjunction with non-porous materials fell more and more into disuse as a large proportion eroded through the conjunctiva and were extruded or had to be removed because of secondary infections.

In 1983 Perry introduced his concept using coral derived hydroxyapatite in combination with penetrating pegs into vascularized porous implant material [20, 21].

17.3 Evisceration/Enucleation – Pros and Cons

For more than 100 years the controversy over enucleation versus evisceration has persisted in the ophthalmic literature. Mules [2], the forefather of implant surgery, first noted that the cosmetic results after evisceration after placing a hollow glass sphere within the scleral cavity were convincing. Two years later, however, Frost published a series of patients who developed sympathetic ophthalmia after evisceration [22].

Going through the literature, and reading the excellent overview by Migliori [23], especially helps with understanding the basis of the controversy and will assist ophthalmologists in recommending the proper procedure.

In a later section of this chapter, suggestions for achieving the best of both surgical procedures will be proposed according to the patients' specific requirements [24, 25].

It is generally accepted that enucleation and evisceration are both suitable procedures for relieving pain, treating an otherwise uncontrollable intraocular infection or for improving the cosmetic appearance. The following factors must be considered in choosing the most appropriate procedure.

17.3.1 Intraocular Malignancy

Evisceration has to be considered as an absolute contraindication when an intraocular tumor is obvious or there is any suspicion of its presence. This is also true for the application of penetrating or lamellar scleral flaps [24–26]. Every possible attempt should be made to preserve the integrity of the eyeball during the enucleation procedure.

17.3.2 Endophthalmitis

Traditionally influenced by reports on uncontrollable orbital infections before the introduction of modern antibiotics, evisceration is preferred over enucleation in order to reduce the chance of subarachnoid and orbital spread of the intraocular infection. This is under question today and even the placement of an implant in these patients seems to be a procedure worth considering as shown by Dresner and Karesh and others [27–29].

17.3.3 Blind and Painful Eye

Patients with these conditions have often undergone prior multiple procedures. To remove an eye can be a complicated surgical process in the presence of scleral buckles and conjunctival shrinkage. The risk of excessive bleeding and uncontrollable scarring of orbital tissues may well make it worth considering an evisceration procedure or at least the preservation of some scleral elements in order to cover an ocular implant [24, 25]. Nevertheless, enucleation and evisceration have both been shown to be able to control pain successfully [30, 31].

17.3.4 Sympathetic Ophthalmia

Sympathetic ophthalmia is an extremely rare but potentially devastating immunologic condition characterized by bilateral granulomatous panuveitis. The precise identity of the antigen is still inconclusive, and every ophthalmologist who has ever come into contact with patients suffering from this condition will consider surgery which leaves potential antigens coming out of the choroid or the retina as being unacceptable. This is especially important to consider as in almost every case enucleation techniques in combination with implant surgery can produce very satisfactory results. It should be stated, nevertheless, that in retrospective studies involving over 3,000 eviscerations, no case of sympathetic ophthalmia has been identified and the authors personally have observed this only in eyes suffering from severe trauma where the sympathetic ophthalmia occurred before removal of the eye [22, 32].

Summary for the Clinician

- **Evisceration and implantation of alloplastic implants seems to give the best motility transmission to the artificial eye**
- **Sympathetic ophthalmia is still not fully understood devastating and blinding disease, so principally enucleation techniques are justified and should be considered in each individual case**

17.4 Orbital Implants – Materials, Shape, Implantation Technique

There are two major groups of orbital implants: (1) integrated vs. non-integrated, and (2) buried vs. exposed. It is generally accepted that no matter what type of implant is used after enucleation in the years to come, the orbital contents will tend to contract posteriorly resulting in the known superior sulcus deformity. This may also be associated with reduced implant motility due to a mild chronic inflammation in some implant materials. This can cause firm fibrous adhesions with the surrounding soft tissue structures [33] (Fig. 17.1).

17.4.1 Non-integrated Implants

This term is used for materials which allow neither ingrowth of granulation tissue nor preformed attachments for the extraocular muscles. They do not have direct contact with the ocular prosthesis. Materials used include silicone, polymethylmethacrylate (PMMA), acrylic and previously also glass, rubber and other materials.

The imbrication of the recti muscles in front of a spherical implant definitely improves implant as well as prosthesis motility. The system can be considered as a ball-and-socket joint. The extent of motion transmission between implant and prosthesis is mainly influenced by two factors:

1. The thickness of tissue material covering the anterior implant surface
2. The depth of the superior and inferior fornices [34] (Figs. 17.2, 17.3A, B).

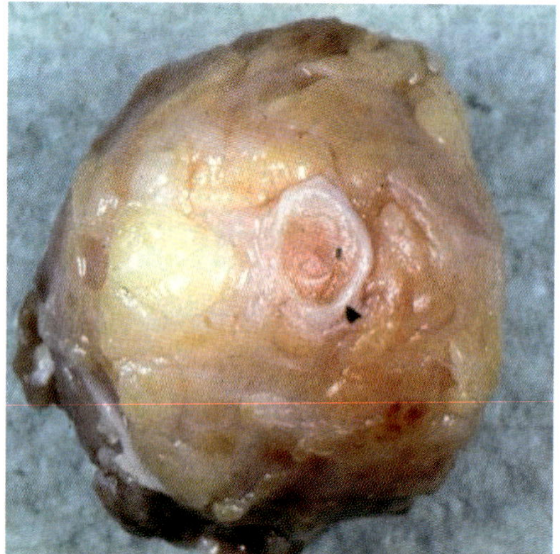

Fig. 17.1. Enucleated Bangerter implant. The implant removal was necessary because of a chronic infection and a non-healing conjunctival dehiscence. Note the firm tissue ingrowth into the nylon meshwork including an attachment of the optic nerve remnant which finally caused a scarred implant with no prosthesis motility [33]

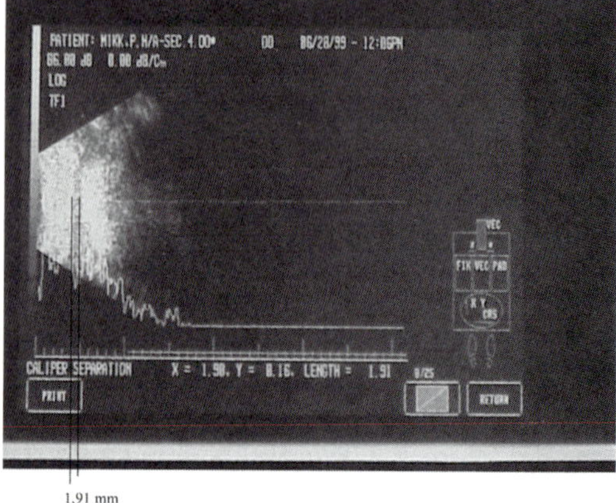

Fig. 17.2. B-scan picture displaying a 1.9-mm soft tissue layer in front of a hydroxyapatite-silicone implant. This amount of healthy tissue in front of the implant allows good motility transmission to the artificial eye [34]

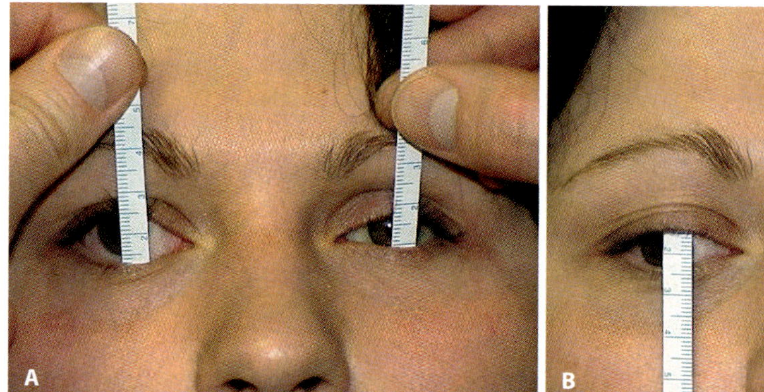

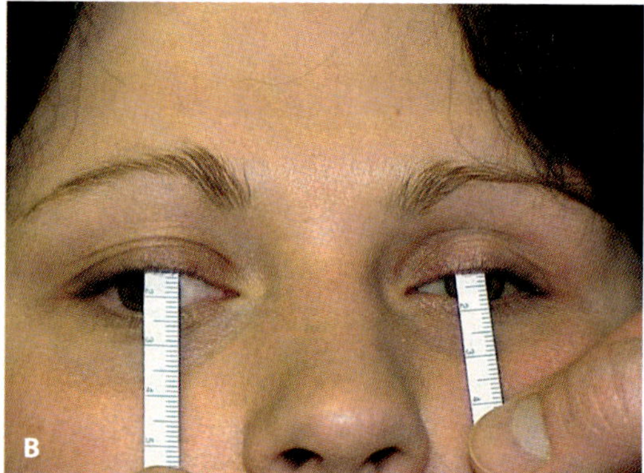

Fig. 17.3. Measuring the depth of the inferior (**A**) and superior (**B**) fornices. Note: The deeper the fornix in front of the artificial eye the better the motility transmission [34]

As a thin tissue layer in front of an alloplastic material does increase the risk of implant erosion, it is worth considering refined techniques of implant covering such as muscle pedunculated scleral flaps in selected patients [25]. It has been suggested that imbrication of the recti muscles over non-integrated implants can result in implant migration caused by contraction of the recti muscles [35, 36].

This phenomenon may also be addressed by a modification of the imbrication technique (Fig. 17.4A–C).

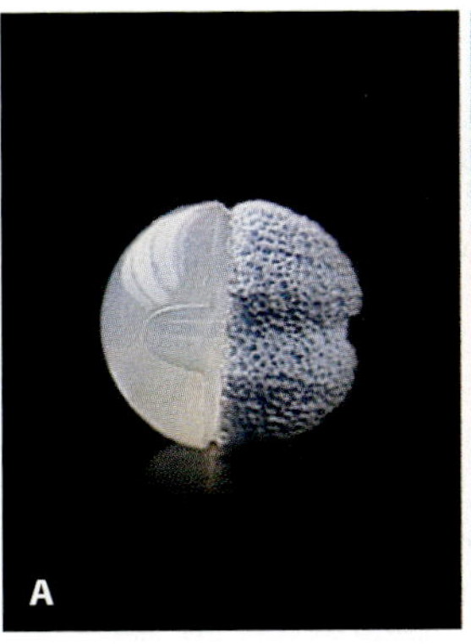

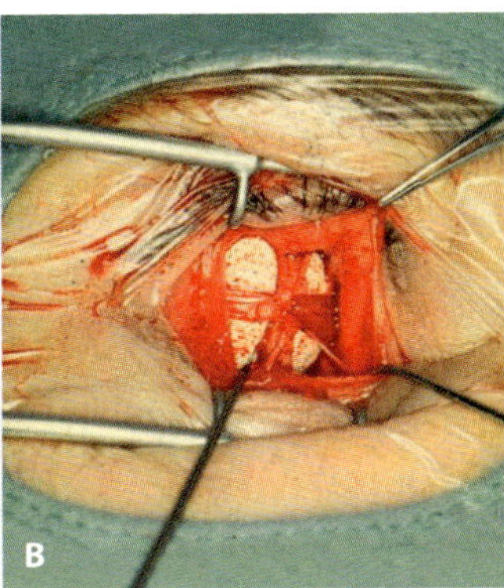

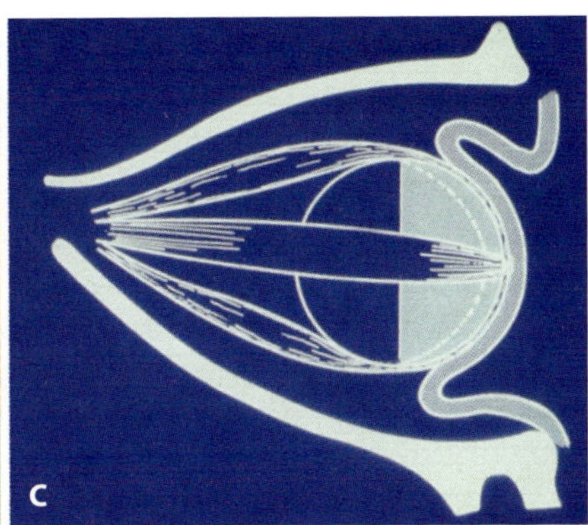

Fig. 17.4. A Hydroxyapatite-silicone implant with grooves to simplify crosswise fixation of recti muscles during surgery. **B** Surgical procedure with muscles in front of the hydroxyapatite part of the implant before closure of Tenon's capsule and conjunctiva [25]. **C** Schematic drawing with the hydroxyapatite-silicone implant in place, creating a joint-like structure between the remnant of Tenon's capsule and the posterior silicone part of the implant [33]

17.4.2 Integrated Implants

Porous materials which allow some tissue ingrowth first were introduced by Bangerter using a nylon meshwork. These materials have been abolished since chronic infections occurred in some of the patients and since the demands for cosmesis were not as high as they are today.

17.4.2.1 Ceramic Materials

The hydroxyapatite orbital implant was introduced by Perry. It was made from modified coral material and reported to be non-toxic, non-allergenic and highly biocompatible [37, 38]. Fully synthetic porous hydroxyapatite ceramics were introduced in 1987 [39] and further modified by adding a posterior segment of the spherical prosthesis produced out of solid silicone [33].*

Large series of synthetic ceramic implants have been published by various authors [40–43]. The first paper dealing with synthetic hydroxyapatite as a porous composition was published by Osborn in 1985 [44]. Specially standardized porous aluminum hydroxite seems to be a new and interesting alternative [45].

17.4.2.2 Porous Polyethylene

Porous polyethylene can be regarded as an integrated implant which allows fibrovascular ingrowth, but not as rapidly as hydroxyapatite [46, 47]. Nevertheless it eventually reaches the center of the alloplastic material [48]. Porous polyethylene implants are smooth enough to be implanted without any other type of wrapping material and are equally suitable for direct muscle suturing at points approximating the original dimensions according to the spiral of Tillaux [49].

Summary for the Clinician

- **Implant materials have been developed to a high standard of biocompatibility**
- **Independently from the chosen materials, muscle attachments are mandatory to transmit motility as well as to stimulate implant integration**

* The first author has a financial interest in this as he is the patent holder of the hydroxyapatite silicone implant.

17.5 Wrapping Materials

The goal of wrapping implants is to allow the precise attachment of the recti muscles to simulate the normal anatomic muscle positions [20, 50] and also to minimize the likelihood of exposure. Hydroxyapatite is particularly difficult to work with because it tends to cling to the surrounding tissue [51].

Porous ceramic implants definitively complicate the implantation technique as these materials behave like a cactus pushed through soft tissue structures – taking anterior portions of tissue far back into the orbit, where they may stimulate migration of the implants towards the conjunctival surface.

The advantage of unwrapped porous material on the other hand may be that there is no barrier to vascularization and of course it is also more cost effective. The theoretical risk of transmitting prion-type disease through non-autogenous donor wrapping material is also eliminated with unwrapped techniques [20].

Autologous materials for wrapping implants include temporalis fascia, fascia lata, dermis and auricular muscle complex. The advantage of these grafts is that we are dealing with living autologous tissue which will exclude foreign body reactions and which will be vascularized rapidly. Synthetic products such as polyglactin 910 (Vicryl®) are advocated by Jordan [52] and have been used in more than 50 patients with success. The discussion of whether it is still worth developing techniques and implants where wrapping can be avoided is still ongoing. Long and co-workers reported in 2003 in a randomized trial that placement of an unwrapped hydroxyapatite implant provides equivalent motility when compared with wrapped spheres of the same material [51].

Summary for the Clinician

- **Biologic wrapping materials are expensive and the risk of disease transmission cannot be totally neglected**
- **It is worth looking for techniques which avoid any biologic material in enucleation surgery**

17.6 Indications for Pegging

Both theoretically and through reviewing the literature on semi-open implants, pegging should improve prosthesis motility. Porous integrated implants after vascularized integration should theoretically reduce the risk of infection and extrusion of pegs as the alloplastic transconjunctivally placed material enters vascularized tissue with a better capacity for local wound healing [53]. Controversy exists, however, regarding the use of the peg and the time that drilling should be performed. Many patients decline the secondary peg procedure because the movement produced by the primary implant was also already satisfactory, especially for eye movements unconsciously performed during conversation [54, 55]. In addition to escalating costs, some studies have reported peg complications in up to 45% of patients [53]. These complications include peg extrusion, secondary infection, audible click and chronic non-specific conjunctivitis [56].

A recent publication [57] has demonstrated in a sophisticated study that at least the wide angle movement of the prosthesis can be improved by the placement of a motility peg in a secondary procedure. Complications may be reduced if peg and sleeve systems with hydroxyapatite coated titanium design are applied.

17.7 Motility Evaluation

In order to compare the transmission quality of implant to prosthesis motility, an objective evaluation should be performed. This can be done via a transparent ruler or with a Kestenbaum spectacle when eye excursions in all directions should be evaluated [58] (Fig. 17.5). More sophisticated techniques have been published adapting newer methods which will allow the most precise simultaneous bilateral motility evaluations [57].

A semiautomated evaluation was described by Klett et al. [34] using digital cameras and offline computer evaluation of the excursion of the prosthesis as well as the implant (Fig. 17.6). For clinical use also the Tranbront/Ruler method seems to be very effective and reproducible [58].

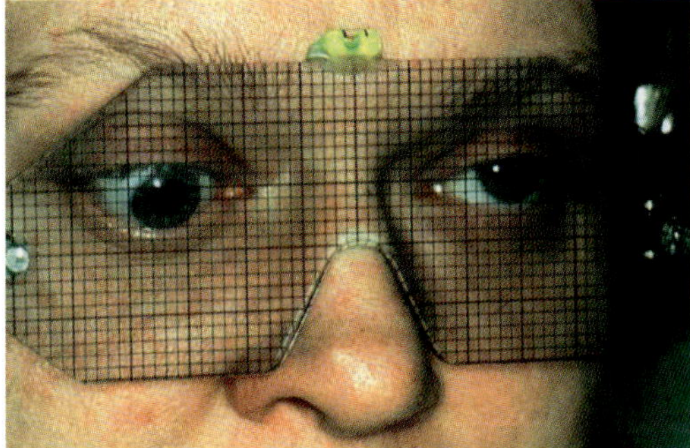

Fig. 17.5. Kestenbaum spectacle to simplify measurements of lid aperture, levator function, implant and prosthesis motility

17.8 Strategies to Improve Prosthesis Motility Without Pegging

Although direct coupling of porous implants to the prosthesis via the motility peg can provide improved prosthesis movement, many patients prefer to avoid a second procedure as Custer and co-workers have pointed out [59].

Nevertheless, it is worth considering the known factors that influence movement transmission between implant and artificial eye. As a primary factor, it is the amplitude of movement of the implant which should be evaluated and techniques applied that can possibly further improve its amplitude. Theoretically, adhesions between the posterior part and the implant may mechanically prevent maximal excursions as demonstrated in Bangerter implants produced from polyamide meshwork as published in 1995 [33]. The posterior part of the hydroxyapatite implant covered by smooth silicone increased prosthesis motility as measured by the Kestenbaum technique [58]. An overall horizontal motility of 8 mm compared to 18 mm in the

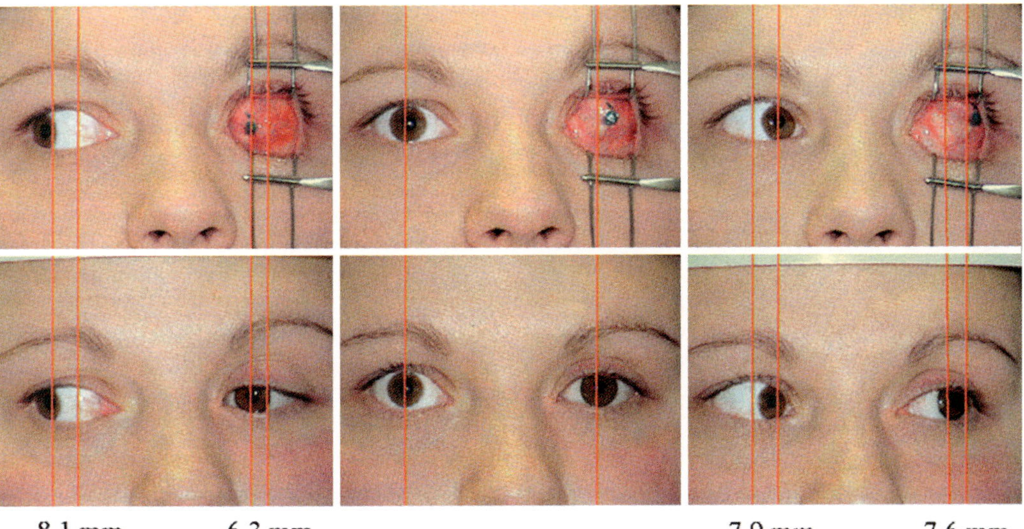

Fig. 17.6. Comparison of implant motility and prosthetic motility after implantation of a 20-mm hydroxyapatite-silicone implant – *upper photos* show the center of the implant overlying conjunctiva marked with *blue*; *lower photos* show patient after insertion of a thin prosthesis with a good motility transmission [34]

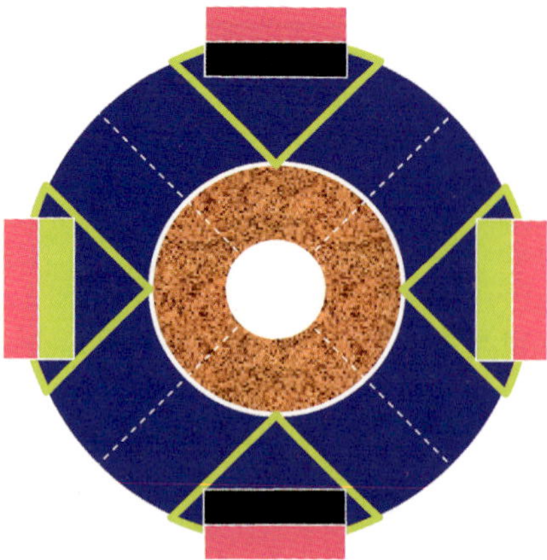

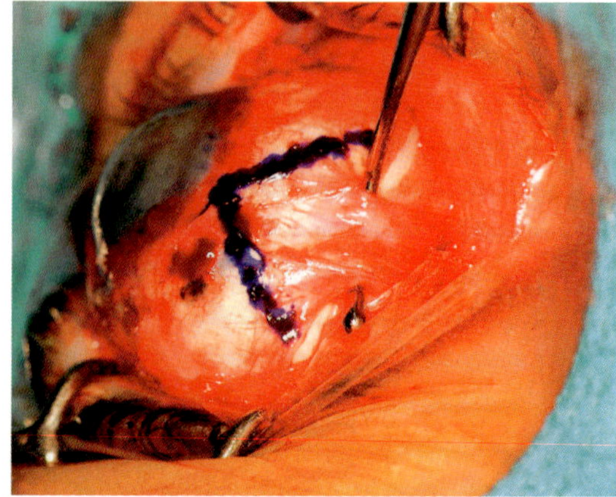

Fig. 17.7. The shape of the triangular scleral flap including the muscle insertion area

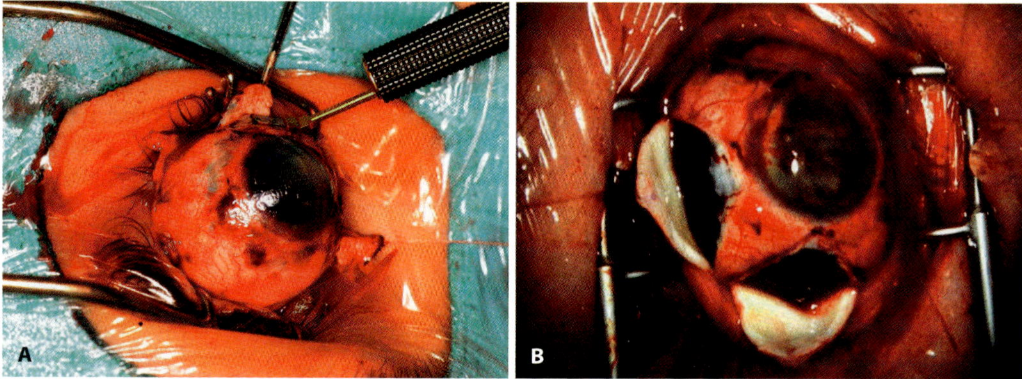

Fig. 17.8. A Lamellar preparation of muscle pedunculated scleral flaps. B Full thickness preparation of muscle pedunculated scleral flaps

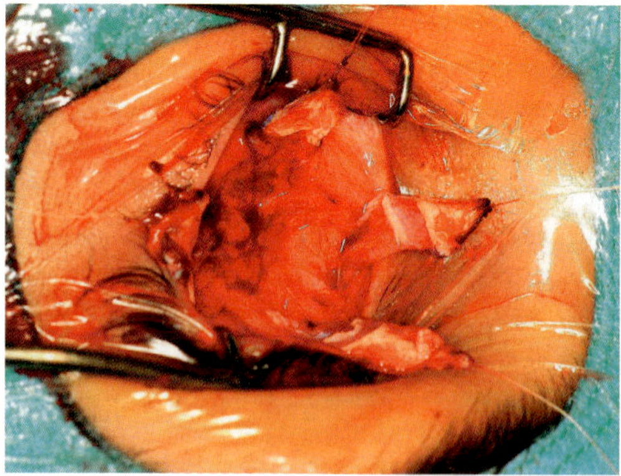

Fig. 17.9. Muscle pedunculated scleral flaps after enucleation

normal eye still did not produce fully satisfactory results. A probably underestimated factor which influences motility transmission is the depth of the conjunctival fornices. This was pointed out recently by Klett et al., who demonstrated a strong correlation between the depth of the superior and inferior fornices and prosthesis motility [34]. In the same paper, the thickness of tissue material covering the implant's anterior surface was also shown to play a role in motility transmission: The thinner the tissue coverage and the deeper the fornices, the better the motility transmission that could be found.

In order to address these two factors, a surgical technique was developed using muscle pe-

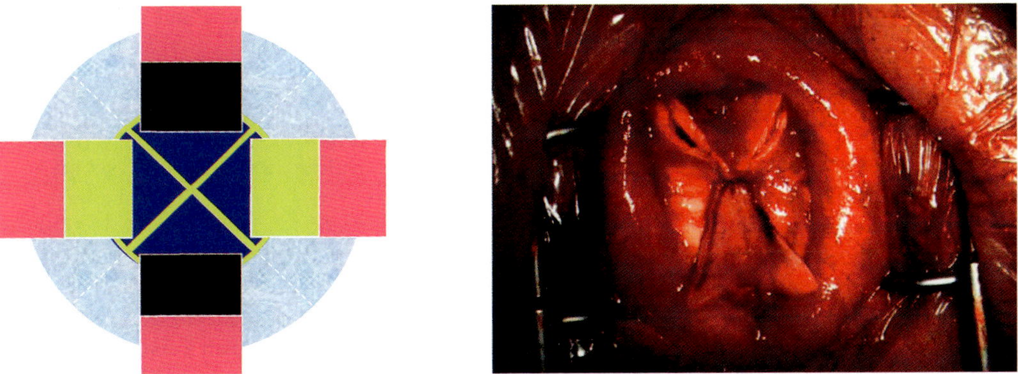

Fig. 17.10. Implant covered by triangular-shaped muscle pedunculated scleral flaps

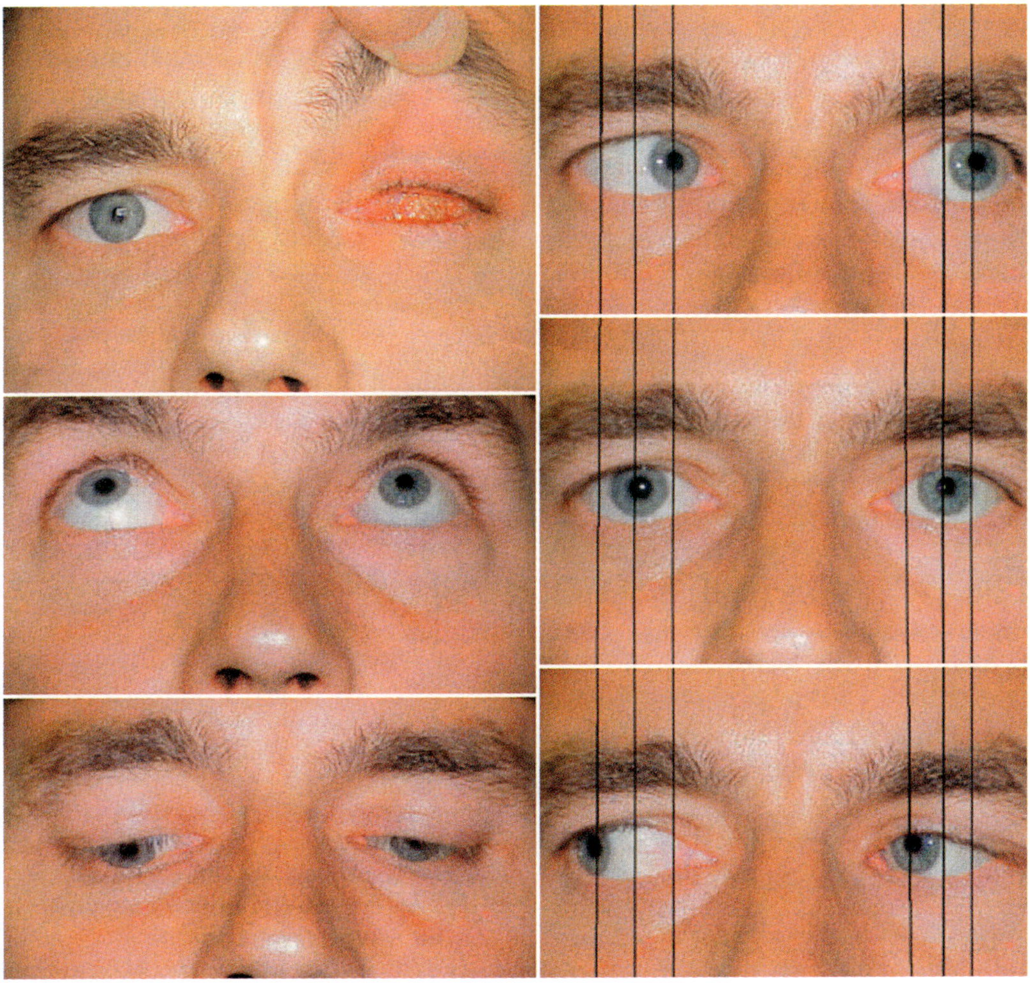

Fig. 17.11. Motility transmission of a 22-mm hydroxyapatite-silicone implant covered with lamellar muscle pedunculated scleral flaps in the left orbit. Differences in all directions of gaze between prosthesis and normal eye are less than 2 mm [34]

dunculated scleral flaps as an autologous covering material for the anterior implant surface. Since 1989 the authors have been using a hydroxyapatite silicone implant which is placed in the muscle cone without any extra covering material. Until recently, the technique as primarily described by Molteno has been applied, covering the implant in place by crosswise suturing of all recti muscles in front of its anterior surface. We have personal experience with this implant in over 300 patients and a considerable number have also been used by our European colleagues.

This product is made out of a porous anterior ceramic part to be integrated in the surrounding tissues and a posterior part from medical grade silicone rubber to create a smooth joint-like structure articulating with Tenon's space. To improve both implant and prosthesis motility and to avoid pegging, which never became popular in Europe, a full thickness and subsequently a lamellar sclera dissection technique was developed (Figs. 17.7–17.10).

Both techniques create muscle pedunculated scleral flaps to smoothly cover the hydroxyapatite silicone implant while avoiding any other alloplastic material. In the lamellar modification the sclera is only partly dissected with an adjustable blade of a diamond knife in a microsurgical procedure. The dissection is continued with a blade for cataract tunnel incisions or a hockey knife. After dissecting the superior and the inferior oblique muscles, the eye is taken out leaving four triangles of the lamellar sclera flaps (Fig. 17.9). This tissue is fully vascularized via its natural blood supply. The implant selected is placed in the muscle cone and the flaps sutured to each other by 6×0 Vicryl®. This forms an implant covering of a cup-like structure with vital and strong connective tissue [25].

Surgery is completed by an absorbable running suture through the conjunctiva and the insertion of a large conformer to support the creation of deep fornices. This procedure is not advocated for tumor-containing eyes. Thus far, more than 40 patients have been treated in this way. In one of them a small defect occurred after 3 months, which was closed without problems. The authors suggest a 22-mm implant and the fitting of a large prosthesis expanding widely into the fornices for optimal motility transmission (Fig. 17.11).

Summary for the Clinician

- **Prosthesis motility is enhanced by deep conjunctival fornices and large orbital implants**

17.9 Suggestions for an Effective Compromise Between Enucleation and Evisceration: Muscle Pedunculated Scleral Flaps

In times where medicolegal aspects play a major role in medicine, muscle pedunculated scleral flaps to cover the implant have been proposed which combine the objectives of evisceration surgery for optimal cosmetic and functional results with a reduced risk for serious complications [25, 26]. This technique, which has become the standard procedure in the authors' hands in eyes where no tumor is suspected, will be described in some detail:

Surgical procedure:

1. Retrobulbar injection of 5 cc local anesthetic with a vasoconstrictor (when the procedure is performed with the patient under general anesthesia, local anesthetic solution can be replaced by saline solution). The infiltration of the retrobulbar space simplifies optic nerve dissection and reduces the chance of intra- and postoperative hemorrhage.
2. Staining of the limbal conjunctiva with a marker pen circular limbal incision dissection of Tenon's space as far posterior as possible
3. At this stage the optic nerve is cut preferentially via the medial inferior quadrant followed by 3 min of posterior orbital compression to stop bleeding
4. Marking of triangular incision lines on the sclera (Fig. 17.7) and a partial thickness scleral incision along the lines with a preadjusted diamond knife (0.3 mm depth of incision)
5. Placement of a 6×0 Vicryl suture at the apex of the scleral triangles
6. Dissection of the scleral triangles up to a line central to the muscle insertions (this step can be performed either full thickness – the

Table 17.1. Prosthesis motility (mm) in patients with hydroxyapatite silicone implant (ref. [25], Table 2)

	Group 1 (*N*=15 with crosswise fixated recti muscles in front of the implant)	Group 2 (*N*=15 with muscle pedunculated scleral flaps)	Improvement of duction (mm)	Normal eye (*N*=30)
Abduction	3.7±1.2	5.4±2.1	1.7	8.7±1.7
Adduction	3.4±1.8	5.0±2.1	1.6	8.2±1.0
Elevation	2.9±1.9	4.2±2.3	1.3	5.6±1.4
Depression	3.2±1.5	4.5±1.2	1.3	6.1±1.2
Average	3.3±1.6	4.8±1.8	1.5	7.1±1.3

choroid generally falls back or can be dissected bluntly with the spatula – or partial thickness using a tunnel blade as applied in cataract surgery; Fig. 17.8a, b)

7. When all scleral flaps are fully separated the "fenestrated" globe is enucleated by dissecting the insertions of the superior and the inferior oblique muscles. Generally this is performed without any extra bleeding.
8. The implant (preferably a hydroxyapatite-silicone implant for the reasons mentioned above) is placed in the muscle cone and the triangular muscle pedunculated scleral flaps are sutured together with 6×0 Vicryl®. This creates a cap-like structure or vascularized covering of the anterior implant surface.
9. Tenon's capsule is approximated with a running 6×0 Vicryl® suture.
10. Conjunctiva is closed in the same way where the blue marker pen color helps to identify the borders to avoid invagination of epithelial surface structures.
11. A rather large conformer is placed in the conjunctival sac to ensure a deep superior and inferior sulcus.

The decision of whether a full thickness or a lamellar scleral flap is dissected does not play a role in the final outcome of implant prosthesis motility. In eyes with thin sclera due to myopia or due to multiple surgical procedures in the past it may be difficult or impossible to perform lamellar flaps. In phthisical eyes we are generally dealing with a thickened sclera where lamellar surgery is mostly straightforward.

Advantages of muscle pedunculated scleral flaps in combination with hydroxyapatite-silicone implants: this concept benefits from the combination of an implant that "per se" needs no extra covering, creating a joint-like structure at its posterior part and an anterior coverage of fully vascularized autologous scleral tissue still attached to its natural blood supply through the recti muscles. This allows a quick vascularization of the anterior porous hydroxyapatite part of the implant and stabilizes the long-term biomechanics of the system.

The departments at Rostock and Tallinn are reviewing more than 60 patients operated on with this new modified technique since 1995 with only two implant exposures, which were easily closed using local tissue without any subsequent recurrence.

Motility of the artificial eye as transmitted by the implant was measured in a series of 15 patients from 1997 to 2001 (Table 17.1). It could be demonstrated that muscle pedunculated flaps increase the horizontal motility by about 3 mm and the vertical motility about 2.5 mm compared with the previous technique, where the muscles were sutured crosswise in front of the implant without any scleral attachments.

Summary for the Clinician

- **Muscle pedunculated scleral flaps are suitable for all non-tumor bearing eyes**
- **They improve implant and prosthesis motility with minimal risk of extrusion**
- **Rehabilitation time is shortened**

References

1. Callahan A (1987) Introduction. In: Vistnes LM (ed) Surgical reconstruction in the anophthalmic orbit. Aesculapius Publishing Co., Birmingham, AL
2. Mules PH (1885) Evisceration of the globe with artificial vitreous. Trans Ophthalmol Soc U K 5:200–206
3. Frost WA (1887) Cited in Lane W: "On the insertion of artificial globes into Tenon's capsule after excising the eye". Trans Ophthalmol Soc U K 7:286
4. Schmidt H (1906) Zur Lösung des Problems der Kugeleinheilung. Z Augenheilk 16:63–80
5. Schmidt H (1910) Zur Lösung des Problems der Kugeleinheilung. Nachtrag 1909. Z Augenheilk 23:321–339
6. Klement R, Trämel G (1932) Hydroxylapatit, der Hauptbestandteil der anorganischen Knochen- und Zahnsubstanz. Hoppe-Seyler's Z Physiol Chemie 230:263–269
7. McLean FC, Urist MR (eds) (1968) Bone fundamentals of the physiology of skeletal tissue, 3rd edn. University of Chicago Press, Chicago
8. Schmidt H (1930) Zur kritischen Würdigung der plastischen Stumpfbildungsmethoden. Verlag von S. Karger, Berlin
9. Aust W, Guist G (1926) Zur Stumpfverbesserung nach Enukleation. Denk W, Schriftleiter. Wiener Klinische Wochenschrift. Organ der Gesellschaft der Ärzte in Wien, p 934
10. Allen JH, Allen L (1950) A buried muscle cone implant. Arch Ophthalmol 43:879–890
11. Suter AJ, et al. (2002) Long term follow up of bone derived hydroxyapatite orbital implants. Br J Ophthalmol 86:1287–1292
12. Ruedemann AD (1946) Plastic eye implant. Am J Ophthalmol 29:947–952
13. Cutler NL (1947) A positive contact ball and ring implant for use after enucleation. Arch Ophthalmol 37:73–81
14. Arruga H (1954) Improved orbital implant. Am J Ophthalmol 38:93–95
15. Durham DG (1949) The new ocular implants. Am J Ophthalmol 32:79–89
16. Gougelmann HP (1970) The evolution of the ocular motility implant. Int Ophthalmol Clin 10:689–711
17. Guyton JS (1949) Symposium: orbital implants after enucleation. Procedures and physiologic factors. Trans Am Acad Ophthalmol 32:1725–1734
18. Hughes WL (1952) Symposium: orbital implants after enucleation. Classification and mechanics involved. Trans Am Acad Ophthalmol Otolaryngol 56:25–27
19. Smit TJ, et al. (1991) Management of acquired anophthalmos: an historical review. In: The post enucleation socket syndrome. Academisch Proefschrift, Amsterdam
20. Perry AC (1990) Integrated orbital implants. In: Bosniak SL (ed) Advances in ophthalmic plastic and reconstructive surgery 8: the anophthalmic socket. Pergamon Press, New York, pp 75–81
21. Roper-Hall MJ (1954) Orbital implants. Trans Ophthalmol Soc U K 74:337–346
22. Cytryn AS, Perman KI (1999) Evisceration. In: Migliori ME (ed) Enucleation, evisceration and exenteration of the eye. Butterworth-Heinemann, Boston, pp 105–112
23. Migliori ME (2002) Enucleation versus evisceration. Curr Opin Ophthalmol 13:298–302
24. Guthoff RF, Schittkowski MP, Klett A (2003) Muscle pedunculated lamellar scleral flaps for implant coverage – a microsurgical modification to improve prosthesis motility. In: ASOPRS Scientific Fall Symposium, 2003. ASOPRS Executive Committee, Anaheim, CA
25. Klett A, Guthoff RF (2003) Deckung von Orbitaimplantaten mit muskelgestielter autologer Sklera. Eine mikrochirurgische Modifikation zur Verbesserung der Prothesenmotilität. Ophthalmologe 100:449–452
26. Schittkowski MP, Klett A, Guthoff RF (2003) A microsurgical modification of implant coverage after enucleation – first experiences with muscle pedunculated lamellar scleral flaps. In: 21st Meeting of the European Society of Ophthalmic Plastic and Reconstructive Surgery, 12–13 Sept. 2003. ESOPRS, Gothenburg
27. Dresner SC, Karesh JW (2000) Primary implant placement with evisceration in patients with endophthalmitis. Ophthalmology 107:1664–1665
28. Shore JW, Dieckert JW, Levine MR (1988) Delayed primary wound closure: use to prevent implant extrusion following evisceration for endophthalmitis. Arch Ophthalmol 106:1303–1308
29. Walter WL (1985) Update on enucleation and evisceration surgery. Ophthal Plast Reconstr Surg 1:243–252
30. Custer PL, Reistad CE (2000) Enucleation of blind, painful eyes. Ophthal Plast Reconstr Surg 16:326–329
31. Shah-Desai SD, Tyers AG, Manners RM (2000) Painful blind eye: efficacy of enucleation and evisceration in resolving ocular pain. Br J Ophthalmol 84:437–438
32. Levine MR, Pou CR, Lash RH (1999) The 1998 Wendell Hughes Lecture. Evisceration: is sympathetic ophthalmia a concern in the new millenium? Ophthal Plast Reconstr Surg 15:4–8

33. Guthoff RF, Vick HP, Schaudig U (1995) Zur Prophylaxe des Postenukleationssyndroms: Das Hydroxylapatitsilikonimplantat. Ophthalmologe 92: 198–205
34. Klett A, Guthoff RF (2003) Wie läßt sich die Prothesenmotilität verbessern? Der Einfluss von Fornixtiefe und Gewebedicke vor einem Hydroxylapatitsilikon-Implantat bei 66 Patienten. Ophthalmologe 100:445–448
35. Allen L (1983) The argument against imbricating the rectus muscles over spherical orbital implants after enucleation. Ophthalmology 90:1116–1120
36. Beard C (1995) Remarks on historical and newer approaches to orbital implants. Ophthal Plast Reconstr Surg 11:89–90
37. Perry AC (1997) Hydroxyapatite: the vascularizing integrated orbital implant. In: Stepherson CM (ed) Ophthalmic plastic, reconstructive, and orbital surgery. Butterworth-Heinemann, Boston, pp 463–479
38. Shields CL, Shields JA, De Potter P (1992) Hydroxyapatite orbital implant after enucleation: experience with initial 100 consecutive cases. Arch Ophthalmol 110:333–338
39. Guthoff RF, Donath K, Osborn JF (1986) Solid hydroxyapatite ceramics as implant material after enucleation. In: XXVth International Congress of Ophthalmology, Amsterdam, 1987. XXV Concilium Ophthalmologicum. Kugler and Ghedini, Rome
40. Jordan DR, Bawazeer A (2001) Experience with 120 synthetic hydroxyapatite implants (FCI3). Ophthal Plast Reconstr Surg 17:221–223
41. Ducasse A, et al. (2001) Tolerance of orbital implants. Retrospective study on 14 years. J Fr Ophthalmol 24:277–281
42. Adenis JP, Dourlhes N (1998) Implants en ceramique. In: Adenis JP, Morax S (eds) Pathologie orbito-palpebrale. Societe Française d'Ophtalmologie. Masson, Paris, pp 675–678
43. Rulfi JY, Adenis JP (2001) Past and present trends in intraorbital biointegrated macroporous material implants. Operative Tech Oculoplast Orbital Reconstr Surg 4:30–35
44. Osborn JF (1985) Implantwerkstoff Hydroxylapatitkeramik. Quintessenz, Berlin
45. Robert PY, Rulfi JY, Adenis JP (2003) Neue Keramikmaterialien zur Verwendung in der Anophthalmuschirurgie. Ophthalmologe 100:503–506
46. Rubin PA, et al. (1994) Comparison of fibrovascular ingrowth into hydroxyapatite and porous polyethylene orbital implants. Ophthal Plast Reconstr Surg 10:96–103
47. Goldberg RA, Dresner SC, Braslow RA, et al. (1994) Animal model of porous polyethylene orbital implants. Ophthal Plast Reconstr Surg 10:101–109
48. Karcioglu ZA, Mullaney PB, Millar LC (1998) Extrusion of porous polyethylene orbital implant in recurrent retinoblastoma. Ophthal Plast Reconstr Surg 14:37–44
49. Karesh JW, Dresner SC (1994) High-density porous polyethylene (Medpor) as a successful anophthalmic socket implant. Ophthalmology 101:1688–1695; discussion 1695–1696
50. Remulla HD, Rubin PA, Shore JW, et al. (1995) Complications of porous spherical orbital implants. Ophthalmology 102:586–593
51. Long JA, et al. (2003) Enucleation: is wrapping the implant necessary for optimal motility? Ophthal Plast Reconstr Surg 19:194–197
52. Jordan DR, Allen LH, Ells A (1995) The use of Vicryl mesh (polyglactin 910) for implantation of hydroxyapatite orbital implants. Ophthal Plast Reconstr Surg 11:95–99
53. Edelstein C, Shields CL, De Potter P, et al. (1997) Complications of motility peg placement for the hydroxyapatite orbital implant. Ophthalmology 104:1616–1621
54. Cepela AC, Teske S (1996) Orbital implants. Curr Opin Ophthalmol 7:38–42
55. Cowper TR (1995) Hydroxyapatite motility implants in ocular prosthetics. J Prosthet Dent 73:267–273
56. Jordan DR, et al. (1999) Complications associated with pegging hydroxyapatite implants. Ophthalmology 106:505–512
57. Guillinta P, Vasani SN, Granet DB, Kikkawa DO (2003) Prosthetic motility in pegged versus unpegged integrated porous orbital implants. Ophthal Plast Reconstr Surg 19:119–122
58. Haase W (1976) Messung der maximalen Bewegungsstrecken der Bulbi. Graefes Arch Clin Exp Ophthalmol 198:291–296
59. Custer PL, Trinkaus KM, Fornoff J (1999) Comparative motility of hydroxyapatite and alloplastic enucleation implants. Ophthalmology 106: 513–516

Current Management of Traumatic Enophthalmos

Richard C. Allen, Jeffrey A. Nerad

Core Messages

- Enophthalmos is a common deformity after orbital trauma
- A thorough knowledge of orbital anatomy aids the clinician in the diagnosis and treatment of traumatic enophthalmos
- Evaluation of the patient with enophthalmos after trauma consists of a complete history and physical examination with special attention to ocular function and periocular and periorbital structures
- Traumatic enophthalmos can be classified as immediate, early, and late. Treatment is dependent upon the timing of the enophthalmos
- The mechanism of traumatic enophthalmos is related to bony volume expansion, primarily, followed by soft tissue contraction and fat herniation or atrophy
- The most common orbital fractures associated with traumatic enophthalmos are orbital floor blow-out fractures and zygomatico-maxillary complex (ZMC) fractures
- Indications for repair in acute trauma include facial asymmetry, a palpable "step" on the orbital rim, enophthalmos, restrictive strabismus, and trismus
- Early surgical correction of orbital fractures offers the best correction of facial deformity. Late intervention is accompanied by increased risk and worse functional result
- There are specific guidelines for the repair of orbital floor and ZMC fractures that are reviewed in this chapter
- Late repair of traumatic enophthalmos should address displaced orbital bones and soft tissue first. If enophthalmos persists, then orbital augmentation should be performed
- Orbital augmentation may be performed with autogenous or alloplastic implants
- Enophthalmos associated with the anophthalmic socket is a common problem addressed by the oculoplastic surgeon. Treatment involves tightening of the lower lid and orbital volume augmentation

18.1 Introduction

Orbital deformity after trauma is a well described entity, and, as with other reconstructive problems, a systematic approach is useful. Early primary repair of traumatic deformity of the orbit is the preferred treatment, but for a number of reasons, late repairs are sometimes necessary, often with less than adequate results [17]. In this chapter, we discuss the most common post-traumatic orbital deformity, enophthalmos. Through a systematic approach of primary and secondary repair, we believe that a satisfactory postoperative result can be obtained.

18.1.1 Anatomy

The anatomy of the orbit has evolved to protect the globe from direct and indirect injury. A strong orbital rim protects the globe. The thin orbital floor and medial wall fracture outward when increased orbital pressure occurs. This "pressure valve" dissipates the energy of impact, often avoiding a ruptured globe. The orbital architecture has predictable strong and weak areas resulting in predictable patterns of fracture.

18.1.1.1 Bony Anatomy

The orbital aperture is a modified oval with sutures between the maxillary, zygomatic, and frontal bones [25]. The small number of bones along the orbital rim and the strength of the individual bones result in predictable fractures along suture lines from blunt trauma. The orbital rim almost always fractures in two or more places, similar to a fracture of the pelvis. Rim fractures are usually associated with an underlying orbital wall fracture due to the extension of the suture lines to the orbital walls.

The four walls of the orbit increase in diameter just posterior to the rim, followed by a slow taper to the orbital apex. The medial wall and orbital floor are the most common walls to fracture. These walls, adjacent to sinuses, are subject to fracture for two reasons: they are thin bones and there is no resistance to fracture on the side of the sinus. The lamina papyracea of the ethmoid bone is the thinnest bone of the body. The orbital floor sustains the typical "blow-out" fracture, either due to buckling of the inferior orbital floor from blunt trauma to the inferior orbital rim or an increase in orbital pressure from blunt trauma to the globe, or a combination of the two. The floor posterior to the rim is first concave and then, just posterior to the globe, convex upward inclining at a 30-degree angle. This results in a constriction to the orbit posterior to the globe. The medial wall of the orbit is joined by the floor posteriorly at a 45-degree angle, resulting in further constriction of the orbit posteriorly. This posterior anatomy is a key determinant of globe position and also a common site of fracture.

The superior orbital rim and roof are relatively strong and resistant to fracture. Orbital roof fractures are often accompanied by other fractures of the skull requiring neurosurgical intervention. A CSF leak is common in this setting. Also, a force to the frontal bone great enough to cause fracture should always increase the suspicion of a traumatic optic neuropathy. A lateral wall fracture, likewise, is rarely an isolated fracture. The anterior portion of the lateral wall is formed by the zygoma. The posterior portion is formed by the sphenoid bone. Both of these bones are thick and rarely fracture, except as part of a zygomatico-maxillary complex (ZMC) fracture. The fracture occurs between the zygoma and the temporal, frontal, and/or maxillary bones along the rim and zygomatic arch. Within the orbit, the ZMC fracture involves the zygomatico-maxillary and zygomatico-sphenoid suture. Most commonly, enophthalmos results when the bony orbital volume is "expanded" due to displacement of the orbital walls.

18.1.1.2 Soft Tissue Anatomy

The soft tissue of the orbit consists of the globe, fat, and muscles surrounded by connective tissue and neurovascular structures. The total volume of the orbit is 30–35 ml. Enophthalmos secondary to trauma from soft tissue changes is thought to be due to fat atrophy but can result from damage to the globe or muscles. Likely, some loss of soft tissue volume occurs in most cases of severe trauma. Minimal changes in volume (approximately 5%) can cause enophthalmos. Soft tissue considerations, which also contribute to globe position, include the relationships between the various ligaments stretched between the bony walls of the orbit [20]. These ligaments act as a sling support for the globe, alterations of which can contribute to enophthalmos.

18.2 Enophthalmos

Enophthalmos is the recession of the globe into the bony orbit. Enophthalmos may be clinically apparent to the examiner and can be measured with a Hertel exophthalmometer, which relies upon non-displaced, symmetrical lateral orbital rims. When measured using an exophthalmometer, enophthalmos is considered to be clinically significant when there is greater than a 2 mm difference in axial displacement between the two globes. Other devices to measure axial displacement have been described that use the external auditory canal or forehead for fixation in situations in which the lateral orbital rims may not be a reliable point of reference [24, 44].

18.2.1 Non-traumatic Causes of Enophthalmos

Although enophthalmos after trauma is most often related to the trauma, there may be pre-existing enophthalmos due to orbital asymmetry, sinus disease, varix, microphthalmia, irradiation, scleroderma, metastatic disease, and neurofibromatosis with absence of the sphenoid wing [6]. Historical review of photographs will often aid in detection of pre-existing facial asymmetry and also aid in the patient's understanding of his or her apparent enophthalmos. Enophthalmos due to metastatic disease is most often seen in the setting of breast cancer where

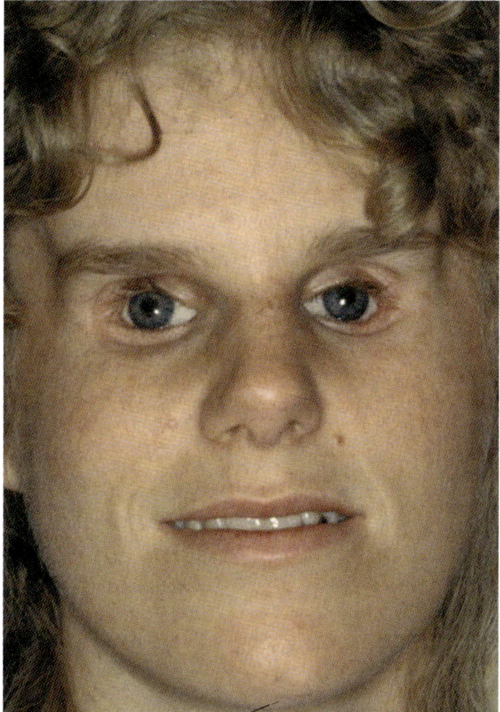

Fig. 18.1. Thirty-five-year-old female with a history of bilateral retinoblastoma, status postorbital irradiation after bilateral enucleation at 2 years of age. Patient exhibits a typical "hourglass" deformity due to bony hypoplasia and orbital fat atrophy. She has had multiple surgical procedures for contracted orbits

sclerotic changes within the fat cause retraction of the globe. Enophthalmos associated with sinus disease ("silent sinus syndrome") was first well described in 1994 [40]. Radiographic studies show an opacified maxillary sinus with destruction of the orbital floor and downward displacement of the globe. Orbital varices are associated with dynamic enophthalmos, which normalizes when the venous pressure increases (Valsalva maneuver). The enophthalmos observed in patients with varices is thought to be secondary to fat atrophy. Microphthalmos associated with enophthalmos is due to diminished soft tissue (globe volume) in the affected orbit. Enophthalmos associated with scleroderma is due to fat atrophy in the involved orbit. The disease is systemic and the finding of enophthalmos points to disease activity in the orbit. Pulsatile enophthalmos (or exophthalmos) is often detected in individuals with an absence of the sphenoid wing. Pulsations from the brain are directly communicated to the orbit, with or without the patient's being aware of movement of the eye. These individuals are almost uniformly diagnosed with neurofibromatosis. Orbital atrophy is frequently seen in individuals with a history of a retinoblastoma treated with radiation in childhood. Bony hypoplasia and loss of orbital fat occur. When bilateral, a characteristic hourglass deformity is seen (Fig. 18.1).

18.2.2 Traumatic Enophthalmos

Traumatic enophthalmos may be classified into early or late. Early enophthalmos is detectable shortly after the injury. Initially, enophthalmos may not be apparent due to associated space-occupying edema and/or hemorrhage. As the swelling decreases, sinking of the eye occurs within 14 days. Late enophthalmos develops weeks to months after the injury. Most often, the enophthalmos will be apparent approximately 1–2 weeks after the injury, when edema has subsided and hemorrhage has been reabsorbed. Therefore, enophthalmos may occur immediately after trauma due to a large bony defect, within 1–2 weeks after swelling decreases, or in weeks to months due to a change in soft tissue architecture usually with an increase in bony volume.

Post-traumatic enophthalmos due to loss of the eye is a special situation. Loss of the globe results in a 6.0–9.0 cc deficit of tissue in the orbit, which when replaced by an implant and prosthesis, only contributes 3–6 cc of volume. In addition, anophthalmic sockets often have a continuing atrophy of fat, which results in additional enophthalmos. Enophthalmos in the anophthalmic socket may manifest primarily as superior sulcus deformity and may also include pseudoptosis and a flattened, almost concave lower lid.

18.2.3 Mechanism of Traumatic Enophthalmos

The mechanism of traumatic enophthalmos can be approached simply through volume considerations. The primary factors are bony volume expansion, soft tissue contraction, and fat herniation [7]. Additional studies have pointed to the relationship of the supporting ligaments to the bony anatomy, which provides an architecture on which soft tissue relationships are maintained [20]. Orbital volume changes of 5% allow clinically significant changes in soft-tissue shape and position and set the stage for enophthalmos [21]. Trauma may result in fractures, which cause an expansion of the bony volume. The periorbita may or may not be disrupted with volume expansion, adding another variable to the resulting enophthalmos. There is a linear correlation between volume changes and enophthalmos. Studies have shown that for every 1 ml of volume expansion, 0.47 mm of enophthalmos results [31]. A 13% or greater increase in orbital volume correlated with greater than 2 mm of enophthalmos. The anatomic changes most commonly responsible for these changes are displacement of the posterior floor and transverse enlargement of the posterior orbit. Trauma also results in a decrease of orbital soft tissue either from fat atrophy or contraction and fibrosis of extraocular muscles and orbital septa after entrapment. Loss of this volume results in additional enophthalmos. The last factor involved in traumatic enophthalmos is the herniation of soft tissue into an adjacent sinus. Again, the fracture may itself result in an expansion of bony volume, or a trapdoor fracture may result in loss of soft tissue into the sinus without an expansion of bony volume. Traumatic enophthalmos will often be due to a combination of the above factors, and treatment addresses each of the factors individually. Restoration of normal orbital volume at primary surgery, however, has the greatest effect in preventing late enophthalmos [30].

18.2.4 Fractures Associated with Enophthalmos

The most common fractures associated with the orbit involve the orbital floor, medial wall, and zygomatico-maxillary complex. Orbital floor fractures result from either a buckling of the orbital floor secondary to blunt trauma to the inferior orbital rim, an increase in the orbital pressure secondary to blunt trauma to the globe, or a combination of both of these factors [10,38]. Twenty to 30% of individuals sustaining an orbital floor fracture will manifest enophthalmos within weeks to months following the injury [41]. Orbital floor fractures result in a direct communication between the orbit and the maxillary sinus, thus increasing the volume of the orbit (Fig. 18.2). There is usually prolapse of orbital soft tissue into the sinus, thus resulting in a loss of soft tissue volume in the orbit. This fracture is usually just medial to the infraorbital groove. Also, tissue will often be entrapped in the fracture, causing atrophy and fibrosis of the tissue with a resultant loss of soft tissue volume. Orbital floor fractures, therefore, frequently result in enophthalmos, depending on the size of the fracture and the amount of tissue that has prolapsed into the orbit or has been entrapped in the fracture.

Medial wall fractures most often result from an increase in orbital pressure following blunt trauma to the orbit. The thin nature of the medial wall with the adjacent ethmoid sinus makes these fractures very common. However, medial wall fractures are not as common as floor fractures since the medial wall is buttressed in many places by septa of the ethmoid sinus. In addition, the greater width of the orbital floor makes it more susceptible to fracture as compared to

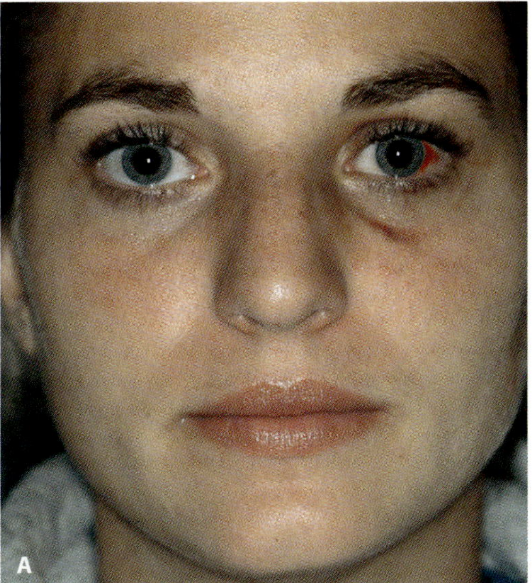

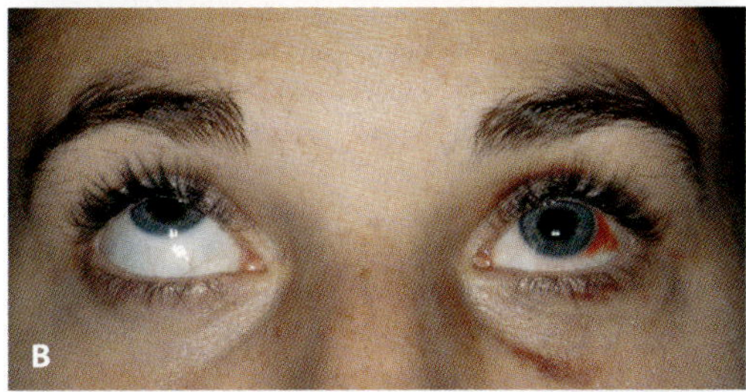

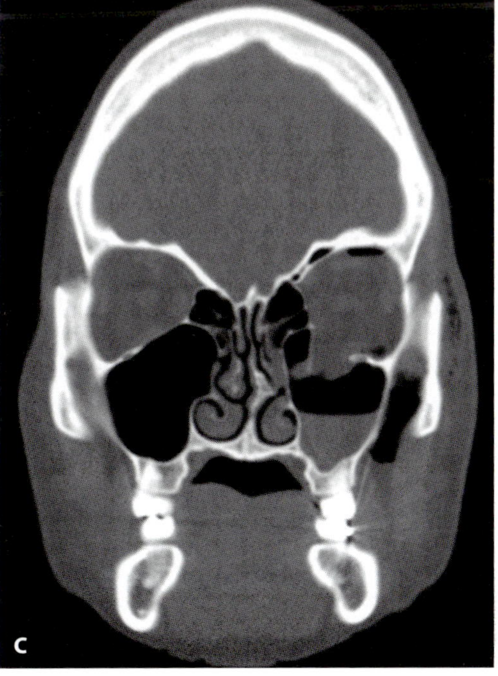

Fig. 18.2. **A** Twenty-four-year-old female, 1 week after periorbital trauma, resulting in an orbital blowout fracture on the left side. The patient has 2 mm of enophthalmos. **B** Ocular motility shows restriction of upgaze of the left eye. Forced ductions demonstrated a restrictive motility disturbance. **C** Coronal CT scan shows an orbital floor fracture with orbital soft tissue prolapsed into the maxillary sinus

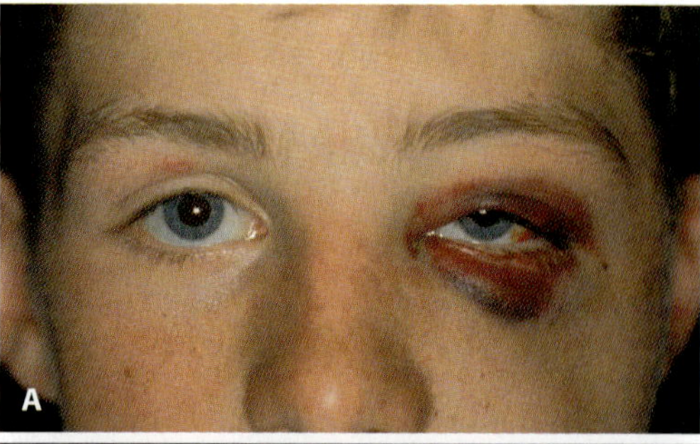

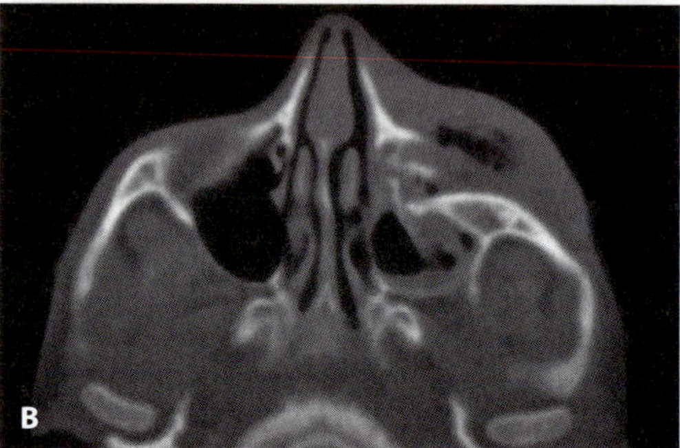

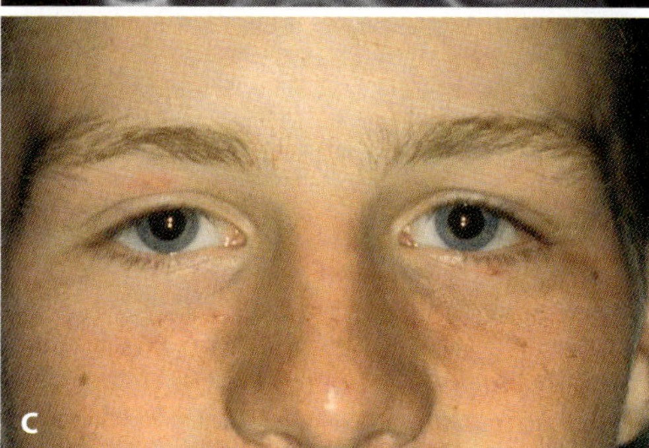

Fig. 18.3. A Fifteen-year-old male, 5 days after periorbital trauma, resulting in a left ZMC fracture. The patient manifests a flattened cheek and downward displacement of the lateral canthus. Hertel measurements were inaccurate due to the displaced lateral orbital rim. **B** Axial CT scan shows the fracture involving the anterior and posterior wall of the maxillary sinus and the zygomatic arch. **C** Three months after open reduction and internal fixation of the fracture with placement of a titanium mesh implant on the orbital floor. The patient's flattened cheek, downward displacement of the lateral canthus, and enophthalmos are improved

the medial wall. The factors causing enophthalmos secondary to medial wall fractures are similar mechanically to those observed with orbital floor fractures.

Zygomatico-maxillary complex (ZMC) fractures result in a rotational displacement of the quadripod segment of the orbitozygomatic region and often have an orbital floor component (Fig. 18.3). Enophthalmos or globe ptosis from these fractures is usually related to the size of the associated floor deformity. In contrast to an orbital floor blow-out fracture, the floor displacement in a ZMC fracture is lateral to the infraorbital groove. There is also an external rotation of the lateral orbital wall, often resulting in an increased intraorbital volume. Other orbital deformities associated with a ZMC fracture include a flat cheek and downward displacement of the lateral canthus.

18.2.5 Evaluation of the Patient with Traumatic Enophthalmos

The oculoplastic surgeon asked to evaluate traumatic enophthalmos may be consulted for the acute trauma or to see the patient after healing has occurred. Evaluation of the patient should be comprehensive and focussed on possible other findings from trauma or other mechanisms of enophthalmos [28]. Evaluation of the patient starts with a complete history and physical. In the acute setting, life-threatening situations need to be ruled out first before the orbit is addressed. In addition, any rupture of the globe must be managed prior to orbital fracture treatment. Any visual complaints should be fully evaluated prior to addressing the concerns of the orbit. The patient's chief complaint should be documented. The patient's complaints may include asymmetry, diplopia, ptosis, or even exophthalmos of the contralateral orbit. Often, the patient may not have a particular complaint, but may be referred due to what was found on a CT scan or other radiological test. A full history should be diligently obtained. Review of old photographs can be helpful in patients with a pre-existing facial or orbital asymmetry. The circumstances of the trauma should explain the

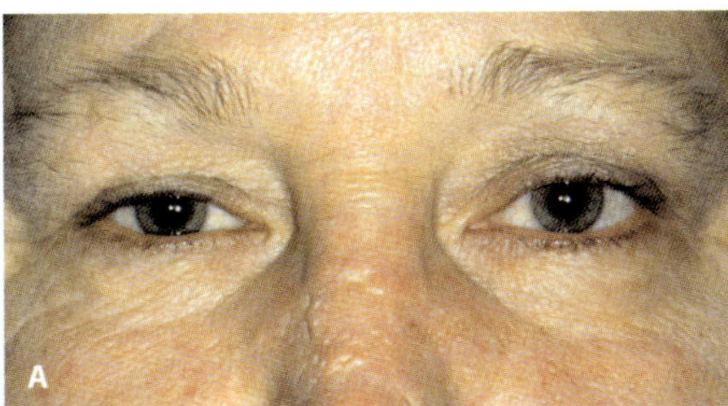

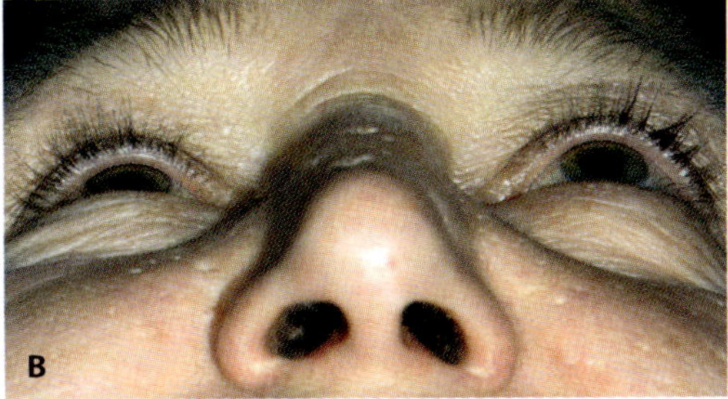

Fig. 18.4. A Fifty-one-year-old female, 3 years after sustaining a right orbital floor fracture. Patient manifests 3 mm of enophthalmos with a Hertel exophthalmometer. **B** Submentovertex projection ("worm's eye view") demonstrates the axial asymmetry

findings on exam. Often, the patient may be obtunded and the history of the event will need to be obtained from any witnesses. While blunt trauma usually results in predictable types of fractures, penetrating trauma will not. The patient's medical history should also be obtained including any history of sinus disease, cancer, prior facial trauma, or surgery. Even though the patient may give a history of trauma, this may be incidental and the enophthalmos on exam may be secondary to a more cryptic cause. A full list of the patient's current medication should be reviewed, with special attention to any medications with anticoagulant properties. The patient's previous ocular history should be obtained with special attention to any previous surgery around the orbit.

A full physical is mandatory. If the patient withstood enough trauma to result in enophthalmos, other injuries should be searched for, often by an emergency room physician or the patient's primary care physician. A full ophthalmic examination should be performed to rule out any globe injury. Special attention should be given to evaluation of a possible open globe, anterior segment inflammation or hyphema, retinal findings, and optic nerve function. Traumatic optic neuropathy must be ruled out. External photographs should be obtained. Lid deformities such as a deep superior sulcus, pseudo-ptosis, and flat or concave lower lid should be documented. Axial displacement of the globe can be evaluated with a Hertel exophthalmometer; however, lateral rim fractures may make these measurements inaccurate. Observation of the orbits from below upward, as in a submentovertex projection ("worm's eye view", Fig. 18.4), or from above downward can be helpful in determining the degree of enophthalmos. Fractures can also result in infraorbital nerve hypoesthesia. Examination of motility is performed. Forced ductions should be evaluated in any patient with an ocular motility problem to determine if the cause is restriction or paresis. Intercanthal measurements should also be obtained.

18.2.5.1 Radiographic Evaluation

Patients with a history of orbital trauma should be evaluated radiologically. The procedure of choice is a CT with fine axial and coronal cuts. Direct coronal cuts are preferred over reconstructions; however, direct coronals require the neck to be hyperextended during the procedure, which often is not possible in patients immediately after trauma who may have neck injury. Plain films, although perhaps useful in the situation in which a CT scan is not available, are not adequate for complete assessment. MRI scans are not useful to image the bony changes associated with fractures. The indications for CT evaluation after trauma include facial asymmetry, severe facial swelling, change in globe position, abnormal motility, subcutaneous/orbital emphysema, and infraorbital hypoesthesia.

18.3 Treatment of Traumatic Enophthalmos

Indications for repair after trauma will affect the timing of the repair. Indications for repair in acute trauma include facial asymmetry (flattening of the cheek, downward displacement of the lateral canthal tendon), a palpable "step" on the orbital rim, enophthalmos, restrictive strabismus, and trismus. The timing of the surgery may be immediate or delayed until swelling has decreased, usually 5–7 days. The special situation of a "white eye" blow-out fracture in children should be repaired on an urgent basis [16, 37]. These fractures result in an ischemic entrapment of the inferior rectus muscle. Indications for delayed repair of fractures which have resulted in enophthalmos include facial asymmetry, globe ptosis, and strabismus as well as repair of the enophthalmos deformity.

18.3.1 Non-surgical Treatment of Traumatic Enophthalmos

Non-surgical options should always be discussed with the patient. If the patient is asymptomatic or unconcerned about any facial asymmetry, observation is an option. Observation may be more attractive to a patient in whom the risk of surgical intervention may outweigh the benefit, as in an elderly patient, a patient with monocular vision, or a patient whose other facial deformities are more significant than the orbital deformity. Other non-surgical options include spectacles to aid in camouflage, a magnifying lens to create an illusion that diminishes the appearance of enophthalmos (if the eye does not see), or a patch.

18.3.2 Surgical Treatment of Traumatic Enophthalmos

Surgical approaches in the treatment of traumatic enophthalmos should address the orbit, strabismus, and lid position [33]. Bony reconstruction or volume replacement should be performed first. Strabismus surgery is performed after all orbital surgery is completed and enough time has elapsed for stable orthoptic measurements (usually 6 months). Lid position is addressed last. This strategy is similar to that for the opposite problem of exophthalmos as seen in Graves' orbitopathy.

18.3.2.1 Camouflage

Surgical repair of enophthalmos may simply camouflage the problem, rather than actually repair the deformity. This is useful in patients who may not tolerate orbital surgery or who prefer a less invasive treatment. The least invasive intervention is the treatment of lid position as in an apparent ptosis (pseudo-ptosis). Some patients may manifest only an asymmetry in lid height with enophthalmos, which may be adequately camouflaged by raising the upper lid. The patient must be aware that lifting the lid may give a cosmetically acceptable result but will not affect the globe position. A simple in-office test to determine if correction of the pseudo-ptosis would be acceptable is to instill 10% phenylephrine drops in the upper fornix to stimulate the sympathetically innervated Muller's muscle. If the upper eyelid elevates well and the patient is satisfied with the cosmetic result, then ptosis repair will usually be acceptable to the patient [29]. Often correction of this alone may give the patient a more pleasing result, rather than a more involved orbital surgery.

18.3.2.2 Early Surgical Repair of Traumatic Enophthalmos

In most cases, early surgical correction of orbital fractures offers the best correction of facial deformity. There is clear evidence that late intervention is accompanied by increased risk and worse functional result [32]. The literature is replete with recommendations and guidelines for early surgical intervention. The guidelines for indications and timing of repair of orbital floor fractures deserve special review. Most surgeons believe that patients with significant diplopia demonstrated to have positive forced duction testing should be repaired within 2 weeks of the injury. Patients with greater than 2 mm of enophthalmos at the time of trauma should also be repaired early. The controversial patients are those who have moderate size fractures, but have no or minimal strabismus and no clinically significant enophthalmos. Hawes and Dortzbach addressed this controversy using CT scanning in trying to predict which patients would develop problems after floor fracture [14]. Their conclusion was that a fracture involving more than 50% of the floor would likely yield enophthalmos. The recommendation was that a patient with a fracture in which more than half of the floor is missing should undergo early repair (within 2 weeks), regardless of whether the patient was symptomatic. But even these guidelines can be difficult to apply clinically due to the difficulty in quantitating "half of the floor" from a CT scan. Also, asymptomatic patients will often be resistant to pursuing a surgery that is not risk free.

Current guidelines for orbital floor fracture repair [4] recommend timing of intervention to be split into three groups: immediate, within 2 weeks, and observation. Immediate intervention is recommended in patients with diplopia with CT evidence of an entrapped muscle or periorbital tissue associated with a non-resolving oculocardiac reflex (bradycardia, heart block, nausea, vomiting, or syncope). This is usually seen in the setting of a "white-eyed blow-out fracture" [16, 37]. Typically this involves a young patient (<18 years old) with a history of periocular trauma, little ecchymosis or edema, marked extraocular motility vertical restriction, and CT examination revealing a small orbital floor fracture with entrapped muscle or perimuscular soft tissue. Immediate intervention may also be pursued in patients with early nophthalmos/hypoglobus causing facial asymmetry. Intervention within 2 weeks is recommended in patients with symptomatic diplopia with positive forced ductions, evidence of an entrapped muscle or perimuscular soft tissue on CT examination, and minimal clinical improvement over time. Repair in this time frame is also recommended in patients with large floor fractures (who would likely develop later enophthalmos), significant hypo-ophthalmos, and progressive infraorbital hypoesthesia [3]. Observation of the fracture is recommended in patients with minimal diplopia (not in primary or downgaze), good ocular motility, and no significant enophthalmos or hypo-ophthalmos.

Indications and timing for repair of other orbital fractures are more straightforward. Midfacial LeFort I, II, and III fractures should be repaired within 7 days. ZMC fractures should be repaired within 1–2 weeks and indications for repair are symptom dependent (flattening of the cheek, displaced lateral canthal tendon, floor fracture component, and trismus). Guidelines for orbital exploration in ZMC fractures are similar to orbital floor fracture repair and include the following [36]: (1) persistent diplopia that fails to improve throughout 7 or more days from the time of injury, accompanied by positive forced duction testing and radiological evidence of perimuscular tissue entrapment; (2) cosmetically significant and clinically apparent enophthalmos associated with abnormal radiological findings (i.e. a large fracture of the floor and substantial herniation of tissue into the maxillary sinus); (3) radiological evidence of significant comminution and/or displacement of the orbital rim; (4) radiological evidence of significant displacement or comminution of greater than 50% of the orbital floor with herniation of soft tissue into the maxillary sinus; (5) combined orbital floor and medial wall defects with soft tissue displacement noted radiologically on CT scans; (6) radiological evidence of a fracture or comminution of the body of the zygoma itself as determined by use of CT scans; and (7) physical or radiological evidence of exophthalmos (secondary) or orbital content impingement caused by displaced periorbital fractures.

Orbital roof fractures should be observed if there is minimal rim fracture; the fracture should be repaired urgently if the trochlea is involved or if there is communication with the CNS [23]. Treatment of medial wall fractures should be repaired within 2 weeks if there is enophthalmos or an entrapped medial rectus muscle [35]. Naso-orbital-ethmoid fractures are repaired depending upon symptoms and should be repaired within 2 weeks; the nasolacrimal system may be damaged, requiring stenting of the lacrimal system or a dacryocystorhinostomy [27].

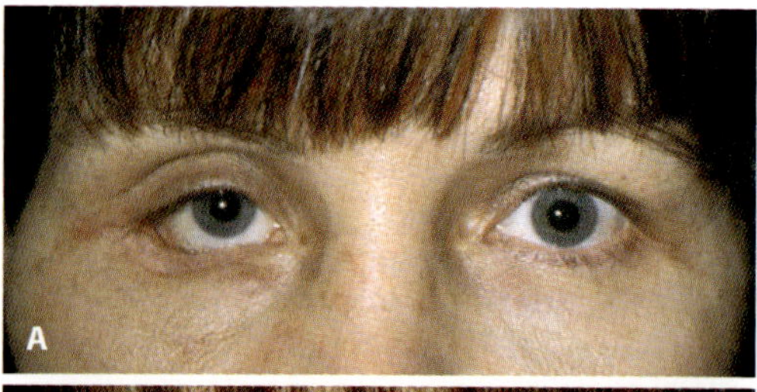

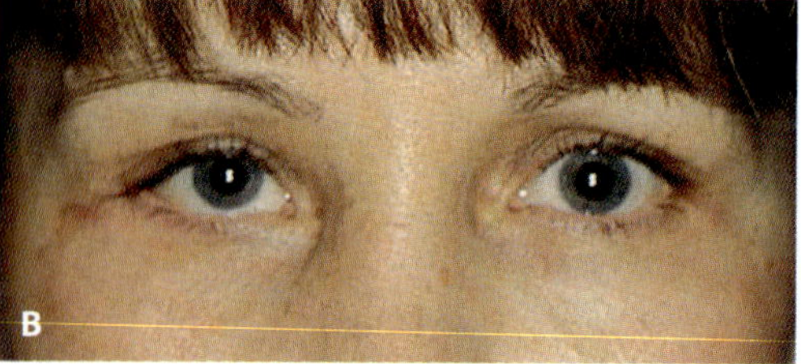

Fig. 18.5. A Forty-year-old female with a history of a right ZMC fracture, status post incomplete repair 6 weeks prior to presentation. The patient has 3 mm of enophthalmos and lower lid retraction. **B** Patient underwent repeat internal reduction and internal fixation of the right ZMC fracture. Placement of a Medpor implant along the orbital floor and lateral canthoplasty were performed along with a lower lid retractor recession. One month after the reoperation, the patient has 1 mm of enophthalmos with residual lower lid retraction

Early repair, as dictated by the above guidelines, treats the structural abnormality. Enophthalmos may be alleviated by simply placing the orbital structures in their anatomically correct positions. However, restoration of orbital anatomy is often incomplete due to the complexity of the fractures, and even when performed with anatomic alignment may still result in enophthalmos due to damage to the soft tissues. Primary post-traumatic orbital deformity is repaired using the following sequence: mobilization of soft tissue from the bone throughout the entire area of fracture, reduction and fixation of the bony orbital rim and walls into their proper position, and reattachment of the soft tissue to the bone at the proper location [12].

Current technique involves rigid fixation of the facial skeleton with titanium microplates [34]. Microplates allow a rigid three-dimensional fixation and have proven to be more effective than fixation using wires [43]. Wiring is imperfect in its ability to support large areas of comminuted bone, often resulting in sagging of the architecture. The identification of stable bone from which to attach fractured bone and knowledge of the buttresses of the facial skeleton aid in guidance of successful internal reduction and fixation [13, 22] (Fig. 18.5). Orbital floor and medial wall defects can be repaired with autogenous and alloplastic implants. We prefer Supramid implants (0.4 mm thickness) for most defects with fixation of the implant to the posterior lip of the orbital rim with one or two titanium screws. Other options include titanium sheets, Medpor sheets (porous polyethylene), and autogenous materials such as bone grafts. Ideal implants should have minimal rates of extrusion, exposure, migration, inflammation, and infection.

18.3.2.3 Late Repair of Traumatic Enophthalmos

Late repair of enophthalmos depends upon the anatomy of the orbit which is presented to the surgeon. Displaced orbital bones and soft tissue should be addressed first. If a primary repair of an orbital fracture is not performed, the initial surgical procedure will release soft tissue from surrounding bone, followed by reconstruction of the bony integrity of the orbit. This may necessitate osteotomies for rim fractures that have healed, especially in the setting of a previous ZMC fracture [19]. Positioning of the bones to their normal anatomic position may be enough to treat the enophthalmos. The axial position of the globes should be assessed intraoperatively to determine if clinically significant enophthalmos is present. If there is still enophthalmos, then orbital volume will need to be added. In cases in which late traumatic enophthalmos is present in the setting of an appropriate repair or non-displaced fractures, then orbital augmentation would be pursued, rather than any further bony or soft tissue manipulation.

18.3.2.4 Orbital Augmentation

Orbital volume augmentation is an effective procedure in reducing enophthalmos. The approach involves placing autogenous or alloplastic implants to push the globe in the direction opposite to the observed dystopia, or positioning of the implants to supplant the area of volume excess. Most commonly, post-traumatic orbits present with enophthalmos with hypoglobus and radiological findings of floor or medial wall expansion (Fig. 18.5). In these cases, implants are usually positioned in a subperiosteal pocket along the inferior and medial walls. Implants placed posterior to the equator of the globe result in forward displacement of the globe. Implants placed inferior to the globe result in elevation of the globe. Most implants are "wedge-shaped;" the wedge is placed with the greater thickness posteriorly in order to push the globe in an anterior vector more than a superior vector.

A number of materials for orbital augmentation have been described. Autogenous materials include costal cartilage and bone implants. Alloplastic materials include porous polyethylene (Medpor) and silicone. There are a number of preformed alloplastic implants available, which are shaped to fit into the orbital floor and push the globe forward. Our current material of choice is donor cartilage, which is available through most local tissue banks. The size and shape of the cartilage pieces can be tailored intraoperatively.

The surgical approach to orbital augmentation is through a transconjunctival incision to gain access to the orbital floor and medial wall. If further exposure is needed for the medial portion of the orbit, a transcaruncular approach may also be employed. Subperiosteal dissection is performed to gain access to the area of the floor and medial wall posterior to the globe. Special attention is paid so that there is no damage to the infraorbital nerve and artery or ethmoidal vessels. After adequate exposure, donor cartilage is shaped to be placed posterior to the equator to the globe, to result in forward displacement of the globe. Placement of two pieces of cartilage on the floor and one piece along the medial wall usually results in a satisfactory position of the globe. Intraoperative observation of the position of the globe is noted to determine if enough volume has been added and the positioning is correct. Observation should be performed from a superior position and it is imperative that the full face is exposed so that symmetry can be assessed.

If there is displacement of the lateral floor due to a previous unrepaired ZMC fracture, positioning an implant deeply along the lateral wall can improve the globe position [11]. In any case where inferior and medial wall augmentation is inadequate, additional volume can be added laterally. The surgical approach laterally can be through a transconjunctival, lateral canthotomy, or upper lid crease incision. Positioning of the implant should not impinge on the superior or inferior orbital fissure. Augmentation along the orbital roof is discouraged due to the probability of inducing an upper eyelid ptosis.

18.3.2.5 CT Quantification of Volume Loss

Volumetric analysis of the enophthalmic socket by CT derived algorithms has been described [2, 8]. This strategy allows a more precise volume restoration with the implant of choice. The volumes of the affected and unaffected orbits are quantified, followed by volume augmentation of the affected orbit with the difference. This strategy has not yet gained popularity, but with continued advancements in orbital imaging and software, this method may come into common use.

18.3.2.6 Complications

Complications of enophthalmos repair are similar to other types of orbital surgery. Blindness is the most feared complication due to globe injury, optic nerve injury, or orbital hemorrhage. Diplopia and ocular motility disturbances may occur due to preoperative factors involving the extraocular muscles or intraoperative factors in which damage, impingement, or entrapment of one or more of the extraocular muscles or structures involved with or connected to the extraocular muscles has occurred. Prophylactic antibiotic therapy may be given to prevent postoperative infection, even though this complication is uncommon. Lacrimal dysfunction secondary to injury to the nasolacrimal duct is also a risk. Lid malposition may occur due to the primary injury or the surgical approach. Lymphedema is common, especially after multiple

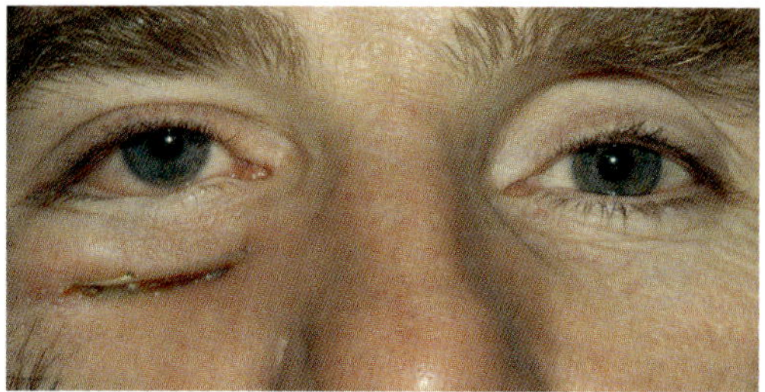

Fig. 18.6. Thirty-nine-year-old male with a history of repair of a right orbital floor fracture with placement of a Supramid implant. Patient returned 2 years after the surgery with an extruding implant (note titanium fixation screw on the edge of the implant)

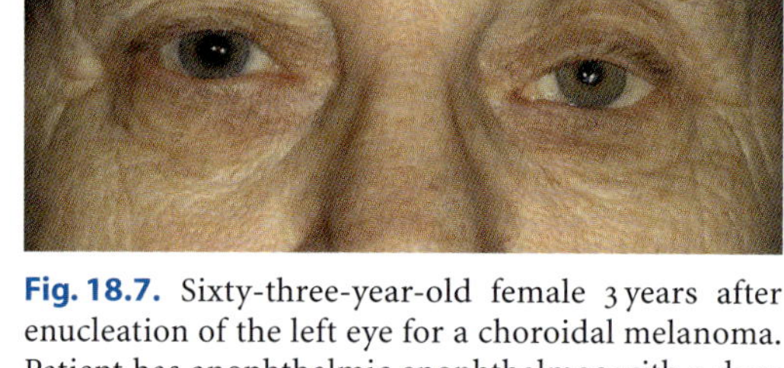

Fig. 18.7. Sixty-three-year-old female 3 years after enucleation of the left eye for a choroidal melanoma. Patient has anophthalmic enophthalmos with a deep superior sulcus and lax lower lid with inferior displacement of her prosthesis

surgeries. Manipulation in the area of the infraorbital nerve may result in hypoesthesia. Pupil irregularities (mydriasis, anisocoria) may occur secondary to ciliary nerve injury. Complications related to the implant include infection, chronic inflammation, migration-extrusion, globe elevation, proptosis, cyst formation, loss of vision from impingement of the implant on the orbital apex, motility restriction, pain, eyelid malposition, and fistula formation [9, 15] (Fig. 18.6).

18.4 Enophthalmos Associated with the Anophthalmic Socket

Enophthalmos associated with the anophthalmic socket deserves special attention [26]. It is probably the most common enophthalmos encountered by the oculoplastic surgeon, and treatment is usually directed purely toward orbital augmentation with lower lid tightening, with no concern for the complications of diplopia or loss of vision. Therefore, the surgeon is able to be more aggressive in these patients in treating their orbital deformity. Anophthalmic enophthalmos most commonly presents with a deep superior sulcus.

18.4.1 Mechanism

As discussed above, the loss of the globe results in a volume deficit of approximately 7 cc of tissue. This deficit is filled by an implant and a prosthesis, which can provide significant volume. Enucleation results in manipulation of the orbit, which often results in continued fat atrophy, with shifting of orbital contents. Evisceration is thought to involve less orbital manipulation with lower rates of postoperative fat atrophy. This continued soft tissue loss results in additional enophthalmos with time, which is often addressed initially by the ocularist, who increases the size of the prosthesis. There is a limitation to the amount to which the ocularist can increase the volume of the prosthesis: a larger prosthesis has poorer motility, and the lower lid may not be able to support the additional weight of the prosthesis, resulting in hypoglobus or periodic luxation of the prosthesis. The eyelid malpositions observed in the anophthalmic socket are caused by inferior and posterior redistribution of the remaining orbital fat and levator muscle retraction by the superior rectus muscle and lid, with the levator displaced from its normal position [41]. Over years, stretching of the lower eyelid may cause the prosthesis to drop, creating a deeper superior sulcus (Fig. 18.7). Prior to the recognition of lower eyelid laxity as the main etiological factor in the anophthalmic "superior sulcus syndrome", the size of the prosthesis was increased to fill the sulcus. Again over time, the increased weight of the prosthesis caused the prosthesis to drop further and the sulcus deepened again. The current treatment of the "superior sulcus syndrome" is to tighten the lower eyelid and replace any orbital volume with a subperiosteal implant, not to increase the size of the prosthesis.

18.4.2 Treatment of Enophthalmos in the Anophthalmic Socket

Treatment of enophthalmos in the anophthalmic socket is directed toward the patient's complaint. If a sagging of the implant or periodic luxation of the implant occurs, a lower lid tightening via a lateral tarsal strip may be appropriate. If the patient notes pseudo-ptosis and wants a minimally invasive procedure, a lower lid tightening with a ptosis procedure (levator advancement) may alleviate the symptoms. If the patient wants the superior sulcus deformity addressed, he or she needs more volume in the orbit. The least invasive procedure would be to augment the prosthesis. As noted above, this often compounds the problem. If the prosthesis is already large, then the patient should have orbital augmentation with either an alloplastic or an autogenous implant. Orbital augmentation is the most appropriate surgery for enophthalmos in the anophthalmic socket [39]. Alloplastic implants that have been described include glass and silicone beads, hydroxyapatite, Medpor, and room-temperature-vulcanized silicone [42]. Autogenous implants include sclera, fat, cranial bone, and cartilage. We commonly use a Medpor enophthalmos wedge implant (Enophthalmos Wedge, Porex Surgical Products Group, Noonan, GA) for an alloplastic implant or donor costal cartilage for an autogenous implant [5]. Cartilage has the advantage of being readily available from tissue banks and easily shaped [18].

Our preferred surgical strategy is orbital volume augmentation with lower lid tightening. A subciliary incision is preferred over a transconjunctival incision due to the risk of shortening the fornix with the transconjunctival incision. Dissection is performed between the orbicularis muscle and orbital septum to the inferior orbital rim. The periosteum is elevated from the orbital floor. The implant is then placed along the orbital floor and medial wall, posterior. There is little concern about placing the implant too posterior since there is no risk of blindness. Anteriorly placed implants may shallow the conjunctival fornix. Care should be taken in any manipulation along the infraorbital groove, in order to avoid postoperative hypoesthesia. Lid tightening is then performed via a lateral tarsal strip [1]. The patient will usually need to have their prosthesis refitted by the ocularist after any orbital manipulation.

Summary for the Clinician

- **Enophthalmos after trauma is a common orbital deformity**
- **Enophthalmos may be noted immediately after trauma, early (within 2 weeks), or late**
- **The most common mechanism of enophthalmos is expansion of the bony orbit**
- **Knowledge of the inherent weaknesses of the orbit and orbital imaging will direct the oculoplastic surgeon to the precise etiology of the enophthalmos, aiding in repair**
- **Current techniques of open reduction with rigid fixation of the facial skeleton and available implants have increased the rate of success in treating orbital deformities**
- **Through a systematic approach to evaluation and surgical repair, as outlined in this chapter, traumatic enophthalmos can be treated successfully with patient and surgeon satisfaction**

References

1. Anderson RL (1981) Tarsal strip procedure for correction of eyelid laxity and canthal malposition in the anophthalmic socket. Ophthalmology 88:895–903
2. Bite U, Jackson IT, Forbes GS, Gehring DG (1985) Orbital volume measurements in enophthalmos using three-dimensional CT imaging. Plast Reconstr Surg 75:502–508
3. Boush GA, Lemke BN (1994) Progressive infraorbital nerve hypesthesia as a primary indication for blow-out fracture repair. Ophthal Plast Reconstr Surg 10:271–275
4. Burnstine MA (2002) Clinical recommendations for repair of isolated orbital floor fractures: an evidence-based analysis. Ophthalmology 109: 1207– 1210
5. Choi JC, Sims CD, Casanova R, Shore JW, Yaremchuk MJ (1995) Porous polyethylene implant for orbital wall reconstruction. J Craniomaxillofac Trauma 1:42–49
6. Cline RA, Rootman J (1984) Enophthalmos: a clinical review. Ophthalmology 91:229–237

7. Converse JM, Smith B (1957) Enophthalmos and diplopia in fractures of the orbital floor. Br J Plast Surg 9:265–274
8. Dolynchuk KN, Tadjalli HE, Manson PN (1996) Orbital volumetric analysis: Clinical application in orbitozygomatic complex injuries. J Craniomaxillofac Trauma 2:56–63
9. Fleming JC, Durboraw CE (1995) Orbital trauma and reconstruction. Curr Opin Ophthalmol 6:70–77
10. Fujino T, Makino K (1980) Entrapment mechanism and ocular injury in orbital blowout fracture. Plast Reconstr Surg 65:571–576
11. Goldberg RA, Saulny S, McCann JD, Yuen VH (2003) Orbital volume augmentation for late enophthalmos using the deep lateral wall. Arch Facial Plast Surg 5:256–258
12. Grant MP, Iliff NT, Manson PN (1997) Strategies for the treatment of enophthalmos. Clin Plast Surg 24:539–550
13. Gruss JS, Mackinnon SE (1986) Complex maxillary fractures: role of buttress reconstruction and immediate bone grafts. Plast Reconstr Surg 78:9–22
14. Hawes MJ, Dortzbach RK (1983) Surgery on orbital floor fractures: influence of time of repair and fracture size. Ophthalmology 90:1066–1070
15. Jordan DR, St Onge P, Anderson RL, Patrinely JR, Nerad JA (1992) Complications associated with alloplastic implants used in orbital fracture repair. Ophthalmology 99:1600–1608
16. Jordan DR, Allen LH, White J, Harvey J, Pashby R, Esmaeli B (1998) Intervention within days for some orbital floor fractures: the white-eyed blowout. Ophthal Plast Reconstr Surg 14:379–390
17. Kawamoto HK Jr (1982) Late posttraumatic enophthalmos: a correctable deformity? Plast Reconstr Surg 69:423–432
18. Linberg JV, Anderson RL, Edwards JJ, Panje WR, Bardach J (1980) Preserved irradiated homologous cartilage for orbital reconstruction. Ophthalmic Surg 11:457–462
19. Longaker MT, Kawamoto HK Jr (1998) Evolving thoughts on correcting posttraumatic enophthalmos. Plast Reconstr Surg 101:899–906
20. Manson PN, Clifford CM, Su CT, Iliff NT, Morgan R (1986) Mechanisms of global support and posttraumatic enophthalmos: I. The anatomy of the ligament sling and its relation to intramuscular cone orbital fat. Plast Reconstr Surg 77:193–202
21. Manson PN, Grivas A, Rosenbaum A, Vannier M, Zinreich J, Iliff N (1986) Studies on enophthalmos: II. The measurement of orbital injuries and their treatment by quantitative computed tomography. Plast Reconstr Surg 77:203–214
22. Manson PN, Clark N, Robertson B, Crawley WA (1995) Comprehensive management of pan-facial fractures. J Craniomaxillofac Trauma 1:43–56
23. McLachlan DL, Flanagan JC, Shannon GM (1982) Complications of orbital roof fractures. Ophthalmology 89:1274–1278
24. Naugle TC (1984) Methodology and measurement with modified lateral orbitotomy. In: Proc VII Cong Eur Soc Ophthal 5:549–550
25. Nerad JA (2001) Oculoplastic surgery: the requisites in ophthalmology. St. Louis, Mosby
26. Paris GL, Spohn WG (1980) Correction of enophthalmos in the anophthalmic orbit. Ophthalmology 87:1301–1308
27. Paskert JP, Manson PN, Iliff NT (1988) Nasoethmoidal and orbital fractures. Clin Plast Surg 15:209–223
28. Patel BCK, Hoffmann J (1998) Management of complex orbital fractures. Facial Plast Surg 14:83–104
29. Putterman AM, Urist MJ (1975) Treatment of enophthalmic narrow palpebral fissure after blow-out fracture. Ophthalmic Surg 6:45–49
30. Ramieri G, Spada MC, Bianchi SD, Berrone S (2000) Dimensions and volumes of the orbit and orbital fat in posttraumatic enophthalmos. Dentomaxillofac Rad 29:302–311
31. Raskin EM, Millman AL, Lubkin V, della Rocca RC, Lisman RD, Maher EA (1998) Prediction of late enophthalmos by volumetric analysis of orbital fractures. Ophthal Plast Recontr Surg 14: 19–26
32. Roncevic R, Stajcic Z (1994) Surgical treatment of posttraumatic enophthalmos: a study of 72 patients. Ann Plast Surg 32:288–294
33. Rubin PAD, Rumelt S (1999) Functional indications for enophthalmos repair. Ophthal Plast Reconstr Surg 15:284–292
34. Rubin PAD, Shore JW, Yaremchuk MJ (1992) Complex orbital fracture repair using rigid fixation of the internal orbital skeleton. Ophthalmology 99: 553–559
35. Segrest DR, Dortzbach RK (1989) Medial orbital wall fractures: complications and management. Ophthal Plast Reconstr Surg 5:75–80
36. Shumrick KA, Kersten RC, Kulwin DR, Smith CP (1997) Criteria for selective management of orbital rim and floor in zygomatic complex and midface fractures. Arch Otolaryngol Head Neck Surg 123:378–384
37. Sires BS, Stanley RB Jr, Levine LM (1998) Oculocardiac reflex caused by orbital floor trapdoor fracture: an indication for urgent repair. Arch Ophthalmol 116:955–956
38. Smith B, Regan WF Jr (1957) Blow-out fracture of the orbit: mechanism and correction of internal orbital fracture. Am J Ophthalmol 44:733–739

39. Soll DB (1971) Correction of the superior lid sulcus with subperiosteal implants. Arch Ophthalmol 85:188–190
40. Soparkar CN, Patrinely JR, Cuaycong MJ, Dailey RA, Kersten RC, Rubin PA, Linberg JV, Howard GR, Donovan DT, Matoba AY, Holds JB (1994) The silent sinus syndrome: A cause of spontaneous enophthalmos. Ophthalmology 101:772–778
41. Stasior OG, Roen JL (1982) Traumatic enophthalmos. Ophthalmology 89:1267–1273
42. Tyers AG, Collin JRO (1982) Orbital implants and post enucleation socket syndrome. Trans Ophthalmol Soc U K 102:90–92
43. Wesley RE (1992) Current techniques for the repair of complex orbital fractures. Miniplate fixation and cranial bone grafts. Ophthalmology 99: 1766–1772
44. Yeatts RP, van Rens E, Taylor CL (1992) Measurement of globe position in complex orbital fractures. I. A modification of Hertel's exophthalmometer, using the external auditory canal as a reference point. Ophthal Plast Reconstr Surg 8: 114–118

Subject Index

A

Adjuvant radiation therapy 45
Allograft contamination, risk 13
Alloplastic implant 223
Aluminium hydroxite 27
Anatomy, conjunctival 21
Anophthalmic socket 248
Aseptic processing 11
Augmentation, orbital 237, 246, 249

B

Balloon dacryocystoplasty 58
Balloon expander 205
Bangerter implant 226
Barrier function of lymph nodes 38
Bicanalicular intubation 85
bilateral anophthalmos 215
BioCleanse 12
Blind microphthalmos 219
Blow-out fracture 237, 238
Bone
- regrowth 58
- tunnelling (in brow suspension) 169
- window 57
Bony orbital decompression technique 97
Breslow thickness 40
Brow lift, endoscopic 163
Buried screw and suture (in brow suspension) 171

C

Cadaveric tissue 9
Caldwell GW 72
Camouflage of enophthalmos 244
Canalicular pump 55
Canalicular stenosis 67
Caruncle 22
- malignancies 33
Caruncular tumour 32
Ceramic material 227
CIN see conjunctival intraepithelial neoplasia
CJF see Creutzfeldt-Jakob disease
Clinical anophthalmos 206
Collarette 83
Composite implant 223
Conformer 205
- in congenital anophthalmos 216
Congenital anophthalmos 205
Conjunctival intraepithelial neoplasia (CIN) 27
Conjunctival neoplasm 21
Contamination 9
Craniofacial surgery in congenital anophthalmos 217
Creutzfeldt-Jakob disease (CJD) 7, 8
Crosswise suturing 232
Cryotherapy in conjunctival lesions 23
CSF leak 79
Cytokeratin 43

D

Dacryocystitis 55
Dacryocystorhinostomy 61
Dacryolith 64, 72
Dermis fat graft in congenital anophthalmos 216
Diplopia 242
Disposable vitrectomy 75
Donor tissue 3

E

En bloc dissection 38
Endonasal dacryocystorhinostomy 71
Endophthalmitis 224
Endotine fixation (in brow suspension) 173
Enophthalmos 239
- traumatic 240
Enucleation surgery 223
Erbium-YAG laser 63
- laserdacryoplasty 66
Escherichia coli 6
Ethmoid forceps 76
Evisceration 224, 225
Excisional biopsy in conjunctival lesions 23
Exophthalmos, contralateral 242
External beam radiation 91
Eyelid length 213

F

Fascia lata 4
Fat atrophy, postoperative 248
Fixation, three-dimensional 246
Flexible endocanalicular endoscopy 61
Forehead muscles, weakening 167
Fracture
- medial wall 241
- orbital roof 245

G

Gamma probe, handheld 42
Ginkgo biloba 73
Gravitational effect 181

H

HBV (hepatitis B virus) 3
HCV (hepatitis C virus) 3, 5
Herniation of tissue 245
HIV (human immunodeficiency virus) 3, 6
Holmium-YAG laser 63
Human immunodeficiency virus see HIV
Hydrogel expander 205, 207
Hypoaesthesia, infraorbital nerve 243
Hypoglobus 245

I

Implant
- alloplastic 237
- hydroxyapatite-silicone 226, 227
- integrated 227
- migration of 228
Incisional biopsy in conjunctival lesions 23
Infectious disease 6
Infraorbital block 73
Infratrochlear block 73
Isosulphan blue dye 37, 41

J

Jones I test 72
Jones tube 72

K

Kestenbaum spectacle 228, 229
Krause fold 65

L

Lacrimal drainage disorder 51
- flow-related 51
- volume-related 51
Laserdacryoplasty 62, 66
Lid fissure development 213
Living donor 9
Lymphoid tumour of conjunctiva 32
Lymphoscintigraphy 39, 41

M

Malignant melanoma of conjunctiva 31
Marsupializing 77
MART-1 (S-100 protein) 43
Melanoma antigen HMB-45 43
Merkel cell carcinoma 37
Microdrill dacryoplasty 62, 68
Microendoscopic technique 61
Microphthalmos 239
Midface 182
- age related changes 183
- anatomy 182
Migration of implant 228
Mini-Mono-Ka 84
Mitomycin-C 78
Monocanalicular lacrimal pathway intubation 83
Monoka intubation 67
Motility
- evaluation 228
- of the artificial eye 233
MRI
- in fractures 243
- predictive value 94
Mucous membrane graft in congenital anophthalmos 216
Muscle pedunculated scleral flap 230, 232
Muscle, entrapped 245
Musculoskeletal tissue graft 15
Myringotomy knife 76

N

Naevus of conjunctiva 28
Neck dissection 44

O

Octreotide scan 94
Ocular surface squamous neoplasia (OSSN) 27
Oculocardiac reflex 245
Orbit expander exchange 212
Orbit expansion 219
Orbital radiotherapy 91
OSSN see ocular surface squamous neoplasia

P

Paediatric EN-DCR 78
Papilloma of conjuncctiva 26
Pegging 223, 228
Periosteum, release 166
Photoablatively 66
Pigmented epibulbar lesion, differential diagnosis 30
Pituitary gland 91
Polyethylene 227
Polyps in the lacrimal sac 64
Preperiosteal dissection (in SOOF lift) 187
Primary acquired melanosis (PAM) 29
Prion disease 3

Prosthesis motility 223
Prosthetic fitting 211
Prosthetics in congenital anophthalmos 218
Pseudo-ptosis 243
Punctal stenosis 63
Pyogenic granuloma 79

R
Radiation-induced retinopathy 94
Radionuclide imaging 40
Radiotherapy in conjunctival lesions 23
Retinoblastoma 239, 240
Rosenmüller fold 64, 65

S
S-100 protein see MART-1
Scalp incision 164
Sclera 16
Scleral flap 226, 232
– lamellar 231
Self-inflating expander 207, 208
Sentinel lymph node biopsy 37
Silent sinus syndrome 239
Socket expander 212
Socket expansion 209
SOOF(suborbicularis oculi fat) lift 181
Squamous cell carcinoma of conjunctiva 27
Staging information 38
Staphylococcus aureus 6
Streptococcus 6
Suborbicularis oculi fat see SOOF
Sump syndrome 77
Superior sulcus syndrome 248
Sympathetic ophthalmia 225

T
Tear meniscus, enlarged 54
Technetium 37
Technetium-99m sulphur 41
Temporalis fascia 228
Temporary tarsorrhaphy 211
Therapeutic lymph node dissection 39
Tight orbit 98
Tissue expansion in congenital anophthalmos 217
Transcanalicular endoscopy 61
– procedure 66
Transillumination 74
Traumatic enophthalmos 237
– treatment 244
Topical chemotherapy in conjunctival lesions 23
Tutoplast 8
Tyrosinase gene 43

U
Unilateral anophthalmos 213

V
Vasconez 163
– forehead lift 163
Vitroptic T 69
Volume loss, CT quantification 247

W
Wait and see 92
Wait and watch 39
Wrapping material 228

Z
Zygomatico-maxillary complex 238, 242